A

R

DO NOT REMOVE
CARDS FROM POCKET

Animal Disease Control

REGIONAL PROGRAMS

Robert P. Hanson, Ph.D.
S. H. McNUTT PROFESSOR
VETERINARY SCIENCE DEPARTMENT
UNIVERSITY OF WISCONSIN, MADISON

Martha G. Hanson, Ph.D.
LECTURER, SCHOOL OF EDUCATION
UNIVERSITY OF WISCONSIN, MADISON

THE IOWA STATE UNIVERSITY PRESS • AMES, IOWA

© 1983 The Iowa State University Press. All rights reserved

Printed by The Iowa State University Press, Ames, Iowa   50010

First edition, 1983

Library of Congress Cataloging in Publication Data

Hanson, Robert P. (Robert Paul), 1918–
    Animal disease control.

    Includes bibliographical references and index.
    1. Veterinary public health—Government policy.
I. Hanson, Martha G., 1920–   . II. Title.
SF740.H37   1983   636.089′4   83–226
ISBN 0–8138–0121–4

70739310

CONTENTS

PREFACE

When it became clear that the confines of a semester course left no time for both the presentation of the concepts and discussion of the applications of epidemiology, we began to develop a new course and a supporting text. The outline was examined in a joint National Research Council-University of Wisconsin Workshop in 1973 entitled "Animal Disease Eradication: Evaluating Programs," and the final format has evolved over the past five years in discussions that we have held with regulatory authorities and research workers in Australia, Brazil, Colombia, England, and the United States.

While we were aware, when we began writing, that much of the literature of applied epidemiology existed in the form of unpublished documents and institutional reports of limited distribution, the volume and the significance of this material came as a surprise. Apart from its value to students, one contribution of this text may be to alert librarians to a need to assess methods of collecting and retrieving the documents and reports that are as essential as refereed publications to such fields of study as applied epidemiology.

This book considers the process used to document program benefits and to weigh the cost of the effort and the record of administrative stewardship. The issue of delegation of responsibility to administrators is central to all programs in which science is applied to human needs. To provide an understanding of the process and the issues involved, we describe how centrally administrated programs are planned, implemented, and evaluated. Consequently, the book should be of interest to all students of agriculture and to individuals in the general public who are concerned with the decision-making processes of regulatory agencies and the funding of government programs.

The authors have found that students grasp the intricacies of decision making systems that interrelate biology, economics, and politics more rapidly if they can work with computer models relating these systems. A 300-sow farrowing operation, described in chapter 4, was programmed by an associate of the authors, Blair McMillan, who had the help of two University of Wisconsin Extension agents--Robert Hall, a veterinarian, and Carl Hirschinger, an expert in swine management. In running the program, students learn the interrelationship of management, disease, and economics. Roger Morris, Director of Clinics, University of Minnesota, and formerly an administrator in the Australian Veterinary Service, has supplied us with two programs for students that illustrate other problems: One concerns the control of mastitis in a dairy herd and the second concerns interventions required to control an epizootic of an exotic disease. Individuals using this book as a course text should consider use of these or similar computer programs as an instructional tool.

ACKNOWLEDGEMENTS

The authors wish to thank the staff of institutions visited in search of information for this book. In Australia: the Bureau of Animal Health, Canberra; Victoria Veterinary Laboratory, Melbourne; South Australia Veterinary Laboratory, Adelaide; and Queensland Veterinary Laboratory, Brisbane. In Brazil: the Centro Panamericano de Fiebre Aftosa, Rio de Janeiro. In Colombia: the Laboratorio de Investigaciones Medica Veterinarias, Bogota; and Centro de Comunicaciones Tibaitata. In the United Kingdom: the Central Veterinary Laboratory, Weybridge; Institute for Animal Disease, Compton; Animal Virus Research Institute, Pirbright; Office of Chief Veterinary, Tolworth; Agriculture Research Council, London; and University of Reading, Reading. In the United States: the Central Offices of the Animal Plant Inspection Service, Washington, D.C., and of Veterinary Services in Hyattsville; National Animal Disease Center, Ames; and Plum Island Animal Disease Center, Greenport.

Individuals who provided special assistance in supplying information or in reading and suggesting changes in the manuscript were: Robert Anderson, John Atwell, Victor Beal, John Brooksby, A. C. L. Brown, Patricia Chain, Kathy Ellis, Peter Ellis, Jaime Estupinan, D.E. Gray, Robert Hall, Sir William Henderson, Cesar Lobo, William Lopez, Hunt McCauley, M. H. McDaniel, Larry Marks, William Moulton, Harry Mussman, J. M. Payne, Graham Purchase and E. C. Sharman.

The authors also wish to acknowledge the assistance of Carolyn Birr, Margo Slater, and Vinni Slotten in typing the manuscript and the manuscript editors of the Iowa State University Press for their help in preparation of the final manuscript.

Animal Disease Control

REGIONAL PROGRAMS

1

Regional Programs

GENERAL OBJECTIVES

The purpose of this book is to describe how the decision-making process can be applied to the control of animal diseases that threaten public welfare. The World Health Organization (1974) defines decision making as a step—by-step process: (1) problem definition, (2) information acquisition, (3) data analysis, (4) judgment, (5) execution, and (6) responsibility bearing. A comparison of the way an independent entrepreneur, a farmer, makes a decision with that of a public agency responsible for controlling disease should illuminate the process. The farmer must undertake all six steps of the process, although advice may be asked of a trusted authority. If the farmer operates under contract or is an employee of an agricultural corporation, the decision making must be shared or relinquished to others.

In the public sector each step of the decision-making process is separate and is carried out by different individuals or groups who imperfectly understand the needs of the individual or group responsible for the next step. While the farmers may not have all the needed information at command or be able to utilize the most useful analytical methods, they have the great advantage of knowing why the decision must be made. It may be to (1) optimize profit regardless of risk, (2) minimize risk, (3) achieve a social or aesthetic goal even though profit is reduced, or (4) forego profit for changes that will be of benefit in the future. Because the individual entrepreneur knows the nature of the decision, no unnecessary information is gathered or useless analyses made. In the public sector, such economies are seldom available to the decision maker because the decision and possible alternatives are subject to the review of advisory groups, whose minds are not known, or possible reversal by an unaccepting public.

Furthermore, the individual knows that the responsibility for the decision cannot be given to anyone else. It is much harder to determine who bears responsibility for decisions that may have been compromises reached in a committee and executed by an agency whose direction may be obscured by actions of successive directors. Yet it is very important that responsibility be assigned and accepted as part of decision making.

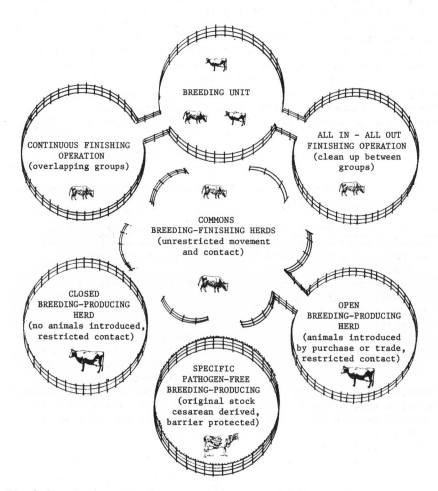

FIG. 1.1.   Herd integrity.

RATIONALE FOR INDIVIDUAL OR COLLECTIVE ACTION

Animal owners who wish to keep their herd free of a disease prevalent in the region can do so (Schwabe et al. 1977) if the herd can be effectively isolated from all other herds (Fig. 1.1). The cost of controlling the diseases in Group 1 of Table 1.1 is reasonable, and successful control enables the owner to produce more animals, use less feed, and obtain a higher price for animals produced. The cost of control depends on the disease and the margin of profit varies from slight to substantial. The reverse is true of diseases in Group 2 in which the cost of control is so large that the margin of profit ranges from insignificant, at best, to substantial loss. Technical modifications in highly intensive husbandry are changing this situation, particularly for breeding stock. The filtered-air, positive-pressure houses for poultry, if operated under strict control, can keep chickens free of exposure to even such highly communicable viruses as those of Marek's disease and Newcastle disease (Drury et al. 1969). However, most animal owners confronted with diseases in Group 2 of Table 1.1 must live with them or

Table 1.1. Characteristics of Parasites That Determine Individual or Regional Control*

Group 1 Individual Herd Control	Group 2 Regional Control
Spread of parasite is stopped by physical barrier such as a fence	Parasite readily passes physical barriers
Rate of spread is slow enough to permit intervention before entire herd becomes infected	Rate of spread is too fast to permit intervention before entire herd becomes infected
Carriers of disease can be detected on the farm	Apparently healthy carriers disseminate the disease that can be detected only by laboratory tests
Parasite does not harm people	Parasite is a human pathogen
Parasite causes low to high morbidity with low or no mortality	Parasite causes high morbidity and high mortality
Highly effective vaccine or treatment is available	Vaccine or treatment is only poorly to moderately effective

*The preferred method of control is indicated by determining which group contains the most characteristics of a given parasite.

urge the government to institute a regional program of control or eradication.

While acting in self-interest is reasonable and usually justifiable, it can have a dark side. In many animal health decisions, the individual producer, in ignorance or full knowledge, may act selfishly to the disadvantage of the neighborhood or society as a whole. In the absence of a cultural or ethical system that deters individuals from taking a course detrimental to the majority, society, through legislative action, has developed procedures for compelling individuals to conform to specified requirements designed to protect the public interest.

The economic benefits gained from controlling most animal diseases may not always be evident, particularly where the offsite costs of disease are large and the onsite costs are small. No one can escape the onsite costs of disease, and consequently everyone recognizes these costs and accepts programs to control them. However, the offsite costs that are passed on to others (a neighbor who loses a herd because a disease-carrying animal was purchased) are not recognized by the seller who gained in the transaction. Similarly, the devaluation of animals and animal products from clean herds that occurs because of neighboring diseased herds is not recognized as an offsite cost by the owners of the diseased herds. The situation is analogous to the problem created by polluting industries that fail to accept responsibility for the cleanup costs that must be paid by neighboring enterprises to prevent contamination of their products. Individuals may seek recourse through the courts, but when a significant number of industrialists or farmers recognize that they are paying for someone else's failure to control pollution or disease, they eventually ask the government to enact measures that will control the problem at the source. Controversy is likely to erupt when individuals who have been escaping offsite disease costs are forced by governmental action to participate in a disease control program they do not feel is beneficial to them.

Disease-control and eradication programs are described in this book as activities of a central government that has the authority to take whatever action is required. Most animal health programs have been carried out in this fashion but an alternative does exist. In place of regulations curtailing every activity that authorities anticipate will spread disease, the seller of a diseased animal is made liable not only for the cost of the unsound animal but also for the cost of cleaning up the disease induced by that animal.

Liability for these offsite costs of disease makes dealing in diseased animals an unprofitable enterprise of high risk. In such a situation, the market becomes a focus of disease control rather than a center for its spread, and the government's role becomes one of providing a system of disease surveillance and giving counsel on methods of control.

A decentralized disease-control program is attractive in many ways: low public cost, ease of introducing innovations for disease detection and control, and strong local support. However, a decentralized program must be specifically tailored to the disease and the production-marketing systems of the host animal. Such a program may not be readily adaptable to all animal disease situations, and some communities are not ready for it. Nevertheless, decentralization should be kept in mind and tried whenever circumstances are favorable.

STRAGEGIES FOR CONTROL OR ERADICATION

Contagious diseases are controlled by creating a physical barrier between diseased and susceptible animals, eliminating the source of infection, or protecting the susceptible animals through use of vaccines or chemicals (Halpin 1975; Brander and Ellis 1977). The concept of barriers goes back over 1,000 years when the first quarantines were employed (Schwabe 1969). The elimination of diseased carriers by slaughter and burial was attempted by Lansci in Italy in 1712 (see Schwabe 1969) and Bates in England in 1714. Vaccines for livestock were introduced beginning in the late 1800s. Chemicals that effectively controlled ticks were used before 1900, but it was not until the middle of this century that anthelmintics, antibiotics, and insecticides came into widespread use (Bushland et al. 1963).

No single procedure can be used to control all diseases. Effective and practical programs must be tailored for each parasite and host because each parasite and host population, and their interaction, has unique characteristics (Thawley et al. 1979).

Control is generally interpreted as meaning reduction of the host-parasite interaction to the point where few animals are seriously parasitized because the number of parasites has been reduced or damage to the host has been prevented (Cockburn 1961; Kaplan 1966). In either situation, loss to the herd owner becomes negligible.

Eradication means the complete elimination of the parasite from a specific region (regional eradication)

(Anderson et al. 1978) or the world (total eradication) (Cockburn 1961; Andrews and Langmuir 1963). In 1979, Arita thought total eradication of smallpox (Henderson 1976) would become a reality in 1980. Whether a strain of smallpox still persists somewhere in monkeys and will reappear in humans remains a question. Total eradication of vesicular exanthema from swine (after the disease was eliminated from the United States, and no cases were detected anywhere in the world for over twenty years) proved to be an illusion when it resurfaced as a disease of marine mammals (Smith et al. 1973). Regional eradication (disease-free zone) of a number of major livestock diseases has been achieved in several parts of the world and has given those countries important economic advantages (Brooksby et al. 1972; McCauley and Stoops 1975). In most instances, eradication has greater economic benefits than control and consequently is sought whenever feasible (Olitsky et al. 1928; Animal Plant Health Inspection Service 1971).

Herd Depopulation

Depopulation means elimination of diseased animals and all normal-appearing individuals in contact with the diseased animals or previously in contact with them during the incubation period. This strategy (Fig. 1.2) disrupts ordinary production and marketing and is used primarily for highly contagious diseases such as foot-and-mouth disease (Sellers et al. 1971), hog cholera, viscerotropic velogenic Newcastle disease (Omohundro 1972), and ectromelia of mice (Anslow et al. 1975). It is also used for difficult-to-diagnose diseases, such as scrapie, that are transmitted through breeding stock (Klingsporn and Hourrigan 1976). Diseases handled by depopulation usually have a short incubation period (foot-and-mouth disease, hog cholera, and viscerotropic velogenic Newcastle disease) but may also be chronic (ectromelia) or have very long incubation periods (scrapie). Any eradication strategy presupposes cooperation of all livestock owners within a specified region. Such cooperation is usually obtained only within an organized program administered by a government with power of condemnation and funds for indemnity.

Removal of Reactors Only

Removal of the reactor can be used to stop the spread of disease and, in some instances, completely eliminate it. This method is particularly effective

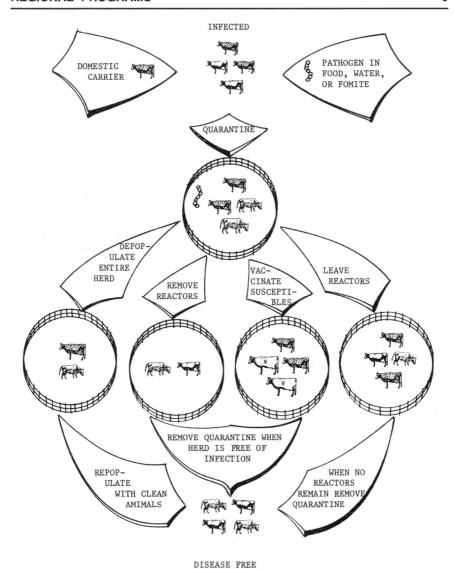

FIG. 1.2. Strategies for eradication of diseases carried by domestic animals.

where the agent is not highly communicable, there is a long incubation period, and the animal becomes a reactor during the incubation stage of the disease. Bovine tuberculosis is an example of such control (Mallman et al. 1964). Removal of reactors only is less disruptive than herd depopulation and has been attempted by some herd owners even in the absence of indemnities. Sometimes, if a control agency's policy to remove reactors only is not successful, the entire infected herd will be depopulated.

Removal of Reactors Combined with Vaccination of Susceptible Animals

When the prevalence of a disease of moderate communicability is high and segregation of herds is inadequate, removal of reactors only will not stop the disease. However, removal of reactors combined with effective vaccination of susceptible animals can halt the spread of disease. In many regions this is the initial approach used in brucellosis eradication because it is the only economically feasible method at the beginning (Food and Agriculture Organization/WHO 1971; World Health Organization 1972). Later, when prevalence of the disease has been reduced and the herds have been closed, vaccination can be discontinued. However, surveillance must be continued, herds with reactors quarantined, and the reactors eliminated until no additional reactors can be detected over a prescribed period of time.

Surveillance Only or Combined With Vaccination.

With a long-term goal of disease eradication, this alternative is possible only for diseases in which diseased animals die or recover without becoming carriers. Quarantine is lifted when surveillance establishes that susceptible animals will not become infected by the movement of recovered animals in commerce. For example, animals recovered from vesicular stomatitis are shipped to market without restriction.

Vaccination

Vaccination is intended to protect an animal against manifestations and debilitating effects of disease. Vaccination may or may not prevent infection and spread of the disease agent to other animals (*Nature* 1967; New 1979a). Appropriate immunogens (purified antigens, inactivated or killed cultures of viruses or bacteria, or modified and living cultures of viruses or bacteria) are given to all susceptible individuals in the herd or flock according to established procedures that may involve a single administration at a certain age or multiple administrations at prescribed intervals over the animal's life span. The direct cost of vaccination varies depending on the price of the vaccine and the labor and equipment required to administer it. Sometimes the vaccine and its administration cause adverse reactions (Lancaster 1964) that vary from a rather common transitory drop in egg or milk production to less common problems such as injection abscesses at the site where vaccine was introduced to rare incapacitating illnesses, and even death. Furthermore, vaccination may increase costs by delaying the scheduled pattern of animal movement between housing units or to pasture or market. The savings provided by an effective vaccine for an enzootic disease that causes heavy losses requires no analysis. When considering use of less effective vaccines or vaccines for diseases that occur infrequently or cause minor losses, the owner must weigh the known costs of vaccination against the probable costs of disease in the immediate future. The unavailability of vaccine because its need was not anticipated is often the greatest limiting factor of its use. (Callis et al. 1975).

Supervised vaccination of susceptible animals to protect them against highly communicable enzootic disease is sometimes employed by a government as the first step in a program that has eradication as its final objective. When the prevalence of the disease has been appreciably reduced by vaccination, authorities further slow the spread by quarantining herds exhibiting active disease. Eventually a program of eradication is announced in which the infected herds are depopulated. In moving step-by-step, authorities recognize that immediate application of an eradication strategy would disrupt the economy, cost a formidable sum, and be strongly resisted by the people support for the program is essential.

Barriers

A barrier is any device or procedure th introduction of a disease onto a premise. T of the barrier depends upon the specific disease To bar domestic carriers of disease, the her closed, all replacements are reared, and the hera confined within single or double fences or in a stable Equipment that may be contaminated, such as livestock trucks and crates, is not permitted in paddocks and pastures. Unfortunately, ordinary fences and sanitary precautions that keep out diseased livestock do not stop wild animals and insect vectors. However, various strategies such as special fences and screens have sometimes provided the needed protection. In some cases, housing structures are designed to exclude disease agents small enough to be airborne (Riley 1980).

For example, the entrance of such highly communicable airborne pathogens as avian bronchitis, Marek's disease, and Newcastle disease has been prevented in poultry houses where entering air is filtered and maintained at positive pressure to prevent infiltration of unfiltered air (Drury et al. 1969).

Certain diseases do not require barriers throughout the entire year. When a seasonal vector is present in the pasture, animals may be stabled continually or, sometimes, for only part of the day during the critical period (Hanson 1952). Stabling only at night has been quite successful in controlling African horse sickness, which is transmitted by a nocturnal vector.

In some cases, environmental alterations are effective in stopping the short distance movement of reservoirs or vectors. Draining a wetland pasture eliminates the snail that serves as the intermediate host of the giant liver fluke, thus preventing that parasitic disease. Pasture spelling (discontinuing use until parasites have died) can also be a useful control measure (Wharton et al. 1969; Lindquist 1970) as can pasture clearing, which sometimes stops the movement of vectors. However, many vectors can fly from 2 to 20 miles and elimination of breeding sites on a single farm is of little practical value to the owner.

If physical barriers between the animal and the disease agent are ineffective, a chemical barrier that will prevent either infection or replication of the parasite may be established in the animal. Such drugs are in widespread use for control of selected protozoan and metazoan parasites and, to some extent, suppression of selected bacteria. A low prophylactic dose is usually administered in feed or water or is sometimes given by injection. Drugs have been ineffectual barriers to viruses.

Elimination of the Carrier or Vector

Controlling disease by eliminating the carrier or vector (Fig. 1.3) requires community action, careful planning, sophisticated methodology, and a commitment to achieve a predetermined goal. The earliest efforts to control disease by this method were probably directed to rabies (World Health Organization 1966). Sporadic and sometimes extensive attempts were made to reduce the diseased fox and wolf populations. The result, at best, was a temporary reduction of the carrier population and a temporary decrease in the incidence of human or live-stock rabies. The reproductive potential of these reservoir animals was too

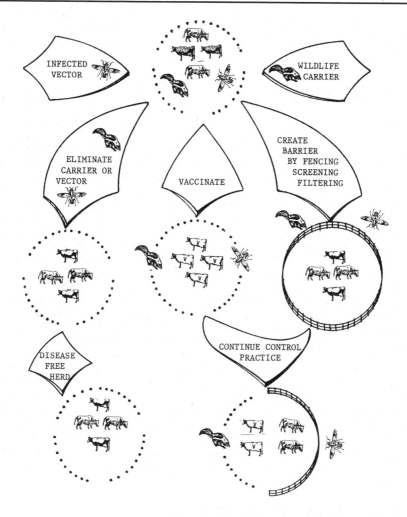

FIG. 1.3. Strategies for control of diseases carried by alternative hosts and vectors.

great for any permanent change to occur (Bogel 1976). Far greater promise is shown by a program for controlling rabies in cattle that destroys only the vampire bats that feed on cattle (Thompson et al. 1972).

The first effective program to eliminate a vector (the tick *Babesia bigemina*) was initiated by the USDA even before the role of the tick as the vector of Texas fever was scientifically established. Texas fever disappeared when this one host tick was eliminated from the United States by use of arachnicide dips and the imposition of control over cattle movement (Curtice 1896). A different approach, suppression of arthropod reproduction by release of sterile males, was success- ful in eliminating the screwworm from southeastern United States (Knipling 1960). Similar programs using sterile males are now being directed against the vector of trypanosomiasis in Africa (Stephen 1975) and the vector of malaria and viral encephalitis in a few selected areas.

Programs to control disease through elimination of the vector or reservoir require a great deal of labora- tory and field research (Mattingly 1962; Smith 1966; Hayes 1979). To be successful, such programs usually require international funding and cooperation over a sustained period.

CONTROLLING DISEASE IN INDIVIDUAL HERDS

Control of disease in herds and flocks is not only practical for many Group 1 diseases (see Table 1.1) but also necessary if the owner is to remain competitive or make a profit. Vaccination and/or barriers are used. The best course is to keep parasites out by creating barriers against their spread. Most infections are introduced by a normal-appearing carrier that, like the Trojan horse, does not reveal the parasite it has until after its addition to the herd (Smithcors 1957; Netto 1973). Consequently, a full history should be obtained on purchased animals to be added to the herd, and the animals should be kept in isolation for an extended period. Better control is gained by maintaining a closed herd in which replacements are reared.

Pathogens can also enter on fomites such as the shoes and gear of service people and visitors. For this reason, access to a herd should be limited. Infection also occurs during animal contact across a common fence or through the use of a single water supply. Double fencing stops the first, and fencing off access to natural waters and wetlands controls the latter. Stabling animals during the critical time of day in the season of vector activity can protect ani- mals from some, but not all, arthropod-borne diseases.

Many parasites induce disease only when the host animal is crowded or its defense is lowered. Manage- ment procedures such as pasture rotation, adjustment of milking order, and use of slatted floors can be effec- tive in controlling the level of infection to which animals are exposed. Regular culling of diseased ani- mals removes individuals that otherwise would heavily pollute their environment and reduces the risk of infection for the rest of the herd.

Susceptible individuals in a herd or flock can be protected by vaccination or by prophylactic treatment with drugs. The latter has become routine for controlling many endoparasites and a few ectoparasites. The primary strategy is to keep infection out or, if infection is present, stop transmission. Therapeutic procedures are seldom routinely practical.

Development of a herd health program requires professional help in appraising the situation, obtaining accurate diagnoses, and selecting a course to follow. While such programs are successful in controlling many problems, they fail to keep out or control highly communicable or exotic diseases and do not protect the herd against diseases arising from widespread environmental pollution.

RATIONALE

The control of exotic and highly communicable diseases is often frustrating for herd owners because (1) they do not have the necessary knowledge, experience, or tools to save their animals; and (2) the effort they do make is negated by the action of a careless or incompetent neighbor, or (3) the realization that their herd could be devastated and they themselves could contract those diseases pathogenic for humans. In addition there are diseases that are not caused by infectious agents but by chemicals in the environment (Walsh 1977) over which the owners have no control. For these reasons, the community (either producers, consumers, or both) demands that the government act in the interest of human welfare (Cockburn 1964; Cockrill 1965).

The government has far greater resources than the individual and possesses the police power that may be necessary to prevent the entry of diseased animals. Quarantine was first employed hundreds of years ago and has major successes to its credit. Police power is also used to stamp out the foci of disease by destroying condemned animals. Through licenses and inspection, a large range of activities can be controlled, thus preventing the dissemination of disease. In addition, government resources can be used to promote the study of disease problems, development of control measures, and creation of organizational structures that can and do eradicate selected diseases from the country.

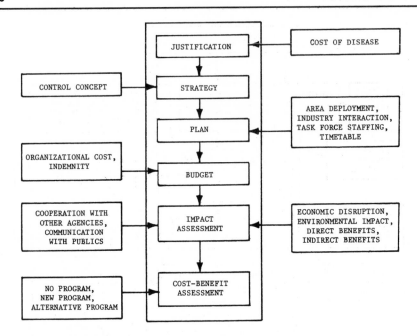

FIG. 1.4. Development of a new disease-control program.

ESTABLISHMENT

Recognizing the Problem

Development of a regional disease control program (Fig. 1.4) starts when responsible professionals in the appropriate branch of government become convinced that a program is both needed and feasible (Estupinan et al. 1977). The need may be established as the result of an academic inquiry or from studies of disease losses initiated at the request of producers. Public health questions and political interest also play a particularly stimulating role in precipitating prompt action (Schwabe and Ruppanner 1972). But in every instance, assessing the problem and establishing the need is the first step in developing a program (Shahan and Perez 1967).

Preparing a Proposal

A proposal for a disease-control program (Fig. 1.5) is seldom written without (1) arranging for one or more studies to determine the feasibility of critical issues, such as the dependability of a diagnostic test, or (2) obtaining a legal opinion on the appropriateness

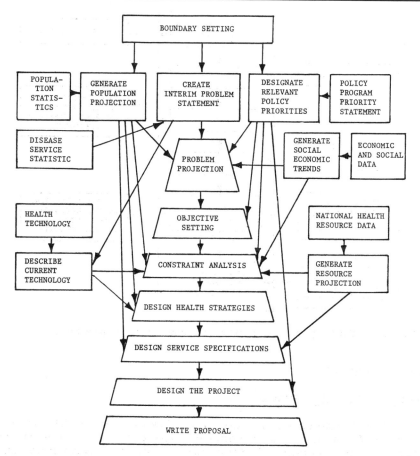

FIG. 1.5. Project formulation activities as suggested by the World Health Organization in 1974.

of a course of action. As these tasks are accomplished, the staff prepares the document that is the basis for authorization and funding (Pan American Health Organization 1966; Ayala 1970; Estupinan 1976). The proposal must be written in language understandable by individuals who are not experts in the field since most of the decisions will be made by generalists, not experts. The proposal tells what is to be done, why, where, and how. Above all, it should give a clear description of the program costs and benefits.

Securing Adoption

Any major disease control program requires both authorization and funding by the legislative branch of

the government.   Before a formal request can be made to
the legislative body, the program must be approved by
the senior officials in the sponsoring agency and the
oversight agency, variously called a budget or management office, in the executive branch of the government.
Here it is judged for soundness and merit in competition with other proposals for human welfare.   Changes
may be negotiated.   Political issues are weighed along
with questions of feasibility and economic merit.
While the favorable and adverse publicity generated by
proponents and opponents of the program may have some
effect on its development, the pressure of public
opinion is particularly efficacious in legislative
halls.

Not all disease programs must go through the full
process.   Some may be authorized by past legislative
action as a standby program to eradicate a highly
contagious exotic disease whenever it enters the
country.   In such cases, provisions may even be made
for emergency funding of such an effort.

ANATOMY OF A PROPOSAL

A document that describes and justifies a major
program will contain a great deal of information.
Inevitably it will be long and many of the people
receiving it will have neither the time nor the persistence to peruse it all.   Nevertheless, each reader
will have certain questions in mind and the answers
should be easy to find.   For this reason, the first
section of the disease-control proposal should provide
a brief statement of objectives and explain the organization of the document so that all readers can easily
find answers to their questions.

The body of the document must contain at least six
sections (Pan American Health Organization 1966; World
Health Organization 1974), each of which is discussed
in the chapters that follow.

Justification

The disease should be described and the significance of the problem explained.   Physical losses should
be given and the cost interpreted in both economic and
social terms.   The relationships between solving the
problem, improving general welfare, and strengthening
the national economy should be made clear.

Control Strategy

The procedures proposed to bring the problem under control should be explained clearly and simply. The rationale for the recommended approach must be easily understood, and its superiority to other approaches should be defended and documented. If, as often happens, some of the proposed procedures are unusual, either individually or collectively, reasons for the procedures' feasibility should be given.

Description of the Region

Each region is unique and the proposed program must be tailored to that particular region's pecularities of climate, topography, and fauna as well as the attitudes and customs of its people (Rosenberg et al. 1979). Careful study of all these matters is essential in planning the program to prevent its failure (Division de Communicacion Social 1974). Careful identification should be made of all the region's significant features, such as natural barriers, that might have bearing on the program.

Assessment of the Infrastructure

Since the proposed program will exist in a world of many other organizations, important institutional relationships and procedures for handling jurisdictional questions must be described. The interrelationships with federal, state, and local governments as well as the many semiautonomous agencies will involve obeying their rules, laying down new rules, or working cooperatively. On some occasions, even international agreements will be affected.

Costs and Benefits

The cost of the program has two parts: implementation and impact. The budget for implementation should include developmental, operational, and evaluation costs (New 1979b). Developmental costs include training, research, and any pilot trials required to establish proven methodology and provide experience for the staff. Operational costs include monies (funds for equipment, materials, salaries, and indemnities) required to carry out the control operation. Evaluation costs cover studies, using accepted criteria, of the program's efficiency to determine degree of success.

It is unlikely that the impact of the program on the economic climate and the natural environment will be entirely favorable. Flow of goods to market is usually disrupted, and control measures may entail use of substances that will harm some nontarget species. Probable adverse impacts of these kinds should be identified and quantitated as accurately as possible. Alleviation methods should also be sought. If none can be found, compensation should be considered.

The benefits of the program to the health and well-being of both human and animal populations as well as the national economy should be identified in considerable detail and quantitative measurements given wherever possible.

Operational Plans

A detailed outline of the program organization, projected timetable, plans for deployment, and general operating procedures should be given so the reader has a clear description of how the program will be carried out and goal achievement measured.

EXAMPLE OF A PROPOSAL

At the request of the Tanzania government, an English team led by John Brooksby prepared a proposal for the creation of a disease-free zone that would permit Tanzania to develop export trade in carcass meat (Brooksby et al. 1972). The team reviewed the epizootiology of foot-and-mouth disease, the control of which was critical to the development of trade. They evaluated the control measures and diagnostic services already in place in Tanzania and then prepared a program for creation of a disease-free zone. The program was based on systematic vaccination of cattle on the ranch of origin plus control of movement of cattle within the country. Implementation of the program required recruiting and training new staff, purchasing and deploying equipment, and constructing a vaccine-filling plant for subsequent operation. A timetable was established and goals set (Table 1.2). Staff needs were determined (Table 1.3), and costs of salaries, equipment, and supplies were estimated (Table 1.4). This study enabled the English team to develop a seven-year budget (Table 1.5).

The Tanzanian proposal illustrates very clearly the need for establishing a timetable and understanding

Table 1.2. Field Operations of Tanzania Disease-free-zone Project

Year	Months	Number Cattle Vaccinated	Number Field Teams	New Teams Equipped	Equipment Replaced
1	12	300,000	6	6	0
2	24	600,000	6	0	0
3	36	900,000	9	3	0
4	48	1,200,000	12	3	6
5	96	2,400,000	24	12	0
6	96	2,400,000	24	0	0
7	44	1,100,000	24	0	3

Source: Adapted from Brooksby et al. 1972.

Table 1.3. Workforce of Tanzania Disease-free-zone Project

	Regional Veterinary Officers	Veterinary Officers	Field Officers	Assistant Field Officers	Field Assistants
Present staff	2	5	15	67	276
Project staff					
Year 1	0	0	0	2	16
2	0	0	0	5	36
3	0	0	0	5	36
4	0	0	0	11	76
5	0	0	0	11	76
6	0	0	0	11	76
7	0	0	0	11	76

Source: Adapted from Brooksby et al. 1972.

Table 1.4. Unit Costs of Tanzania Disease-free-zone Project

Items	Costs, Tanzania Dollars
Vaccine	1,990,000 per million doses
Vaccine-filling plant	
Capital investment	2,722,450 total
Training program	45,000 total
Salaries	161,400 per yr
Depreciation	178,875 per yr
Miscellaneous	106,000 per yr
Variable costs	variable
Field campaign	
Capital costs	
Vehicle and equipment (syringes, cooler, camping gear)	40,000 per team
Crushes (animal-handling equipment)	5,000 each
Base refrigerator	2,200 each
Ear tags	115 per 1000
Capital replacements (every 4 yr)	40,000 per team
Recurrent costs	
Salaries (per mo)	8,537 per team
Maintenance (per mo)	2,270 per team
Control operations	variable

Source: Adapted from Brooksby et al. 1972.

Table 1.5. Seven-year Budget for Tanzania Disease-free-zone Project

Items	Year 1	Year 2	Year 3	Year 4	Year 5	Year 6	Year 7
Vaccine	752,000	1,445,400	1,504,400	2,260,440	4,158,960	4,233,000	3,096,520
Vaccine-filling plant							
Capital investment	245,520	2,749,175	...	...	...	...	...
Training programs	41,983	7,517	...	...	...	...	...
Salaries	...	...	177,540	177,540	177,540	177,540	177,540
Depreciation	...	...	196,762	196,762	196,762	196,762	196,762
Miscellaneous	...	...	116,000	116,000	116,000	116,000	116,000
Variable costs	...	...	30,360	48,620	97,350	99,550	70,180
Field campaign							
Capital costs							
Vehicles and equipment	264,000	...	132,000	132,000	528,000	...	...
Crushes	275,000	275,000	330,000	137,500	...	...	...
Base refrigerators	4,840	...	...	2,420	9,680	...	...
Ear tags	40,480	4,048	57,937	9,487	111,320	2,530	2,530
Capital replacements	...	...	...	264,000	...	...	132,000
Recurrent costs							
Salaries (per mo)	112,695	225,390	338,085	450,780	901,560	901,560	413,215
Maintenance (per mo)	29,964	59,928	89,892	119,956	239,712	239,712	109,868
Control operations	137,280	158,400	158,400	337,920	337,920	337,920	337,920
Total (Tanzanian dollars)*	1,903,762	4,924,858	3,131,376	4,253,325	6,874,804	6,304,574	4,652,535

Source: Brooksby et al. 1972.
*10% contingency calculated in costs.

such logistic problems as queueing, inventory, and replacement. The budget varied from year to year as new kinds of activities were added and field work was expanded or reduced. For example, the major capital expenditure for the vaccine-filling plant occurred in the second year of the budget, but hiring staff did not occur until the third year. Salaries for the field campaign increased each year for five years, but field equipment costs fluctuated as new teams were activated and worn-out equipment was replaced.

This proposal reflected a good understanding of Tanzanian ranching and marketing procedures as well as the effect that climatic, geographic, and cultural patterns can have on program goals. The proposal was wisely built on existing institutions and added only what was necessary to achieve the objective.

REFERENCES

Anderson, R. K.; Berman, D. T.; Berry, W. T.; Hopkins, J. A.; and Wise, R. 1978. Report National Brucellosis Technical Commission. Anim. Plant Health Insp. Serv., USDA, Washington, D.C.

Andrews, J. M., and Langmuir, A. D. 1963. The philosophy of disease eradication. *Am. J. Public Health* 53:1-6.

Animal Plant Health Inspection Service. 1971. Programming, planning, and budgeting model for cattle fever tick eradication program. PPB Code 1-2-164. USDA, Hyattsville, Md.

Anslow, R. O.; Ewald, B. H.; Pakes, S. P.; Small, J. D.; and Whitney, R. A., Jr. 1975. Control of infectious diseases among rodent stocks. *Science* 189:248.

Arita, I. 1979. Virological evidence for the success of the smallpox eradication programme. *Nature* 279: 293-298.

Ayala, P. P. 1970. Planning of a foot-and-mouth disease control program. *Pan Am. Sanit. Bur. Sci. Publ.* 196:41-57.

Bates, T. 1714. A brief account of the contagious disease which raged among the milch cows near London in the year 1714 and the methods that were taken for suppressing it. *Philos. Trans. R. Soc. London.*

Bogel, K. 1976. Assessment of fox control operations on wildlife rabies. In Wildlife Diseases, ed. L. A. Page. New York: Plenum Press, pp. 487-490

Brander, G. C., and Ellis, P. R. 1977. Animal and

Human Health--The Control of Disease. London:
Bailliere Tindall.

Brooksby, J. B.; Stubbins, A. J. G.; and Petrzik, J.
1972. Report to the government of Tanzania: Control of foot-and-mouth disease and the establishment of a disease-free zone. TA3146. FAO, UN,
Rome.

Bushland, R. C.; Radeleff, R. D.; and Drummond, R. O.
1963. Development of systemic insecticides for
pests of animals in the United States. *Annu. Rev.
Entomol.* 8:215-238.

Callis, J. J., Graves, J. J., McKercher, P. D., and
Uskavitch, R. 1975. Report on worldwide foot-
and-mouth disease vaccine production (Feb.).
Restricted doc., Plum Island Anim. Dis. Cent.,
Greenport, N.Y.

Cockburn, T. A. 1961. Eradication of infectious
diseases. *Science* 133:1050-1058.

Cockburn, W. C. 1964. The implications of large-scale
programmes for the control of infectious
disease. In *Global Impacts of Applied
Microbiology*. New York: John Wiley and Sons, pp.
456-461.

Cockrill, W. R. 1965. IV. The principles and application of international disease control. *Vet. Rec.*
77(48):1438-1448.

Curtice, C. 1896. On the extermination of the cattle-
tick and the disease spread by it. *J. Comp. Med.
Vet. Arch.* 17:649-655.

Division de Comunicacion Social. 1974. Plan de
divulgacion de la campana contra la brucelosis.
Instituto Colombiano Agropecuario, Bogota,
Colombia, Nov.

Drury, L. N.; Patterson, W. C.; and Beard, C. W. 1969.
Ventilating poultry houses with filtered air under
positive pressure to prevent airborne diseases.
Poult. Sci. 48:1640-1646.

Estupinan, J. A. 1976. Animal health program for controlling and eradicating foot-and-mouth and other
diseases in Colombian livestock. World Meat
Congr. Proc., Buenos Aires, Argentina, Aug. 3-6

Estupinan, J. A.; Lobo, C. A.; and Reyes, M. 1977.
Establishment of pilot areas for the control and
eradication of foot-and-mouth disease in Colombia.
8th Pan Am. Congr. Vet. Med. Zootech. Proc. Santo
Domingo, Dominican Republic.

Food and Agriculture Organization/World Health Organization. 1971. Joint FAO/WHO expert committee on
brucellosis: Fifth report. WHO Tech. Rep. Ser.
464. Geneva.

Halpin, B. 1975. Patterns of Animal Disease. Baltimore: Williams & Wilkins Co.

Hanson, R. P. 1952. The natural history of vesicular stomatitis. *Bacteriol. Rev.* 16:179-204.

Hayes, R. O. 1979. Concepts and techniques for control of arthropods and arthropod-borne diseases. Paper read at Conf. Concepts Tech. Control Erad. Anim. Dis. Sept. 10-14, Auburn, Ala.

Henderson, D. A. 1976. The eradication of smallpox. *Sci. Am.* 235(4):25-33.

Kaplan, M. 1966. The problems of choice between control and eradication. Joint WHO/FAO Expert Comm. Zoonoses, Geneva, Dec. 6-12.

Klingsporn, A. L., and Hourrigan, J. L. 1976. Progress in the scrapie eradication program. *U.S. Anim. Health Assoc. Proc.* 80:376-392.

Knipling, E. F. 1960. The eradication of the screwworm fly. *Sci. Am.* 203(4):54-61.

Lancaster, J. E. 1964. Newcastle disease: Control by vaccination. *Vet. Bull.* 34:57-76.

Lindquist, W. D. 1970. Nematodes, Acanthocephalids, Trematodes, and Cestodes. In Diseases of Swine, 3rd ed., ed. H. W. Dunne. Ames, Ia.: Iowa State Univ. Press, pp. 717-718.

McCauley, E. M., and Stoops, D. 1975. Abstracts of animal disease control programs and their socioeconomic impact. World Bank Work. Pap., Jan., Int. Bank Reconstr. Dev., Washington, D.C.

Mallmann, W. L.; Mallmann, V. H.; and Ray, J. A. 1964. Bovine tuberculosis: What we know, do not know, and need to know in order to eradicate. *U.S. Livest. Sanit. Assoc. Proc.* 68:327-332.

Mattingly, P. F. 1962. Mosquito behavior in relation to disease eradication programmes. *Annu. Rev. Entomol.* 7:419-436.

Nature. 1967. Slaughter or vaccination? 216:1057-1059.

Netto, L. P. 1973. Carriers in foot-and-mouth disease. *Biol. San Paulo* 39:14-16.

New, J. C., Jr. 1979a. The effect of vaccination programs on endemic foot-and-mouth disease. In A Study of the Potential Economic Impact of Foot-and-Mouth Disease in the United States, eds. E. H. McCauley, N. A. Aulaqi, J. C. New, Jr., W. B. Sundquist, and W. M. Miller. Tech. Rep. 1. Washington, D.C.: USGPO, pp. 9-21.

————. 1979b. Technical and cost dimensions of theoretical control programs against foot-and-mouth disease in the United States. In A Study of the Potential Economic Impact of Foot-and-Mouth

Disease in the United States, eds. E. H. McCauley, N. A. Aulaqi, J. C. New, Jr., W. B. Sundquist, and W. M. Miller. Tech. Rep. 3. Washington, D.C.: USGPO, pp. 33-62.

Olitsky, P. K.; Traum, J.; and Schoening, H. W. 1928. Report of the Foot-and-Mouth Disease Commission of the United States Department of Agriculture. Tech. Bull. 76. USDA, Washington, D.C.

Omohundro, R. E. 1972. Exotic Newcastle disease eradication. *U.S. Anim. Health Assoc. Proc.* 76:264-269.

Pan American Health Organization. 1966. Guide for the preparation of projects for control of foot-and-mouth disease. Doc. 2, Aftosa, Pan Am. Health Organ., Washington, D.C., Aug. 8-9.

Riley, R. L. 1980. Part I. History and epidemiology: Historical background. *Ann. N.Y. Acad. Sci.* 353: 3-9.

Rosenberg, F. J.; Astudillo, V. M.; and Goic-M., R. 1979. Regional strategies for the control of foot-and-mouth disease: An ecological outlook. In Veterinary Epidemiology and Economics. Int. Symp. Vet. Epidemiol. Econ. Proc. 2:587-596. Canberra: Aust. Gov. Publ. Serv.

Schwabe, C. W. 1969. Veterinary Medicine and Human Health, 2nd ed. Baltimore, Md.: Williams & Wilkins Co.

Schwabe, C. W., and Ruppanner, R. 1972. Animal diseases as contributors to human hunger problems of control. *World Rev. Nutr. Diet.* 15:184-224.

Schwabe, C. W.; Riemann, H. P.; and Franti, C. E. 1977. Epidemiology in Veterinary Practice. Philadelphia: Lea & Febiger.

Sellers, R. F.; Herniman, K. A. J.; and Donaldson, A. I. 1971. The effects of killing or removal of animals affected with foot-and-mouth disease on the amounts of airborne virus present in looseboxes. *Br. Vet. J.* 127:358-365.

Shahan, M. S., and Perez, E. 1967. Report of survey in Panama and Central America of preventive practices against foot-and-mouth disease and readiness for control and eradication of the infection in the event of its occurrence in this currently free region. Restricted doc., Pan Am. Health Organ., Washington, D.C., Aug.-Sept.

Smith, A. W.; Akers, T. G.; Madin, S. H.; and Vedros, N. A. 1973. San Miguel sea lion virus isolation, preliminary characterization and relationship to vesicular exanthema of swine virus. *Nature* 244: 108-110.

Smith, E. H. 1966. Advances, problems and the future of insect control. In Scientific Aspects of Pest Control. NAS-NRC Publ. 1402. Washington, D.C.

Smithcors, J. F. 1957. James Mease, M.D., on the diseases of domestic animals. *Bull. Hist. Med.* 31(2):122-131.

Stephen, L. E. 1975. African trypanosomiasis. In Diseases Transmitted from Animals to Man, 6th ed., eds. W. T. Hubbert, W. P. McCulloch, and P. R. Schnurrenberger. Springfield, Ill.: Charles C. Thomas, pp. 745-764.

Thawley, D. G.; Wright, J. C.; and Solorzano, R. F. 1979. An evaluation of options for the control and eradication of pseudorabies in the USA swine herd. In Veterinary Epidemiology and Economics. Int. Symp. Vet. Epidemiol. Econ. Proc. 2:597-606. Canberra: Aust. Gov. Publ. Serv.

Thompson, R. D.; Mitchell, G. C.; and Burns, R. J. 1972. Vampire bat control by systemic treatment of livestock with an anticoagulant. *Science* 177:806-808.

Walsh, J. 1977. Seveso: The questions persist where dioxin created a wasteland. *Science* 197:1064-1067.

Wharton, R. H.; Harley, K. L. S.; Wilkinson, P. R.; Utech, K. B.; and Kelley, B. M. 1969. A comparison of cattle tick control by pasture spelling, planned dipping, and tick-resistant cattle. *Aust. J. Agric. Res.* 20:783-797.

World Health Organization. 1966. WHO expert committee on rabies: Fifth report. WHO Tech. Rep. Ser. 321. Geneva.

————. 1972. A socio-economic assessment of controlling brucellosis in a developing country. WHO Consultations on Socioeconomic Aspects of Zoonoses. Reading, UK, Nov. 21-25.

————. 1974. Health project formulation: A manual of procedures. WHO Proj. Syst. Anal. 71.1, Rev. 2, Draft 2. Geneva, June.

2

Cost of Animal Disease

DISEASE LOSSES AND THEIR MEASUREMENT

For more than 3,000 years, cattle herders have complained of losses from diseases that cause either the death of promising young stock, fat cattle, and strong bullocks (Schwabe 1969) or dysfunctions such as barrenness, sores, and unsoundness (Fig. 2.1). The effects of disease can be observed directly in three ways: (1) death, (2) loss of function, and (3) altered

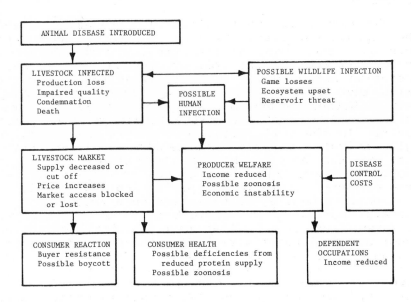

FIG. 2.1. Possible consequences of disease introduction.

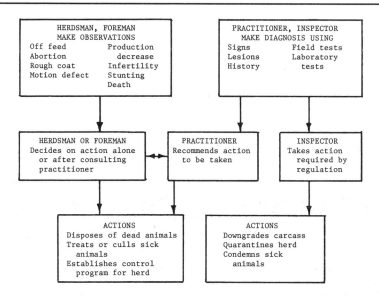

FIG. 2.2. Observations and diagnosis of disease and options for action.

appearance (Fig. 2.2). These are physical losses that can be measured.

Mortality

In nature and to the livestock producers as well, the reproducing animal is more important than the new-born or aged. Many species produce large numbers of young anticipating the loss of all but a fraction to predation and disease. This is illustrated by cotton-tails that have four litters of four to five young a year. Without heavy mortality of the young, cotton-tails would be a plague on the landscape in only a few years. In the wild, predation removes the older, less agile animals; on farms and ranches producers harvest most of the animals before they become old. Only people and pets live long enough to experience death from diseases of the post-reproductive individual.

Until recently, farmers have been tolerant of high neonatal mortality in cattle and swine, but the death of productive animals that have required considerable labor and feed has always been a matter of deep concern and has been recorded frequently (Bierer 1974; Davis 1979). Currently, this concern has motivated some livestock producers to keep mortality records of the herd by age categories (National Research Council 1968).

Morbidity

        In recent years, producers have realized that the
effects of disease are as important as mortality losses
(Committee on Morbidity and Mortality Statistics 1947).
The important dysfunctions are infertility, unsoundness, cessation of growth, and reduced production of
eggs or milk.
        Infertility arises from failure to produce fertile
sperm or eggs, failure to accomplish fertilization, or
failure of the fetus to mature (absorption and abortion).   Breeders   report   their   losses   as   abortion,
failure to breed, or a problem of increased breeding
intervals (repeat breeder).
        Cessation of milk production or lay (Gordon 1967;
Ellis 1975) and the production of abnormal milk or eggs
is induced by diseases of the reproductive organs and
many   systemic   infections   (Ellis   and   Kendall   1964;
Halvorson 1971; Pilchard 1972).   Such losses are readily quantitated (McCauley 1979a).   Record keeping systems are usually based on the herd or flock, but some
managers, particularly of dairys, keep breeding and
milk production records of individual animals (Kaneene
and Mather 1982).
        If   disease   causes   inappetence,   malabsorption,
diarrhea, or energy sapping fever, animals stop growing
and begin to lose weight.   For example, parasites that
take blood for nourishment do it at the expense of
growth of the host (Ross 1970; Copeman and Hutchinson 1979; Dobson and Cargill 1979; Gordon, 1979).   The
diseased or parasitized animal may be permanently
stunted, or maturity may be delayed.   In all these
instances, the feed efficiency of the animal is reduced
(Betts and Beveridge 1953; Ciordia et al. 1972; Fitzgerald 1980) and more feed and labor are required to
bring it to market (Ames et al. 1969).   This loss is
most serious in rapidly maturing animals such as broilers and turkey poults, substantial in feeder pigs and
feedlot steers, and less serious in young animals such
as beef calves that have a chance to catch up while
still on pasture.   In intensive operations producers
keep accurate records of feed consumed and days to
market (feed efficiency) to measure the impact of
disease.
        Disease-induced unsoundness, inability to move
normally because of locomotive malfunction (such as
lameness and paralysis) or sensory impairment (such as
blindness and deafness), destroys the value of work and
pleasure animals.   Although disease in pleasure animals
is a problem in developed nations, disease in draft

animals used to till the soil and transport goods causes much greater problems in developing nations (National Research Council 1977). In tropical wetlands and the difficult terrain of mountainous areas where no substitute for work animals has yet been found, diseases that impair locomotion can bring all food production to a standstill (Cockrill 1974). Unfortunately, reports of workdays lost because of animal disease are rare, and no studies were located in the literature examined.

Disease may induce changes not only in the physical appearance of the animal, such as unkempt hair coat or loss of hair, but also in its behavior, such as listlessness or irritability. The carcass may contain lesions or have an unattractive appearance. These losses are measured directly at sale or slaughter when the animal or its carcass is downgraded. The Meat Inspection Service in the United States and the United Kingdom provides statistical information on the prevalence of abscesses, tumors, and condemnations, in whole or part, of animals subjected to inspection (Pickard 1952; Taylor 1974). The culminative impact of such things as warble fly holes in hides, foot rot, and jowl abscesses can be very substantial (Special Swine Abscess Committee ca. 1964).

Disease can also result in the loss of domestic market for animals and animal products of herds that are infected with zoonoses as well as the loss of foreign markets when certain diseases are diagnosed in just one herd in the region.

Role of the Owner-Operator in Detection of Disease

Early detection of disease is critical in the control of communicable diseases. It depends upon the ability of every individual who has any responsibility for animals to recognize a change in their well-being and report the observation in an appropriate fashion. The ability to perceive must be structured and the criteria that distinguishes an abnormal from a normal animal must be learned. In addition, it is important to know the conditions that make it difficult for animals to maintain the physiologic and immunological homeostasis necessary for health. With an understanding of animal needs, stressful conditions can be reduced without resorting to overcompensation that is not cost effective, as may happen in the management of pets. The following four points outline these directives.

Understanding of responsibility. Set standards for all tasks and establish schedules for their completion. Be sure that all personnel responsible for the animals are acquainted with the standards and schedules and the reason for them.

Structure perception. Record production and developmental events. Record abnormalities such as inappetence or lameness. Observe each animal (appropriately identified) with a checklist of items and maintain ongoing records. Report critical items to the responsible individual. Review and analyze records regularly. Cull animals on the basis of disease predisposition and subnormal productivity or lack of desired confirmation.

Recognition of stressful conditions. Maintain adequate nutrition. Deprivation of either food or water and abrupt changes in dietary constituents can result in malnutrition as serious as the omission of an essential nutrient. Provide space for natural functions to avoid crowding that leads to harassment or limits access to food, water, or shelter. Fill environmental needs by providing protection from excessive insolation and heat, severe cold, and wind chill.

Reduction of opportunities for transmission. Using fences, screens, and chemicals, isolate the animals as far as practical from other species that may be reservoirs or vectors of disease. Segregate the animals into discrete units of modest size and avoid contact both during and after assembly. Quarantine individuals before adding them to a unit. Remove animal wastes regularly or design the facility to separate animals from wastes that might contaminate their food, water, or air.

SYSTEMS FOR REPORTING LOSSES

A committee of the National Academy of Science concluded in 1974 that the primary problems in assembling meaningful statistics on disease losses were a lack of uniformity in reporting losses and a central organization for gathering and systematizing the data (Hutton and Halvorson 1974). Miller discussed a modified system in 1979. Beal (1980) emphasized that quality control of the statistics being gathered is necessary if results are to be useful. Because of the variety of record keeping systems used in specific disease control programs, it is not possible to compare their results or utilize other information collected in a haphazard fashion for other diseases. Until a comprehensive national scheme for collecting animal disease statistics is established, McCallon (1981) urges adoption of the Minnesota plan for collecting data from a sample of livestock enterprises that are appropriately stratified for such important variables as herd type and size and geographic location.

Procedures also differ from country to country (Poppensiek et al. 1966; Gregory 1976; Khera 1979). Almost no quantitative information is gathered in some countries; a great body of such information is collected in others. For instance, a nationwide attempt to organize animal health statistics is presently under way in Australia (Roe 1979). The districts feed information into a computer center where analysts interpret and disseminate the information for use by disease-control officials.

Current systems of gathering information (Table 2.1) can be divided into (1) government statistics that are automatically gathered under controls that insure a degree of accuracy, (2) government statistics that are automatically gathered without control over accuracy, and (3) special statistics. The first two types are required by regulation or law. The third is usually voluntary, but, if required, no penalty exists for noncompliance although a reward system may be employed.

Program Statistics

Statistics of the first category above include information on disease programs that incorporate a system of gathering data on reactors, diseased, and condemned animals. In such programs, populations are known for each governmental jurisdiction and each owner. Consequently, statistics concerning losses from diseases covered by control programs (such as brucellosis (Table 2.2), tuberculosis, and sometimes foot-and-mouth disease) are quite accurate in many countries. Professionally supervised meat inspection services can supply good information of the second category on problems perceived at antemortem and postmortem examination of animals offered for slaughter (Table 2.3). Reasons for condemnation of animals and rejection of carcass parts are routinely collected (Willeberg 1979) and reported in most nations. These reporting systems are relatively free of sampling bias of the market-age animals, although it is possible that animals known to be

Table 2.1.   Source of Information on Prevalence of Animal Disease

Source	Example
Government statistics with accuracy control	
Reports of diseases from official control or eradication programs give a valid measurement of prevalence and incidence by region because total populations are known and regular, reliable procedures of detection are employed.	The U.S. Cooperative State-Federal Brucellosis Eradication Program Report. Table 2.2.
Reports of diseases following meat inspection of animals marketed through regulated plants provide a reliable estimate of prevalence for a defined segment of a known population.	The U.S. Federal Meat and Poultry Inspection Service Report. Table 2.3.
Government statistics without accuracy control	
Reports of animal diagnostic laboratories operated by private and public institutions do not give reliable estimates of prevalence because of sample bias and lack of population data, but reliable indication of presence is provided.	The Wisconsin Animal Diagnostic Laboratory Annual Report. Table 2.4. The New York State Veterinary College Report. Table 2.5.
Voluntary statistics	
Reports by farmers and veterinarians of diseased and dead animals on farms are usually invalid as a measure of prevalence or incidence because they are compiled with reference only to populations observed and without allowance for the nature of sampling bias.	The Minnesota Infectious Disease Report. Table 2.6.
Compilations by national and international groups of information obtained from the above sources.	The FAO-WHO-OIE Animal Health Yearbook. Table 2.9. The Pan-american Foot-and-Mouth Disease Center Vesicular Disease Report. Table 2.10.

diseased are diverted to small slaughtering operations that are not inspected and withholding for economic reasons occurs. Analyses of mandatory, systematically collected reports permit epidemiologists to estimate

Table 2.2. Statistics Reported for a Brucellosis Eradication Program in the United States (Animal Disease Eradication Division) (1962)

STATE OR TERRITORY	BRUCELLOSIS BLOOD TESTS										BRUCELLOSIS RING TESTS							MODI- FIED CERTI- FIED COUN- TIES	CERTI- FIED BRUCEL- LOSIS- FREE COUN- TIES	TOTAL CERTI- FIED COUN- TIES
	LOTS	CATTLE	INFECTED LOTS NUMBER	PER-CENT [a]	PER-CENT [b]	REACTOR CATTLE NUMBER	PER-CENT [a]	PER-CENT [b]	CALVES VACCI-NATED	HERD TESTS	ESTIMATED CATTLE REPRESENTED	SUSPICIOUS HERD TESTS NUMBER	PER-CENT	NEGATIVE TESTS	PER-CENT	ESTIMATED CATTLE IN NEGATIVE HERDS			
Alabama	1,294	24,028	189	14.6	10.9	567	2.40	1.30	6,129	467	20,548	22	4.7	445		19,580	26		26
Alaska	3	9	0	0.0	0.0	0	0.00		19							-	0		-
Arizona	179	1,404	6	3.4	3.4	7	1.50	0.50	1,405							-	40		40
Arkansas	5,075	19,707	206	4.0	1.3	179	0.68	0.06	8,707	1,485	37,125	69	4.6	1,416		35,500	68		68
California	5,483	28,498	38	4.7	2.3	179	0.68		37,017	2,470	263,038	111	4.5	2,359		267,622	56	15	56
Colorado	928	13,668	28	3.0	2.6	61	0.15	0.37	19,668	134	2,938	5	3.7	129		2,803	35		35
Connecticut	400	3,510	1	0.3	0.3	1	0.03	0.01	1,832	614	9,824	5	0.8	609		9,744	8		8
Delaware	135	4,008	8	4.3	4.3	12	0.30	0.30	392							-	3		3
Florida	1,013	22,110	139	13.7	10.9	440	1.99	0.88	4,538	344	63,716	85	24.7	259		27,746	30		30
Georgia	18,613	26,305	190	1.0	1.0	386	1.06	0.40	5,014	1,350	75,600	62	4.6	1,288		72,128	159		159
Hawaii	163	3,040	13	8.0	8.0	42	1.38	1.38	138							-	0		0
Idaho	673	9,760	21	3.0	0.7	11	0.42	0.09	24,842	2,505	37,575	25	1.0	2,480		37,200	40		40
Illinois	2,938	34,681	106	3.6	1.1	229	0.66	0.21	12,259	6,371	76,488	39	1.0	6,335		76,020	79	13	79
Indiana	2,976	18,855	67	2.3	0.9	121	0.64		8,670	4,580	107,355	45	1.0	4,535		106,300	92	13	92
Iowa	5,469	37,598	135	2.5	1.1	344	0.91	0.25	18,336	7,397	103,558	207	2.8	7,190		100,660	24		24
Kansas	3,023	55,514	300	10.0	1.6	805	1.50	0.64	31,935	3,501	70,020	119	3.3	3,382		67,640	46		46
Kentucky	5,456	28,773	216	4.4	20.8	350	1.22	0.74	10,629	3,790	18,950	55	11.5	3,735		18,675	87		87
Louisiana	3,708	25,243	432	11.2	0.2	852	2.97	2.04	11,600	252	11,823	29	11.5	223		13,084	6		6
Maine	249	3,892	1	0.2	0.8	3	0.08	0.01	2,348	1,191	38,626	7	0.5	1,184		38,424	16	15	16
Maryland	1,124	25,553	13	1.1		16	0.06	0.04	3,613	607	13,778	3		604		13,710	23		23
Massachusetts	318	5,593	9	9.1	3.4	51	0.97	0.33	2,204	541	10,820	11	2.0	530		10,600	11		11
Michigan	2,051	19,880	29	5.9	3.2	212	1.07	0.44	8,877	1,724	28,446	25	1.5	1,699		28,033	83		83
Minnesota	5,202	102,402	107	2.6	0.4	234	0.23	0.04	11,117	21,539	430,780	90	10.4	21,449		428,980	87	13	87
Mississippi	7,076	16,041	256	3.5	1.1	492	3.07	0.04	2,892	182	9,011	19	10.4	163		8,661	43	13	43
Missouri	3,240	43,246	137	4.2	1.1	279	0.65	0.19	29,978	9,177	105,535	62	0.7	9,115		104,823	93		93
Montana	1,317	6,766	12	0.9	0.7	25	0.37	0.26	38,612	285	2,850	4	1.4	281		2,810	54		54
Nebraska	2,658	35,889	138	5.2	2.4	371	1.03	0.55	55,715	3,081	31,725	25	0.8	3,056		31,465	54		54
Nevada	175	2,686	3	1.7	1.0	0	0.15	0.05	1,551	123	4,740	1	0.0	122		4,684	17	10d	17
New Hampshire	766	10,657	0	0.0	0.0	0	0.00	0.00	1,554	623	18,669	0	0.0	623		18,669	0	7	10
New Jersey	862	15,909	24	2.8	1.0	36	0.23	0.05	1,481	1,523	64,868	34	2.2	1,489		63,378	21		21
New Mexico	1,386	3,218	6	0.4	0.4	30	0.90	0.70	5,226	162	1,134	1	0.6	161		1,127	32		32
New York	1,075	14,758	98	9.1	0.5	155	1.05	0.08	28,482	2,599	165,682	58	0.6	2,581		164,696	62	3	62
North Carolina	1,580	25,533	21	2.6	0.5	69	0.26	0.08	1,279	499	65,975	18	0.7	498		65,755	100	6	100
North Dakota	1,219	21,075	51	3.0	3.0	145	0.69	0.17	48,944	8,693	8,183	1	0.2	8,445		8,166	44		44
Ohio	2,727	27,505	106	4.2	0.9	235	0.85		7,387		117,269	248	2.9			113,923	69		69
Oklahoma	1,866	31,918	288	15.4	8.6	729	2.28	1.34	17,589	1,571	23,565	73	4.6	1,498		22,470	6		6
Oregon	2,998	15,267	54	1.8	1.0	92	0.60	0.12	26,582	2,417	62,350	78	3.2	2,339		60,130	36	3	36
Pennsylvania	2,711	41,490	38	1.4	0.5	77	0.19	0.04	13,009	2,417	131,406	32	0.7	2,748		130,366	67		67
Rhode Island	139	916	0	0.0	0.0	0	0.04	0.04	16	15	300	0		15		300	5		5
South Carolina	613	8,807	22	3.6	3.6	64	0.73	0.73	1,299							-	41		41
South Dakota	2,401	41,103	155	6.5	2.7	439	1.07	0.91	56,566	3,506	65,842	63	1.8	3,443		64,696	26		26
Tennessee	5,372	8,854	104	1.9	1.6	189	2.13	0.44	15,444	1,123	12,353	38	3.4	1,085		11,935	95		95
Texas	2,942	35,243	285	9.7	8.1	670	1.90	1.27	41,124	634	19,020	56	8.8	578		17,340	75		75
Utah	830	4,107	15	1.8	0.6	18	0.44	0.08	7,157	1,574	39,350	16	1.0	1,558		38,950	29		29
Vermont	234	4,775	20	8.5	1.0	40	0.84	0.08	3,506	1,731	46,737	10	0.6	1,721		46,467	11		11
Virginia	3,235	29,587	45	1.4	0.5	109	0.37	0.11	6,118	5,125	51,250	137	2.6	4,988		49,880	83	20	83
Washington	2,478	14,666	19	0.8	0.5	35	0.24	0.10	16,075	1,036	20,340	14	1.4	1,022		20,040	39	10	39
West Virginia	1,055	12,889	14	1.3	1.0	30	0.23	0.20	366	330	2,310	0	0.5	330		2,310	55		55
Wisconsin	2,874	32,180	49	1.7	0.4	75	0.13	0.10	37,899	10,169	264,394	53	0.0	10,116		263,016	61		71
Wyoming	261	5,372	62	2.0		0	0.13	0.10	37,552	30		0		30		30	15		15
Puerto Rico	200	11,331	62	31.0	15.2	129	1.14	0.53	1,379	289	13,535	20	8.7	209		12,802	77c		77
Virgin Islands	2	2	0	0.0	0.0	0	0.00	0.00								-	3o		3
TOTAL	**116,075**	**1,047,904**	**4,395**	**3.8**	**1.8**	**9,842**	**0.94**	**0.26**	**723,672**	**131,800**	**2,792,781**	**2,075**	**1.6**	**129,725**		**2,703,438**	**2,233**	**103**	**2,336**

(a) Percent of herd and cattle blood tests only.
(b) Percent of herd and cattle infection and tests and BRT negative herds and cattle.
(c) Modified Certified States
(d) Certified Brucellosis-Free States

Table 2.3. Number of Carcasses Condemned by U.S. Federal Meat and
Poultry Inspection, Calendar Year, 1978

Cause of Condemnation	Cattle	Calves
Degenerative and dropsical conditions:		
Emaciation	6,006	1,918
Miscellaneous	1,888	158
Infectious diseases:		
Actinomycosis, actinobacillosis	2,595	13
Caseous lymphadenitis	...	...
Coccidioical granuloma	22	...
Swine erysipelas	...	...
Tuberculosis nonreactor	...	3
Tuberculosis reactor	85	...
Tetanus	9	9
Miscellaneous	234	20
Inflammatory diseases:		
Eosinophilic myocitic	4,646	7
Mastitis	1,194	8
Metritis	1,757	24
Nephritis, pyelitis	3,845	312
Pericarditis	5,484	157
Peritonitis	4,648	1,583
Pneumonia	13,942	6,593
Uremia	1,192	70
Miscellaneous	1,996	853
Neoplasms:		
Carcinoma	3,303	7
Epithelioma	16,833	38
Malignant lymphoma	7,945	128
Sarcoma	325	10
Miscellaneous	816	16
Parasitic conditions:		
Cysticercosis	347	...
Myiasis	3	10
Miscellaneous	227	4
Septic conditions:		
Abscess, pyemia	11,460	578
Septicemia	8,879	3,155
Toxemia	4,030	1,289
Other:		
Arthritis	1,936	3,309
Central nervous system disorders	118	36
Contamination	...	...
Deads	10,003	27,363
Icterus	499	3,467
Injuries	4,446	1,342
Moribund	2,351	1,892
Pigmentary conditions	317	44
Pyrexia	207	31
Residue	110	44
Sexual odor	...	...
Miscellaneous general	292	212
Other reportable diseases	56	10
Total	124,046	54,723

Source: Food Safety and Quality Service 1978.

the prevalence and incidence of disease and, depending upon the adequacy of records, determine the effects of managerial factors, such as herd size and purchase of replacement stock, on the risk of disease.

However, epidemiologists using these program statistics must be careful not to make unwarranted assumptions about their uniformity. Regulatory changes may result in the inclusion of animals previously with-held from testing, and criteria for placement of ani-mals in the reactor group may change because the test protocol has been altered or the positive titer has been raised or lowered. False positives that were of little significance early in a program may make up the majority of positives later, rendering the data obtain-ed late in a program of much less value. For these reasons care must be taken in preparing tables and charts that show trends in disease-control programs (Beal 1980).

Voluntary Reporting Programs

Disease reports are also obtained from diagnostic laboratories (Tables 2.4 and 2.5). Unfortunately, data from laboratories that are dependent upon submissions determined by proximity to the laboratory, by economic value of the animal, or changing policy cannot provide a true picture of disease prevalence. A typical policy change occurred when a laboratory director rejected all specimens from skunks suspected of having rabies be-cause most specimens had been rabid; consequently all skunks were administratively considered rabid. As a result, rabid skunks were not listed in subsequent reports of the laboratory, although the disease pro-bably persisted. Faulty conclusions can also be drawn from the appearance of a new disease in a laboratory report. This usually reflects the addition of a new test to the diagnostic repertoire and not the appear-ance of a disease new to the area.

Disease reports are also obtained from veterinar-ians and farmers who answer questionnaires about the presence of disease on farms (Table 2.6). In some regions where tradition dictates or monetary incentives exist, veterinarians provide reasonably good reports of scheduled or reportable diseases. The system is very uneven in most countries and difficult to sustain (Poppensiek et al. 1966). Because of these inconsis-tencies and biases, the reports are of dubious value (Beal 1977).

Even when diagnosticians and voluntary practit-ioner reporters are conscientious, information on the

Table 2.4. Segment of an Annual Report from a State Animal
Disease Diagnostic Laboratory, 1976-1977. Mink, Miscellaneous
Test Summary, Aleutian Disease (number positive, 1,482;
number negative, 32, 396)

Diagnosis or Findings	Number of Herd Diagnoses	Total Animals in Herds	Number of Animals Sick or Dead
Agalactia	1	9,000	2
Aleutian disease	1	10,700	4
Bacterial isolations			
Clostridium septicum	1	10,000	17
Escherichia coli	6	3,001	41
Escherichia coli-hemolytic	2	2	2
Proteus species	5	50,000	16
Pseudomonas species	2	6,000	200
Salmonella			
blockley	1	1	1
Staphylococcus aureus	9	2,003	9
Streptococcus-alpha hemolytic	1	1	1
Streptococcus equi	1	4,000	85
Streptococcus species	1	1	1
Botulism	2	14,530	150
Bronchopneumonia	1	10,000	200
Cystitis	2	2	2
Deficiency disease			
Malnutrition	2	7,004	10
Starvation	1	6,000	2
Degeneration	1	2,600	2
Distemper	2	5,004	94
Edema	1	10,000	3
Emaciation	1	150	14
Endocarditis	1	10,000	11
Enteritis	1	1	1
Fatty liver disease	1	1	1
Hemorrhage	3	3	3
Hypoglycemia	1	1	1
Metritis	1	900	1
Myocarditis	1	10,000	10
Necrosis	2	1,600	33
Nephritis	1	28,000	81
Nephrosis	1	1	1
Pneumonia	1	1,400	26
Pregnancy disease	1	1,500	700
Septicemia	1	1	1
Urinary calculi	2	42,001	91
No visible lesions	1		
Normal animal tissue	1		
Specimen unsuitable	1		

Source: Wisconsin Department of Agriculture, Trade, and
Consumer Protection 1977.

Table 2.5. Segment of a Report from a State Animal Disease Diagnostic Laboratory. Summary of Accessions

DIAGNOSIS	Dogs	Cats	Cattle	Sheep	Swine	Horses	Miscellaneous
CONGENITAL AND INHERITED DEFECTS							
Anomaly, brain	3	1	4	...	...	...	
Anomaly, cardiac	1	1	1	2	...	1	
Anomaly, circulatory	...	...	1	...	...	...	
Anomaly, eye	...	...	1	...	...	...	
Anomaly, genital	...	...	2	...	1	...	
Anomaly, intestinal	2	...	1	2	...	...	
Anomaly, kidney	4	1	3	...	...	...	
Anomaly, muscoloskelatal	...	1	5	1	1	3	
Anomaly, pulmonary	...	...	1	...	...	...	
Hip dysplasia	3	...	...	...	...	...	
NUTRITIONAL, METABOLIC AND DEGENERATIVE DISEASES							
Acetonemia	...	...	3	...	...	...	
Amyloidosis, hepatic	...	...	1	...	...	...	
Amyloidosis, renal	...	...	1	...	...	...	
Anemia, idiopathic	...	...	1	...	...	...	
Anemia, nutritional	...	...	...	...	8	...	
Arthropathy, degenerative	...	...	...	...	...	...	
Diabetes mellitus	3	...	...	...	...	...	
Goiter	...	...	...	1	...	...	
Heat stroke	...	...	...	...	2	...	
Hyperplasia, Parathyroid (Secondary)	5	...	...	...	1	...	
Hypocalcemia	...	...	...	...	1	...	1 Rabbit
Hypothyroidism	1	...	...	...	...	...	
Hypovitaminosis E (muscular dystrophy)	...	...	9	5	...	...	1 Goat
Inanition	1	...	19	15	15	1	1 Monkey 2 Rats 4 Goats 1 Rabbit 1 Guinea Pig
Liver, necrosis, dietary	...	...	...	...	1	...	
Parturient paresis	...	...	4	...	...	...	
Rickets	...	...	1	...	...	...	
Toxemia, feedlot	...	...	1	...	...	...	
Toxemia, pregnancy	...	...	...	10	...	...	1 Guinea Pig
POISONING							
Poisoning, arsenic	...	...	4	...	...	...	
Poisoning, copper	...	...	...	1	...	...	
Poisoning, unidentified	1	...	...	...	...	...	
Poisoning, ethylene glycol	1	...	...	...	...	...	
Poisoning, lead	1	...	9	...	...	...	
Poisoning, nitrate	...	...	...	2	...	...	
Poisoning, sodium chloride	...	...	...	...	1	...	
SPECIFIC INFECTIOUS DISEASES							
Aspergillosis	...	...	1	1	...	1	
Atropic rhinitis	...	...	...	...	4	...	
Blackleg	...	...	1	...	...	...	
Contagious ecthyma	...	...	...	1	...	...	
Cocciomycosis	1	...	...	...	...	...	
Distemper, canine	39	...	...	...	...	...	
Enteritis, infectious calf (calf scours)	...	...	36	...	...	...	
Enteritis, infectious feline (panleukopenia)	...	7	...	...	...	...	
Enterotoxemia	...	...	1	15	...	...	

Source: New York State Veterinary College 1961.

population observed and its relationship to the overall population of the region is usually unavailable. Beal discussed this problem in papers presented in 1977 and 1980. Using information on anaplasmosis reported by practicing veterinarians to their state animal disease official as well as information gathered through a well-designed probability sample of animals in the market cattle test program, Beal showed that Arkansas, which had three times as many cases as Oregon on the probability sample survey, reported 19 times as many cases as Oregon in the state disease report (Table 2.7). Nationally, these state disease reports gave a very misleading picture of the prevalence of anaplas-

Table 2.6. Segment of Voluntary State Animal Health Report. Minnesota Infectious Disease Reports for Swine Herds, 1st Calendar Quarter 1973 (no. cases/thousand animals)

Piglets	Swine	Disease
4.81	16.41	Abscesses
		Abortion or reproductive diseases
		Brucellosis
	48.72	Leptospirosis
		MMA (metritis, mastitis, agalactiae)
	58.97	Pseudorabies
		SMEDI (stillbirths, mummifications, embryonic deaths, infertility)
	5.64	Etiology undetermined
		Arthritis diseases
1.89		Corynebacteria
2.27		Erysipelas
0.09		Mycoplasma arthritis
0.09		Streptococcal arthritis
17.18	23.08	Etiology undetermined
		Dermatitis and external parasites
		Exudative epidermatitis
101.55	163.08	Mange: specify etiology if determined
74.09	103.08	Pediculosis
		Ringworm
		Swinepox
		Etiology undetermined
		Diarrheal diseases
65.22		Colibacillosis
0.28		Edema disease

Piglets	Swine	Disease
		Enterotoxemia
		Salmonellosis
		Transmissible gastroenteritis
0.19		Vibrionic dysentery (bloody scours)
82.21	25.64	Etiology undetermined
		Eperythrozoonosis
		Neurologic diseases
		Listeriosis
		Rabies
		Tetanus
0.19		Viral encephalomyelitis (vomiting and wasting disease)
		Etiology undetermined
		Parasitism—internal
		Lungworms
3.78		Roundworms
		Other: specify etiology if determined
		Etiology undetermined
		Respiratory diseases
29.82		Atrophic rhinitis
		Bull nose
16.99		Mycoplasma pneumonia
		Polyserositis
21.42	0.51	Sporadic pneumonia
85.13	2.56	Swine influenza
10.67		Etiology undetermined

Source: Diesch et al. 1974.
Number of piglets observed, 10,595; number of pigs observed, 1,950.

Table 2.7. Comparison of Two Surveys for Anaplasmosis in Arkansas
            and Oregon, 1968-1972

	Arkansas	Oregon
Statistic descriptor		
Number of farms	31,115	15,661
Number of cows	1,300,000	690,000
Average number of cows per farm	42	44
USDA probability sample survey of		
market cattle test samples		
Incidence rate	21.7	13.4
Number infected	282,490	92,805
Ratio of 2 states	3	1
State report based on information		
from practicing veterinarians		
giving 5-yr total for 1968-1972		
Number infected	12,984	682
Ratio of 2 states	19	1

Source: Beal 1977.

mosis. California, which on the probability sample
survey had 10 percent of the infected animals in the
United States, reported less than 1 percent, and
Arkansas, which had 5 percent in the sample survey,
reported 36 percent of the cases in the country (Table
2.8). The problem lies not only in the varying efforts
of the states in promoting reporting but also in skew-
ness of sampling and failure to relate the cases
detected to the populations at risk.
     Nevertheless, voluntary systems, if well designed
and administered, can provide good information. The
Minnesota animal disease-reporting program (Diesch
et al. 1974) uses a panel of veterinarians and livestock owners that make internal checks on each other,
and in all instances, the number of cases in the popu-

Table 2.8. Percent of Infection of Anaplasmosis in United States,
            1968-1972

Area	State Report of Infection Based on Information from Practicing Veterinarians	Report of Infection Based on USDA Probability Sample Survey of Market Cattle
United States	100.0	100.0
Arkansas	36.4	5.3
California	0.7	10.4
Louisiana	14.2	4.3
Missouri	2.1	6.5
Oregon	1.9	1.6
Texas	11.3	19.3

Source: Adapted from Beal 1980.

lation observed is related to the population at risk
(Table 2.6). The stratified random sample of on-the-
farm information collected by Minnesota has few biases
and is obtained at modest cost. A validation study
(University of Minnesota 1981) established the relia-
bility of statistics gathered. The low cost of voluntary systems is very attractive to disease-control
officials (Simpson and Wright 1979; Simpson et al.
1979).

Disease losses are more difficult to assess in
wildlife populations than livestock populations because
the population at risk is only rarely known within an
accuracy of 50 percent and significant death losses may
go undetected, particularly in nongregarious species
(Chapman 1957). Only catastrophic mortalities from
such diseases as botulism, fowl cholera, and duck virus
enteritis in waterfowl are likely to be observed (Davis
et al. 1971; Page 1976). Even when census techniques
determine that the population has decreased, there is
usually no indication whether the losses were juveniles
or adults or resulted from a failure of the breeding
population to reproduce (Keith 1963). Only sustained
in-depth studies of selected wildlife populations
provide reliable information.

Compilation of Disease Reports

National and international agencies publish
reports of disease after assembling data from a multi-
tude of dissimilar sources and varied validity. The

Table 2.9. Segment of an International Animal Disease Report
FAO–WHO–OIE

Disease	Species	UK–GB	UK–NI	Eire	Denmark	Norway
Anthrax	bov	+V*	(−)73*	(−)*	+*	(+)Qi*
B. anthracis	eq	−*	−*	−*	−*	−Qi*
	ov	(+)*	−*	−*	−*	−Qi*
	sui	(+)V*	−68*	−*	−*	−Qi*
Blackleg	bov	+/V	+TtV	+V	−	+Qi
Cl. chauvoei	ov	+/V	+TtV	+V	−	−
Enterotoxemia	ov	+/V	++TtV	+V	−	+
Cl. welchii						
Botulism						
Cl. botulinum		av,pel:(+)	−,0000	−	bov:+	pel:(+)

Source: *Animal Health Yearbook* 1978.
Code: 0000 never occurred; − not present; (−) probably not
present; 68, 73, year last observed; (+) exceptional occurrence;
+/ reduced but still exists; + low incidence; ++ moderate
incidence; * notifiable; Qi, quarantine measures and movement
control; Tt, therapeutic treatment; V, vaccination; av, avian;
bov, bovine; eq, equine; ov, ovine; pel, fur-bearing; sui, swine.

Animal Health Yearbook of FAO/WHO/OIE (Table 2.9) attempts to provide information on all the important diseases in a major livestock species. The monthly report (Table 2.10) of the Pan American Foot-and-Mouth Disease Center on vesicular diseases, is more successful because it is limited to diseases in one control program. Information regarding location of disease, populations involved, and type of virus is solicited each week from leaders of vesicular disease-control programs in South and Central America. Reporting procedures are standardized, and an international laboratory serves as a diagnostic reference facility (Astudillo and Deppermann 1980). Geographic prevalence is shown on a uniform grid of districts that clearly depicts distribution of disease within each country (Fig. 2.3).

Table 2.10. Segment of an Animal Disease Report on Vesicular Diseases in South America

Country Province	Affected Herds	Diagnosis					
		FMD			Ves.	Stom.	
		0	A	C	NJ	IND	Neg
Argentina	25	6	4	1	–	–	5
Buenos Aires	5	–	3	–	–	–	2
Cordoba	3	1	1	–	–	–	–
Corrientes	4	–	–	1	–	–	–
Entre Rios	8	5	–	–	–	–	1
La Pampa	1	–	–	–	–	–	1
Sante Fe	4	–	–	–	–	–	1
Colombia	434	59	15	–	7	1	18
Antioquia	16	8	–	–	–	–	1
Bolivar	10	–	1	–	–	–	–
Boyaca	61	13	1	–	–	–	2
Caldas	9	2	–	–	1	–	–
Casanare	3	2	1	–	–	–	–
Cauca	4	1	–	–	2	–	–
Cordoba	5	1	1	–	1	–	1
Cundinamarca	280	26	5	–	1	–	4
El Cesar	7	–	1	–	–	–	–
Huila	1	–	1	–	–	–	–
La Guajira	1	–	–	–	–	–	–
Magdalena	1	–	–	–	–	–	1
Meta	3	1	–	–	–	–	2
Narino	2	–	–	–	–	–	1
Norte de Santander	5	2	1	–	–	1	1
Risaralda	3	1	–	–	–	–	2
Santander	9	1	2	–	–	–	1
Sucre	2	–	–	–	–	–	1
Tolima	9	1	–	–	1	–	1
Valle	3	–	1	–	1	–	–

Source: Pan American Foot-and-Mouth Disease Center 1980b.

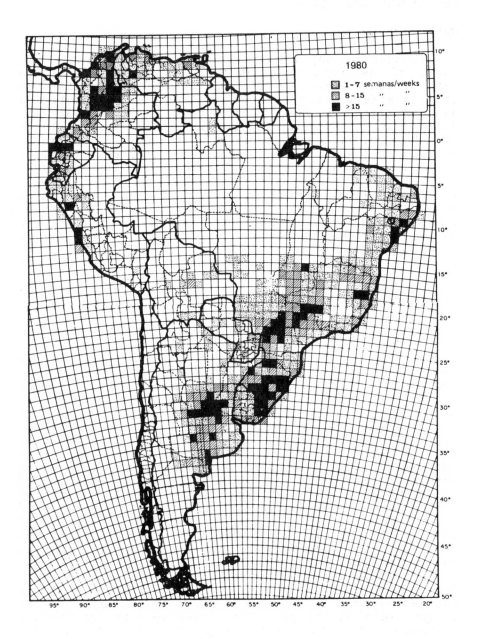

FIG. 2.3. Geographical distribution of vesicular disease
(Pan American Foot-and-Mouth Disease Center 1980a).

ESTIMATING THE COSTS

Nature of Costs

Losses of any kind must always be interpreted in terms of the population at risk. Ten birds with the same kind of lesion in a flock of 20 is far different from 10 affected birds in a flock of 20,000. Neither a diagnostician nor an epidemiologist will become very excited about a nonlethal disease that has a prevalence of 0.5 percent, particularly when the cost of the individual is low. Fifty percent prevalence is another matter. Establishing the size of the herd, flock or population in a region to determine the prevalence or incidence of a disease is dependent upon information obtained from both the owner of the herd and the census reports. If the census information is old or has failed to cover the species for which information is needed, a survey like the one conducted in Tierra del Fuego (see chapter 3) is required. Leech (1971) discussed some of the problems in obtaining good animal population information, and Khera (1979) dealt with the problem of deriving animal health indices from available data.

The primary cost of a disease can be calculated from a knowledge of its morbidity and mortality rates. Death of the animal, although important for a few diseases, is less significant to livestock producers and the country in general than disease-induced disability because the latter occurs more frequently. Direct costs from disease-induced disability result from condemnation of all or part of a carcass, downgrading of the saleable product, delay in maturation, feeding inefficiency, and an increased breeding interval (Maurer 1975). Indirect losses result from health service costs, increased capitalization for maintaining a large but less-productive breeding herd, increased labor costs for handling diseased animals, and loss of market opportunities. Monetary values can be assigned to both direct physical losses and indirect losses, and from these combined values the economic loss can be calculated (Halvorson 1971; Bell 1973).

However, totalling losses and their costs may not be enough. Economists point out that elimination of a disease may not mean that the producer will receive all or even part of the gain that might be expected because increased productivity may depress market prices and benefit the consumer or enhance international trade balances to the benefit of the nation. In such instances, the farmer would receive none of the benefit.

Furthermore, some losses may be ephemeral. McCauley (1979b) argues that calves that suffer a weight loss early in their development can compensate for that loss by time for market. However, a weight loss later in development cannot be regained, and any compensatory attempt represents a major cost in feed. Where a program for the control of a specific disease is instituted in an animal population, it will encompass animals that receive less than optimal care and suffer from other diseases. Consequently, elimination of a single disease or nutritional deficiency should not be expected to bring that population to optimal production (Hawkins 1979; Hugh-Jones 1979).

Systems for Estimating Costs

A realistic estimate of the benefits that would be obtained if effective control eliminated disease losses should be based on studies of herds that are comparable in their breeding, management, and sanitation (Hugh-Jones 1979). Two kinds of studies can provide such an estimate. In one, a number of herds are followed over a period of time until the disease status of a given herd changes by natural events from diseased to free or free to diseased. Accurate records (i.e., milk production and quality of milk or pounds of meat marketed) are kept on the health and productivity of each herd (Morris 1971; Gordon 1979), and the differences between diseased and disease-free herds are determined. The other approach pairs diseased and healthy herds according to size, general management, and breeding. Productivity of each pair of herds is then compared. In either type of study, at least one year of production records must be available for comparison. Even one year is inadequate to measure the long-term effects of disease such as infertility. Problems of bias exist with both methods and should always be considered and discussed when results are presented.

IMPACT OF COSTS ON PRODUCTION AND MARKETING

Major unanticipated disease losses can lead to several responses (Hugh-Jones 1979). Some farmers will apply for additional credit to reestablish production, but others will refinance to spread or defer credit payments. Planned improvements or expansion are invariably put off because most farmers facing a decrease in income become more conservative about credit. Certain farmers shift to an alternative farm enterprise (corn

only instead of a hog-corn operation) and some older
farmers may retire earlier than planned.

Losses can seriously impair the flow of goods to
market. The scarcity that results forces up the price;
a benefit to unaffected producers but a detriment to
consumers. Ordinarily, buyers facing high prices reduce their consumption, at least initially, and attempt
to find a satisfactory alternative. Unfortunately for
the producer, some of the individuals who turn to an
alternative product do not go back to the first product
when it again becomes available.

Even control of disease can affect the producer
adversely. The poultry industry's rapid adoption of
Marek's vaccine, which stemmed mortality (Purchase and
Schultz 1979) put more pullets into the laying houses
in 1971 than had been planned. The resulting increase
in the egg supply flooded the market and depressed the
price of eggs. The consumer, not the producer,
benefited.

When diseases cause interruptions and diminutions
in the supply of goods, the processor and jobber face
increased processing costs and possible penalties
resulting from failure to meet scheduled deliveries.
The processor and jobber may also lose a market to an
alternate product.

Animal disease presents the consumer with scarcity, higher prices, and often an inferior product.
The unavailability of animal protein, for which no substitute is available, can lead to malnutrition among
some socioeconomic groups.

OTHER IMPACTS

Zoonoses and Malnutrition

Some of the major diseases of livestock are
zoonoses. Brucellosis and bovine tuberculosis cause
debilitating and sometimes fatal disease in farmers and
consumers of meat and milk products. Hydatidosis and
Rift Valley fever cause serious disease problems in
human populations of endemic areas. More than 50
diseases caused by viruses, bacteria, rickettsia, pro-
tozoa, and helminths can be transmitted from animals to
humans (Hubbert et al. 1975). Some are acquired by
close association with the infected animal, others by
consumption of meat, milk, or eggs produced by infected
animals. In Iran a leading source of brucellosis in
the human population is a rennet cheese made from milk
of infected sheep. In the United States a similar
source of infection has been unpasteurized cow's milk.

Trichinosis results from the consumption of undercooked
pork, and anthrax in wool sorters has been traced to
batches of wool from infected sheep.

While death can result from such diseases as
rabies, bovine tuberculosis, and several of the encephalitides, the important loss faced by human populations is incapacitation--particularily from chronic
illnesses like undulant fever and schistosomiasis. In
such situations, health insurance, if available, is
inadequate to pay for farm labor and family needs.

The impact of zoonoses on human health plays an
important role in establishing priorities for the
eligibility of a disease for regional control. The
emphasis on zoonoses control is also shown by the
amount of funds allocated for this purpose and the
order in which major disease-control programs are
adopted.

Diseases that are not zoonoses can also affect
human health. Catastrophic animal losses drive up the
price of animal protein, disrupt patterns of its distribution, and essentially remove it from the diet of
the poor (Maurer 1975; National Research Council 1977).
The result in some segments of the population, particularly among children, is protein malnutrition or
kwashiorkor.

Impoverishment of the Environment

Animals provide companionship and pleasure to
people who enjoy singing birds, running horses, track-
ing dogs, soaring hawks, and kittens' antics. There is
no agreement on the value of these things, but the
prices paid for some companion animals indicates the
value their owner places on them--more than $1,000 for
a parrot (Animal Plant Health Inspection Service 1978),
$3,000 for a hunting dog, $5,000 for a pleasure horse,
and several hundred thousand dollars for a racehorse.
The death of a parakeet belonging to an old woman or a
cur dog belonging to a small boy may cause depression
that can impair the physical health of these individuals. The public outcry following an oil spill that
sickens and kills most of the marine birds along a
stretch of coast indicates the value that the public
places on seeing healthy wildlife at the beach, be it
wheeling gulls or diving pelicans.

Waterfowl and deer hunters, who purchase licenses
for the right to pursue their sport, have demanded that
the government protect game from devastating diseases
and provide improved habitat (Page 1976). The economic
value of game has been estimated on the basis of

license fees, cost of hunting equipment, and other costs accrued in pursuit of the sport. Decreases in game populations are quickly reflected in the reduced income of both the government from loss of hunting fees and private enterprise from decreased hunting outlays.

Some estimates of the value of unhunted wild animals can be obtained by prorating the income derived by government and industry from use of parks and forest lands for viewing wildlife (birds, bears, bison). Although these estimates are difficult to make, some authorities value these species as equal to that of game.

REFERENCES

Ames, E. R.; Rubin, R.; and Matsushima, J. K. 1969. Effects of gastrointestinal nematode parasites on performance in feedlot cattle. *J. Anim. Sci.* 28:698-704.

Animal Disease Eradication Division. 1962. Summary of brucellosis eradication activities in cooperation with the various states. Agric. Res. Serv., USDA, Washington, D.C.

Animal Health Yearbook 1978. Rome: FAO/WHO/OIE.

Animal Plant Health Inspection Service. 1978. Eradication of exotic Newcastle disease in southern California 1971-74. APHIS 91-34, USDA, Hyattsville, Md.

Astudillo, V. M., and Deppermann, R. 1980. Animal disease information and surveillance system. Centro Panamericano Fiebre Aftosa Bltn. 39-40: 17-30.

Beal, V. C., Jr. 1977. Animal disease reporting. Anim. Plant Health Insp. Serv., USDA, Hyattsville, Md., Aug.

————. 1980. Recordkeeping systems and computer applications in disease prevention and control with emphasis on having a valid purpose for their existence. Paper read at Work Conf. Teach. Prev. Med., Epidemiol., Public Health, Feb. 4-6, Fort Worth, Tex.

Bell, D. 1973. The socio-economic impact of the V.V.N.D. problem on the poultry industry of southern California. Agric. Ext., Univ. Calif., Davis, Calif.

Betts, A. O., and Beveridge, W. I. B. 1953. Virus pneumonia in pigs: The effect of the disease upon growth and efficiency of food utilization. *Vet. Rec.* 65:515-521.

Bierer, B. W.   1974.   History of Animal Plagues of
    North America: With an Occasional Reference to
    Other Diseases and Diseased Conditions.   Copyright
    1939.   Washington, D.C: USDA.
Chapman, D. G.   1957.   Problems of estimation of wild-
    life mortality rates.   Biometrics 13:548-549.
Ciordia, H.; Baird, D. M.; Neville, W. E.; and
    McCampbell, H. C.   1972.   Internal parasitism of
    beef cattle on winter pastures: Effects of
    initial level of parasitism on beef production.
    Am. J. Vet. Res. 33:1407-1413.
Cockrill, W. R.   1974.   The Husbandry and Health of the
    Domestic Buffalo.   Rome: FAO.
Committee on Morbidity and Mortality Statistics.   1947.
    Report of the committee on morbidity and mortality
    statistics.   U.S. Livest. Sanit. Assoc. Proc. 51:
    228-238.
Copeman, D. B., and Hutchinson, G. W.   1979.   The
    economic significance of bovine gastrointestinal
    nematode parasitism in North Queensland.   In
    Veterinary Epidemiology and Economics.   Int. Symp.
    Vet. Epidemiol. Econ. Proc. 2:383-387.   Canberra:
    Aust. Gov. Publ. Serv.
Davis, G. B.   1979.   A sheep mortality survey.   In
    Veterinary Epidemiology and Economics.   Int. Symp.
    Vet. Epidemiol. Econ. Proc. 2:106-110.   Canberra:
    Aust. Gov. Publ. Serv.
Davis, J. W.; Anderson, R. C.; Karstad, L. H.; and
    Trainer, D. O.; eds.   1971.   Infectious and Para-
    sitic Diseases of Wild Birds.   Ames, Ia.:   Iowa
    State Univ. Press.
Diesch, S. L.; Martin, F. B.; Johnson, D. W.; and
    Christensen, L. T.   1974.   The Minnesota disease
    reporting system for food producing animals.   U.S.
    Anim. Health Assoc. Proc. 78:3-27.
Dobson, K. J., and Cargill, C. F.   1979.   Epidemiology
    and economic consequence of sarcoptic mange in
    pigs.   In Veterinary Epidemiology and Economics.
    Int. Symp. Vet. Epidemiol. Econ. Proc. 2:401-407.
    Canberra: Aust. Gov. Publ. Serv.
Ellis, E. M., and Kendall, H. E.   1964.   The public
    health and economic effects of vesicular stomati-
    tis in a herd of dairy cattle.   J. Am. Vet. Med.
    Assoc. 144:377-380.
Ellis, P. R.   1975.   The economics of animal health.
    In Economic Factors Affecting Egg Production, eds.
    B. M. Freeman and K. N. Boorman.   Edinburgh,
    Scot.:   Br. Poult. Sci. Ltd., pp. 71-82.
Fitzgerald, P. R.   1980.   The economic impact of cocci-
    diosis in domestic animals.   In Advances in Veter-

inary Science and Comparative Medicine, Vol. 24, eds. C. A. Brandly and C. E. Cornelius. New York: Academic Press, pp. 121-143.

Food Safety and Quality Service. 1978. Statistical summary: Federal meat and poultry inspection for calendar year 1978. Meat Poult. Insp., USDA, Washington, D.C.

Gordon, H. McL. 1979. The influence of helminthosis on the growth of prime lambs to market weight. In Veterinary Epidemiology and Economics. Int. Symp. Vet. Epidemiol. Econ. Proc. 2:388-392. Canberra: Aust. Gov. Publ. Serv.

Gordon, R. F. 1967. The economic effect of disease on the poultry industry. Vet. Rec. 80:101-107.

Gregory, M. W. 1976. Study of the creation of a system for providing information on the prevalence and cost of animal disease. Cent. Vet. Lab., Minist. Agric., Fish., Food, Weybridge, UK.

Halvorson, L. C. 1971. Estimation of economic losses and costs arising from bovine mastitis. Board Agric. Renewable Resour., NAS-NRC, Washington, D.C.

Hawkins, C. D. 1979. Methods of measuring the effects of a disease on the productivity of sheep. In Veterinary Epidemiology and Economics. Int. Symp. Vet. Epidemiol. Econ. Proc. 2:490-505. Canberra: Aust. Gov. Publ. Serv.

Hubbert, W. T.; McCulloch, W. F.; and Schnurrenberger, P. R.; eds. 1975. Diseases Transmitted from Animals to Man, 6th ed. Springfield, Ill.: Charles C. Thomas.

Hugh-Jones, M. E. 1979. Some effects of foot-and-mouth disease in Brasilian cattle. Paper read at 2nd Int. Symp. Vet. Epidemiol. Econ., May 7-11, Canberra, Aust.

Hutton, N. E., and Halvorson, L. C. 1974. A Nationwide System for Animal Health Surveillance. Washington, D.C.: NAS.

Kaneene, J. B., and Mather, E. C., eds. 1982. Cost Benefits of Food Animal Health. East Lansing, Mich.: Michigan State Univ. and W. K. Kellogg Found.

Keith, L. B. 1963. Wildlife's Ten Year Cycle. Madison, Wis.: Univ. Wis. Press.

Khera, S. S. 1979. Use of existing sources of information for estimation of animal health indices. In Veterinary Epidemiology and Economics. Int. Symp. Vet. Epidemiol. Econ. Proc. 2:203-206. Canberra: Aust. Gov. Publ. Serv.

Leech, F. B. 1971. A critique of the methods and re-

sults of the British national surveys of disease
in farm animals. II. Some general remarks on
population surveys of farm animal disease. *Br.
Vet. J.* 127:587-592.

McCallon, W. R. 1981. A proposed survey for meat and
milk production efficiency. Personal communication.

McCauley, E. H. 1979a. Estimation of the physical
loss in animals infected with foot-and-mouth
disease. In A Study of the Potential Economic
Impact of Foot-and-Mouth Disease in the United
States, eds. E. H. McCauley, N. A. Aulaqi, J. C.
New, Jr., W. B. Sundquist, and W. M. Miller.
Tech. Rep. 2. Washington, D.C.: USGPO, pp.
23-32.

————. 1979b. Impact of disease and feed restriction
on animal growth performance: A review. In A
Study of the Potential Economic Impact of Foot-
and-Mouth Disease in the United States, eds. E. H.
McCauley, N. A. Aulaqi, J. C. New, Jr., W. B.
Sundquist, and W. M. Miller. Tech. Rep. 8.
Washington, D.C.: USGPO, pp. 133-147.

Maurer, F. D. 1975. Livestock, a world food resource
threatened by disease. *J. Am. Vet. Med. Assoc.*
166:920-923.

Miller, W. M. 1979. An information system for animal
disease epidemics. In A Study of the Potential
Economic Impact of Foot-and-Mouth Disease in the
United States, eds. E. H. McCauley, N. A. Aulaqi,
J. C. New, Jr., W. B. Sundquist, and W. M. Miller.
Tech. Rep. 11. Washington, D.C.: USGPO, pp.
185-200.

Morris, R. S. 1971. Economic aspects of disease control programmes for dairy cattle. *Aust. Vet. J.*
47:358-363.

National Research Council. 1968. Prenatal and Post-
natal Mortality in Cattle. NAS-NRC Publ. 1685.
Washington, D.C.

National Research Council. 1977. Supporting Papers:
World Food and Nutrition Study, vol. 1.
Washington, D.C.: NAS-NRC.

New York State Veterinary College. 1961. Report of
the New York State Veterinary College at Cornell
University for the year 1960-1961. Legislative
Doc. (No. 89) 1962, State of New York.

Page, L. A., ed. 1976. Wildlife Diseases. New
York: Plenum Press.

Pan American Foot-and-Mouth Disease Center. 1980a.
Situation of the foot-and-mouth disease control
programs in South America. Rio de Janeiro,
Brazil.

————. 1980b. Occurrence of vesicular diseases in the Americas. Foot-and-Mouth Dis. Vesicular Stomatitis Epidemiol. Rep. 12(1):1. Rio de Janeiro, Brazil.

Pickard, J. R. 1952. Tuberculosis condemnations. *U.S. Livest. Sanit. Assoc. Proc.* 56:144-148.

Pilchard, E. I. 1972. Economic importance of mastitis research in the United States. *Agric. Sci. Rev.* 10(2):30-35.

Poppensiek, G. C.; Budd, D. E.; and Scholtens, R. G. 1966. A Historical Survey of Animal Disease Morbidity and Mortality Reporting. NAS-NRC Publ. 1346, Washington, D.C.

Purchase, H. G., and Schultz, E. F., Jr. 1979. The economics of Marek's disease control in the United States. *World's Poult. Sci. J.* 34:198-204.

Roe, R. T. 1979. Features of the Australian national animal disease information system. In Veterinary Epidemiology and Economics. Int. Symp. Vet. Epidemiol. Econ. Proc. 2:26-34. Canberra: Aust. Gov. Publ. Serv.

Ross, J. G. 1970. The economics of Fasciola hepatica infections in cattle. *Br. Vet. J.* 126:(4)xiii-xv.

Schwabe, C. W. 1969. Prevention, control, and eradication of disease. Veterinary Medicine and Human Health, 2nd ed. Baltimore: Williams & Wilkins Co., pp. 374-440.

Simpson, B. H., and Wright, D. F. 1979. The use of questionnaires to assess the importance of clinical disease in sheep. In Veterinary Epidemiology and Economics. Int. Symp. Vet. Epidemiol. Econ. Proc. 2:97-105. Canberra: Aust. Gov. Publ. Serv.

Simpson, B. H.; Talbot, L.; Davidson, R. M.; and Wright, D. F. 1979. The use of sentinel farms as a source of information on the epidemiology of clinical diseases. In Veterinary Epidemiology and Economics. Int. Symp. Vet Epidemiol. Econ. Proc. 2:87-92. Canberra: Aust. Gov. Publ. Serv.

Special Swine Abscess Committee. Ca. 1964. Swine abscesses: A request for research funds. Livest. Conserv. Inc., Chicago, Ill.

Taylor, S. M. 1974. The cost of liver fluke in Northern Ireland. *Agric. North. Irel.* 49:264-268.

University of Minnesota. 1981. Validation study of the Minnesota food animal disease reporting system. U.S. Animal Plant Health Inspection Service and College of Veterinary Medicine Cooperative Study, St. Paul, Minn.

Willeberg, P. 1979. Epidemiological applications of Danish swine slaughter inspection data. In Veterinary Epidemiology and Economics. Int. Symp.

Vet. Epidemiol. Econ. Proc. 2:161–167.   Canberra:
    Aust. Gov. Publ. Serv.
Wisconsin Department of Agriculture, Trade and Consumer
    Protection.   1977.   Report of Wisconsin Animal
    Health   Laboratories   1976–1977.   Bull.   402,
    Madison, Wis.

3

Climate, Land, and People

REGIONAL CHARACTERISTICS

The foot-and-mouth disease eradication program employed successfully by USDA in 1925 in California (Mohler 1925) had to be modified in 1954 in Mexico where the climate, the land, and particularly the people were different (Machado 1968). But even within a country, changes are necessary when the program is moved from one region to another. For example, a brucellosis-eradication program that had been success-ful in the north central and northeastern states in the sixties ran into serious difficulties in the South in the early seventies (Anderson et al. 1978). Although a difference in herd management was the primary reason for the problem, the roots were far deeper. In the South, replacement animals are usually purchased rather than reared on the farm. Moreover, the southern cattle auction, which is incompatible with the concept of closed herd development, is an integral part of the social fabric and not subject to change by government fiat. The discontinuation of vaccination after the initial phase of the program, as was done in the North, was disaster in the open herds of the South.

Rarely can a successful program be transferred from one region to another without some modification. The ease of adjusting the program to a new locale depends on the number of modifications required. Consequently it is important to identify, as soon as possible, any of the region's unique features that may necessitate program changes so that effective altera-tions can be made (Pan American Foot-and-Mouth Disease Center 1979). This chapter is concerned with the sources of information about regional characteristics

and the identification of those parts of the program
that require modification.

In order to show the interrelationships of information gathered from a variety of sources, the illu-
strations used pertain to an area in southwestern
Wisconsin (encircled area in Fig. 3.1).

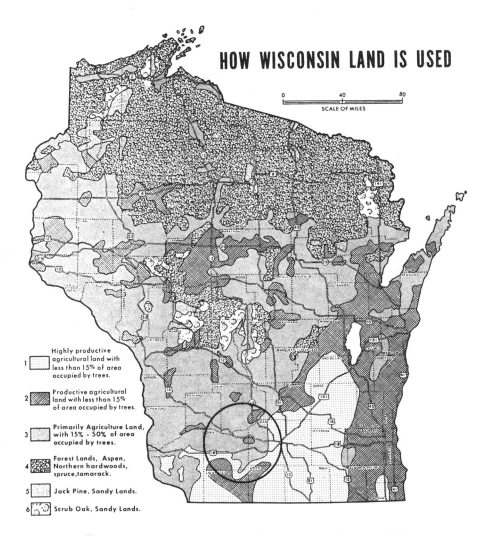

HOW WISCONSIN LAND IS USED

1   Highly productive agricultural land with less than 15% of area occupied by trees.

2   Productive agricultural land with less than 15% of area occupied by trees.

3   Primarily Agriculture Land, with 15% - 50% of area occupied by trees.

4   Forest Lands, Aspen, Northern hardwoods, spruce, tamarack.

5   Jack Pine, Sandy Lands.

6   Scrub Oak, Sandy Lands.

FIG. 3.1. Agricultural use of land in Wisconsin; circled
area depicted in Fig. 3.8 (Wisconsin Department of Public
Instruction 1962).

CLIMATE AND LAND

Information Sources and Interpretation

Regional meteorological records. Meteorological services in every country around the world have cooperated in developing and analyzing records based on observations made at fixed stations for periods of 50 to 100 years or more. The network of stations ranges from good to inadequate not only in its coverage of regions within a nation but also in the extensiveness of the records kept. Particularly important for agricultural and epidemiological purposes is a parameter such as evapotranspiration which may be more significant in its effect on animal physiology and parasite survival than inches of rainfall. Information about worldwide meteorological activity has been strengthened by use of weather satellites that continuously monitor conditions over large ocean expanses. In addition, detailed records for specific locations are available from appropriate government agencies. In the United States, the National Oceanic and Atmospheric Administration issues *Climatological Data* monthly. This publication covers the entire nation but is available in sections that deal with a single state (Table 3.1).

Seasons and weather (Fig. 3.2) affect the mobility and activity of both reservoirs and vectors of pathogens (Birch 1957). Cold, particularly freezing temperatures, aridity, drought, and low humidity immobilize invertebrate vectors, and cold-blooded reservoirs hibernate, estivate, or die. Warm-blooded reservoirs migrate, hibernate, or make physiologic adjustments to survive adverse environmental periods.

Transmission of a disease will cease abruptly when the vector dies, a reservoir is no longer present, or access to a contaminated food or water source is eliminated (Fig. 3.3). On the other hand, climate and weather can facilitate transmission of disease by providing ideal conditions for the proliferation or movement of a vector and, sometimes, survival of the pathogen (Levine 1963; Ollerenshaw and Smith 1969) or its transport (Hemmes et al. 1960). In other instances, the mechanism mediating the prevalence and severity of disease remains unknown (Hope-Simpson 1981). Soft, moist, steady winds having laminar flow are reputed to carry virus aerosols for many miles and then set them down on vegetation in a light rain (Smith 1964; Smith and Hugh-Jones 1969). Hurricanes that displaced salt marsh mosquitoes inland along the Atlantic

Table 3.1. Extract from the Climatological Report for Wisconsin (April 1978); Monthly Summarized Station and Divisional Data

STATION	TEMPERATURE									NO. OF DAYS				PRECIPITATION				SNOW. SLEET		
	AVERAGE MAXIMUM	AVERAGE MINIMUM	AVERAGE	DEPARTURE FROM NORMAL	HIGHEST	DATE	LOWEST	DATE	DEGREE DAYS	MAX. 90° OR ABOVE	MAX. 32° OR BELOW	MIN. 32° OR BELOW	MIN. 0° OR BELOW	TOTAL	DEPARTURE FROM NORMAL	GREATEST DAY	DATE	TOTAL	MAX. DEPTH ON GROUND	DATE
FAIRCHILD RANGER STA	54.3	33.1	43.7		75	1	21	21	634	0	0	16	0	4.02	1.60	.72	9	1.0	1	11
HATFIELD HYDRO PLANT	58.0	29.3	43.7	-1.2	75	28	18	21	633	0	0	22	0					.0	0	
LA CROSSE FAA AP	55.8	36.0	45.9	-1.7	74	28	26	21	565	0	0	7	0	4.01	1.38	.81	9	T	0	
MATHER 5 NW	53.5M	30.4M	42.0M	-2.4	78	1	23	21	684	0	1		0	3.53	.70	.84	6	T	T	20
MENOMONIE	58.0	33.0	45.5	-.4	74	27	21	21	576	0	0	16	0	3.81	1.05	.85	6	3.0	T	3
MONDOVI	56.9	33.6	45.3		75	1	21	21	586	0	0	12	0	3.44		.78	6	T	T	3+
RIDGELAND 1 NNE	55.3	29.8	42.6		73	28+	17	21	666	0	0	20	0	3.02	.16	.74	6	T	T	5+
RIVER FALLS	55.6	33.2	44.4	-.9	71	28	21	21	608	0	0	13	0	3.02	.48	.98	6	1.5	T	2
SPARTA	55.1M	33.2M	44.2M	-2.7	79	1	25	22+	614	0	0	14	0	3.83	1.15	1.25	6	.3	T	3+
TREMPEALEAU DAM 6	56.2	35.3	45.8		72	28	24	2	568	0	0	8	0	2.86	.27	.61	5	.0	0	
DIVISION			44.4	-1.5										3.50	.83			.6		
CENTRAL 05																				
CLINTONVILLE	51.2	31.0	41.1		73	29	24	22+	709	0	0	18	0	4.07		.82	9	T	0	
CODDINGTON 1 E	52.6	28.9	40.8	-2.8	72	28	18	21+	720	0	0	23	0	4.34	1.60	.79	9	T		2
DALTON	54.8M	33.9M	44.4M		73	1	25	21+	611	0	0	15	0	3.24		1.08	6	.4	T	2
HANCOCK EXP FARM	55.3	32.2	43.8	-1.5	77	1	22	21	632	0	0	15	0	4.25	1.54	1.19	4	T	T	4+
MARSHFIELD EXP FARM	53.4	31.2	42.3	-1.3	72	28	18	18	675	0	0	16	0	4.02	1.25	1.34	9	.0	0	
MAUSTON 1 SE	58.2	28.0	43.1		78	28	20	22+	653	0	0	22	0	5.31	2.38	1.44	6	T	0	
MONTELLO	55.9	33.7	44.8	-1.1	73	28	26	21+	599	0	0	11	0	3.71	.71	1.25	6	T	0	
NECEDAH	56.6	30.0M	43.3M		75	1	20	22+	629	0	0		0	3.86		.90	9	T	0	
NEW LONDON	53.5	31.8M	42.7M	-3.0	75	28	24	21	653	0	0		0	3.96	1.02	.76	7	T	T	14+
PINE RIVER 3 NE	53.4	31.4	42.4		75	28	23	15	671	0	0	16	0	5.44		1.13	6	T		2
PITTSVILLE	54.7	31.7	43.2		74	1	23	21	649	0	0	18	0	3.82		1.06	10	T	0	
ROSHOLT	52.7	29.5M	41.1M		72	28	19	2	740	0	0	17	0	4.95		1.02	9	T	0	
STEVENS POINT	52.6	31.3	42.0	-3.1	75	1	19	3	685	0	0	18	0	4.29	1.53	1.08	10	1.0	1	18
WAUPACA	51.9	32.4	42.2	-3.4	73	29	21	2	676	0	0	12	0	4.90	1.95	.84	9	.0	0	
WISCONSIN RAPIDS	53.5	30.1	41.8	-2.5	77	28	20	5	688	0	1	20	0	4.63	1.84	1.80	9	T	0	
DIVISION			42.6	-2.4										4.32	1.49			.1		
EAST CENTRAL 06																				
APPLETON	50.4	32.3	41.4	-3.5	70	28	27	17+	702	0	0	15	0	3.91	.89	1.00	6	T		2+
CHILTON	52.7	32.3	42.5		73	1	25	22+	670	0	0	17	0	3.00		.83	6	T	0	
ELDORADO 1 SSW	52.4M	33.7M	43.1M	-2.8	72	28	26	22	655	0	0	14	0	5.02	2.47	2.76	4	1.5	0	
FOND DU LAC	50.9	32.7	41.8	-4.4	70	28	26	2+	691	0	0	14	0	5.29	2.77	1.92	3	T	T	2
GREEN BAY WSO AP //R	49.4	31.2	40.3	-3.5	73	28	26	22+	733	0	0	19	0	3.44	.75	.89	6	T		3
KEWAUNEE 5 S	47.7	33.2	40.5	-2.2	63	28+	25	16	730	0	0	12	0	3.29	.51	.74	4	.0	0	
MANITOWOC	52.6M	32.6M	42.6M	-1.5	66	28+	25	16	666	0	0	13	0	3.94	1.24	.90	6	T	0	
OSHKOSH	52.1	32.1	42.1	-3.1	71	28	26	30+	680	0	0	15	0	4.26	1.52	1.12	6	T		2
PLYMOUTH	51.7	32.2	42.0	-2.8	75	28	22	22	684	0	0	14	0	4.57	1.53	1.66	4	.4	T	2
SHEBOYGAN	51.7	35.4	43.6	-.7	69	1	30	22+	636	0	0	10	0	3.94	1.24	1.05	4	.0	0	
STURGEON BAY EXP FARM	49.7	33.3	41.5	-.9	69	28	26	17+	698	0	0	13	0	3.06	.24	.62	6	T	1	4+
TWO RIVERS	49.5	34.0	41.8		64	12	28	22+	691	0	0	10	0	3.29		.73	6	.0	0	
WASHINGTON ISLAND	45.8	28.0	36.9		62	27	16	3	836	0	0	25	0	2.35		.75	10	.7	0	
DIVISION			41.5	-2.8										3.80	1.05			.2		
SOUTHWEST 07																				
BARABOO	55.5	30.5	43.0		73	28	23	16+	654	0	0	21	0	4.35	1.33	.81	18	T	T	2
DARLINGTON	57.5	34.5	46.0	-1.7	73	28	26	15	561	0	0	11	0	3.84	.47	1.11	6	T	0	
DODGEVILLE 1 NE	57.2	35.0	46.1	-.7	73	1	22	2	558	0	0	10	0	4.35	1.29	1.44	6	T	T	2
GENOA DAM 8	56.5	36.9	46.7		70	29+	28	21	540	0	0	6	0	3.99	1.17	1.36	6	.0	0	
HILLSBORO																				
LANCASTER 4 WSW	59.1	36.6	47.9	.0	75	1	27	2	509	0	0	7	0	4.83	1.71	1.50	6	T		2
LONE ROCK FAA AP //R	57.7	34.2	46.0		80	1	23	17	564	0	0	11	0	3.81		.93	4	.0	0	
LYNXVILLE DAM 9	58.8	37.5	48.2		73	27	29	17	497	0	0	6	0	3.80	.94	1.10	6	T		2
PLATTEVILLE	58.9	35.6	47.3		75	1	28	15	524	0	0	10	0	4.93	1.63	1.65	6	.2	0	
PRAIRIE DU CHIEN	61.3	37.1	49.2	-.2	78	1	29	22+	469	0	0	7	0	5.50	2.56	1.87	4	.0	0	
PRAIRIE DU SAC 2 N //	54.7	35.9	45.3	-1.3	74	28	28	2	584	0	0	5	0	4.35	1.69	.62	24+	.3	T	2
REEDSBURG	57.4	34.4	45.9		76	28	25	22	565	0	0	12	0	4.40		.95	4	.2	T	3+
RICHLAND CENTER	57.4	34.3	45.9	-2.0	79	1	26	22+	566	0	0	13	0	4.94	1.85	1.46	6	.8	T	2
VIROQUA	55.0	33.7	44.4	-1.6	72	28	24	15	614	0	0	14	0	3.76	.93	1.32	6	.0	0	
DIVISION			46.3	-1.1										4.37	1.38			.1		
SOUTH CENTRAL 08																				
ARBORETUM-UNIV OF WISC	58.0	32.6	45.3		81	1	20	22+	584	0	0	14	0	5.55		1.28	6	.0	0	
ARLINGTON UNIV FARM	55.2	33.9	44.6		72	28	26	12	605	0	0	13	0	2.98		1.10	6	.5	T	2
BEAVER DAM	53.3	32.9	43.1		73	28	25	18	657	0	0	15	0	3.49		.77	6	T	T	2
BELOIT	59.8	37.1M	48.5M	-1.2	74	1	30	22+	496	0	0	7	0	4.14	1.30	.98	6	.0	0	
BRODHEAD	60.4	34.9	47.7	.1	76	1	24	22	515	0	0	11	0	3.66	.44	.75	5	.0	0	
CHARMANY UNIV FARM	55.4	34.0	44.7		80	1	23	15	601	0	0	11	0	5.00		1.30	6	T	0	
FORT ATKINSON	56.9	34.9	45.9	-1.9	78	1	26	22+	566	0	0	10	0	3.49	.73	.83	6	T	0	
HORICON	55.5	33.5	44.5		74	1	26	2	609	0	0	14	0	3.80		1.40	6	T	T	2

Source: National Oceanic and Atmospheric Administration 1978.

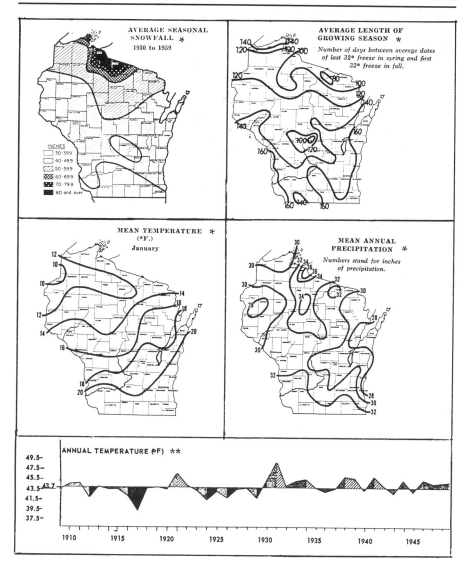

FIG. 3.2. Effect of weather and seasons (*Wisconsin Legislative Reference Bureau 1974; **Wang and Suomi 1958).

seacoast have spread vectors with encephalitis virus among susceptible horse populations from New Jersey to the Carolinas (Hess and Holden 1958; Hayes and Hess 1964). Once every decade or two, precipitation in the arid center of Australia has created a transient bridge of ponds and vegetation that permitted birds and mosquitoes to carry Murray Valley encephalitis virus

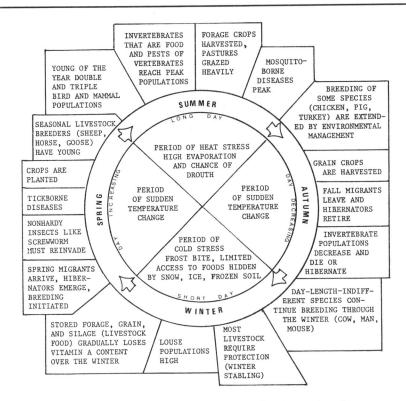

FIG. 3.3. Seasonal cycle and animal populations in the temperate zone of the northern hemisphere.

from an enzootic area in Queensland south to susceptible human and animal populations in Victoria (Anderson 1952). Severe river floods occur in many humid parts of the world every decade or so, and in the Mississippi Valley floods have uncovered and spread anthrax spores (Van Ness 1971). Extreme droughts, like the one that lasted several years in the Sahel region of Africa, recur at irregular intervals of 20 to 200 years. Because droughts force animal populations to crowd around the remaining waterholes in arid Africa, susceptible animals are exposed to high levels of parasites shed by carriers (Temple and Thomas 1973). Similarly, waterfowl crowd into the open spring-fed ponds of the northern United States when other bodies of waters have frozen over. Enteric pathogens are concentrated in the environment by such actions, and the probability that the crowded animals will ingest an infective dose is greatly increased (Walker et al. 1969). Significant year-to-year variations in the

weather can be expected in most regions of the world
(Fig. 3.2) with associated changes in the probability
of disease.

Climate and weather directly affect growth and
productivity of animals as well as their distribution
(International Livestock Environment Symposium Proceedings 1974). The greater adaptability of certain breeds
of livestock to the tropics is well recognized and is
determined by their greater resistance to ectoparasites
or hemoprotozoan diseases and the debilitating effects
of heat. In cold regions, protection from the weather
and occasional supplemental heat is required to prevent
hypothermia or frostbite. In hot regions, protection
from the sun and the use of sprinkling systems enable
swine to grow and chickens to continue laying (Wilson
1974).

Meteorologic changes can also affect the disease
susceptibility and resistance of the host by altering
internal physiology, influencing the immunologic system, and sometimes, impairing respiratory secretions
and the integrity of the skin (Marshall 1959; Thaxton
and Siegel 1970; Tromp 1973; Hyslop 1974; Siegel 1974).

Topographical and physical features. The availability
of detailed and accurate geographical information has
improved greatly since the introduction of aerial
photography. Not only can physical relief be obtained
by use of stereophotography, but sensitivity of film
has made it possible to differentiate vegetation types
and, sometimes, distinguish diseased from healthy crops
and measure grain production (Idso et al. 1977). Constructed features, such as roads, bridges, and buildings, are easy to identify. By using infrared film,
occupied buildings can be distinguished from unoccupied
ones. In certain kinds of open landscapes, wildlife,
such as antelope in a savanna or geese on ponds, are
frozen on film and can be counted (Watson 1969).

Maps for specific uses are prepared by a number of
government agencies in every country. In the United
States the U.S. Coast and Geodetic Survey prepares
relief maps (Fig. 3.4) using the conventional brown
contour line to show 20-foot elevation changes. These
quadrangles, scaled at 1 to 62,500, cover an area of
approximately 200 square miles. Detailed information
useful to field crews is given on all natural and some
constructed features.

The information provided by the geological survey
on bed rock and surface deposits (Fig. 3.5) helps the
user understand soils and the distribution of plants
and animals. Detailed surface-soil maps that enable

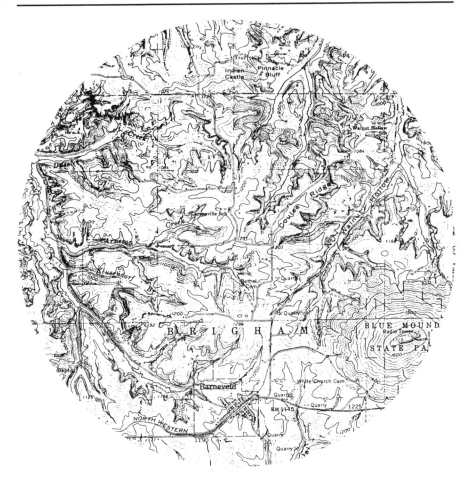

FIG. 3.4. A segment of a physiographic map using contour
lines to show elevation; located within small circle of Fig.
3.8. (Geological Survey 1962).

farmers to plan field use are available in many regions
(Fig. 3.6).

Ecological information. Since vegetational maps are
not standardized, some show vegetational types
(prairie, Fig. 3.7) and others show distribution of
specific plants (such as *Geum triflorum*). Occasionally, quantitative information is presented on
vegetational stands (Curtis 1959). General information
about the range of birds and mammals (Fig. 3.7) is
reasonably good throughout the world but local detail

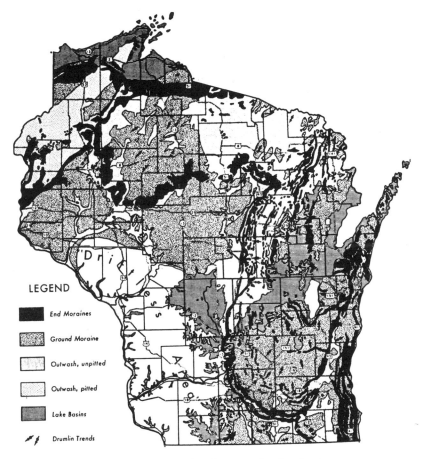

FIG. 3.5. Map of Wisconsin showing geologic features
(Wisconsin Legislative Reference Bureau 1964).

and information about rarer species is harder to obtain
(Darlington 1957). Much less is known about the range
of lower animals, particularly invertebrate species
that may be reservoirs or vectors of pathogens. Fortunately, reasonable deductions can often be made about
the local range of an arthropod vector and transmission
by combined use of meteorologic, topographic, soils,
and vegetational maps (Van Ness and Stein 1956; Audy
1958). Black flies, for example, are found near small
fast streams and salt marsh mosquitoes along the sea
coast, features that are readily identified on topographical maps. The movement of a rabies epizootic in
the fox population in Europe has been related to landscape features (Bacon and Macdonald 1981).

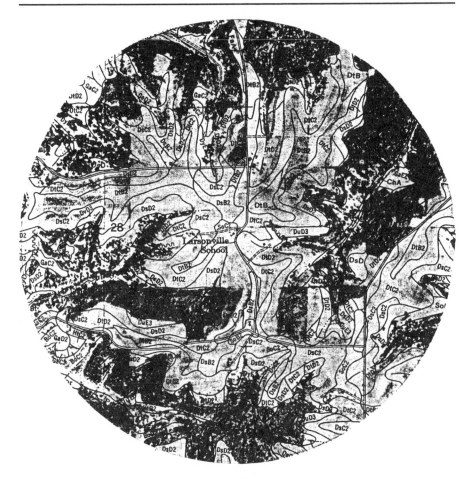

FIG. 3.6. A segment of a map showing soil types; located
within small circle of Fig. 3.8 (Soil Conservation Service
1962).

When consideration is given to controlling a
reservoir or vector by reducing populations or creating
barriers to its movement, information is needed about
its population size and distribution in the region
(Seber 1973; Pan American Foot-and-Mouth Disease Center
1979). The effect of climate on population numbers and
the seasonal movement of vectors and reservoirs is
particularly important (Hansen and Yuill 1976). For
example, the program for eradication of the screwworm
in the southeastern United States was initiated in the
wake of one of the coldest winters experienced in that
region (Knipling 1960). Because of the cold, the fly
was extirpated from much of its normal winter range.

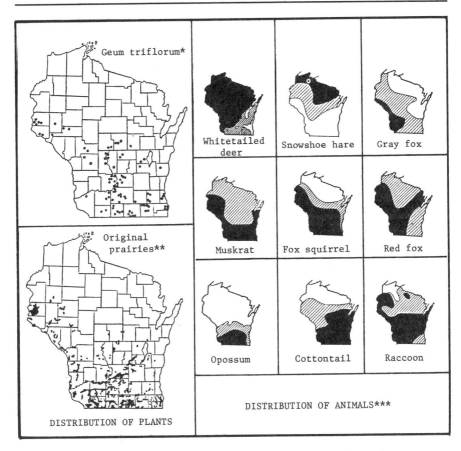

FIG. 3.7. Ecologic maps giving plant and animal distribu-
tions. Plants: dot or spot = present; animals: black =
common, hatched = fairly common, white = rare or none
(*Mason and Iltis 1958; **Location of orginal prairies from
John Curtiss, The Vegetation of Wisconsin [Madison: The
University of Wisconsin Press; copyright 1959 by the Board
of Regents of the University of Wisconsin System]; ***Hine
1968.

Starting the control program at this point and preventing the fly from moving back into its larger summer
range greatly reduced the cost of control. The retreat
of a vector or reservoir in the face of drought or cold
is an event that should be utilized by program planners. Conversely, planners must also anticipate
seasons that will be unusually favorable to vectors or
reservoirs. During such a period in the southwestern
United States, the screwworm leaped over barriers that

were too narrow and reinvaded an area previously freed
of the fly (Richardson 1978). Defenses were inadequate
to the rear of the barrier and the fly spread rapidly.
Program planners had not anticipated the need for more
effective barriers, and the resulting losses were very
high.

Political features and economic records. None of the
maps previously discussed provide up-to-date information on constructed features or political jurisdictions. State or provincial highway maps that are
published annually (Fig. 3.8) are the best source of

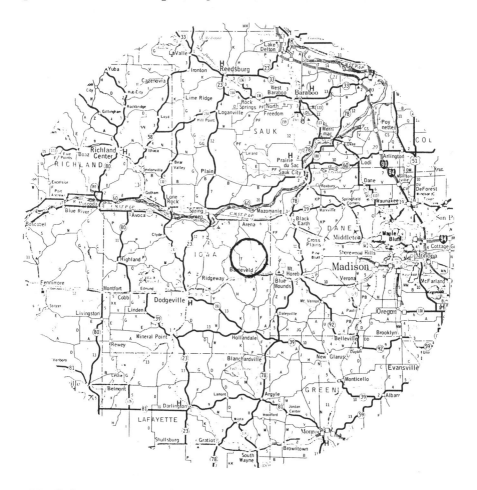

FIG. 3.8. A segment of the official highway map of
Wisconsin; located within circle of Fig. 3.1 (Wisconsin
Department of Transportation 1980-81)

information on major roadways. For lesser roads, location of farm holdings, and often the ownership of
farms, the county plat book (Fig. 3.9), which is
published by regional entrepreneurs and regularly
updated, should be used.

Statistical information on livestock populations
can be obtained from the agricultural census conducted
periodically by the central government. Data is organized by state and county units and summarized in a
series of publications that report animals on farms by
age cohort and size of herd. Trends are analyzed in

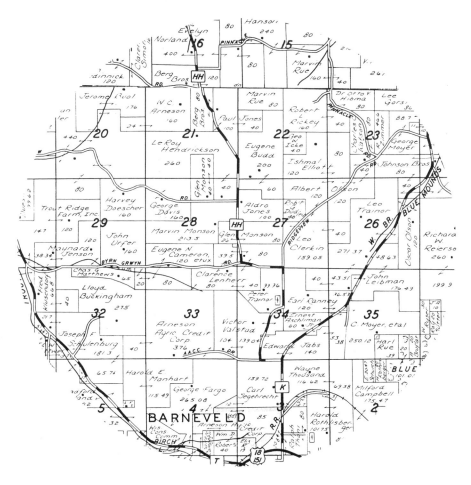

FIG. 3.9. A segment of the Iowa County, Wisconsin plat
book; located within small circle of Fig. 3.8 (Permission to
reproduce this map was granted by Rockford Map Publishers,
Inc.).

studies conducted by agricultural economists (Fig.
3.10) and demographers (Figs. 3.11, 3.12, and 3.13) at
state experiment stations and other institutions
(Friend 1979; Worden 1979).   Marketing areas and
marketing trends may also be examined.   In areas where
information on animal populations is lacking, disease-
control officials may be required to gather it
(Malaga-Cruz et al. 1979).

The flow rate of animals to market in terms of
seasonality, direction, age cohort, and particularly
the number that go to livestock auctions and other
markets from which they return to farms rather than
going on to slaughter, has great epidemiologic significance (Schnurrenberger et al. 1965).   Since farm-
market-farm loops that are unknown to program planners
can seriously weaken the program, every effort should
be made to obtain such information.

Unfortunately, all sections of the world are not
covered in equal detail or with equal accuracy, nor do
all nations make the data collected readily available.
For example, the republics of the USSR compile and keep
statistics on agriculture, but they do not publish

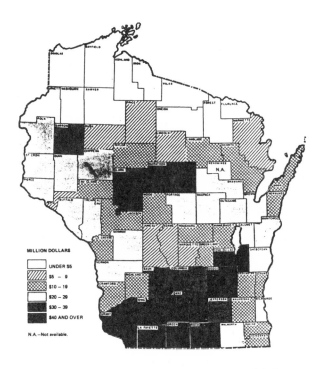

FIG. 3.10. Value of Wisconsin farm products sold by county
in 1969 (Wisconsin Legislative Reference Bureau 1973).

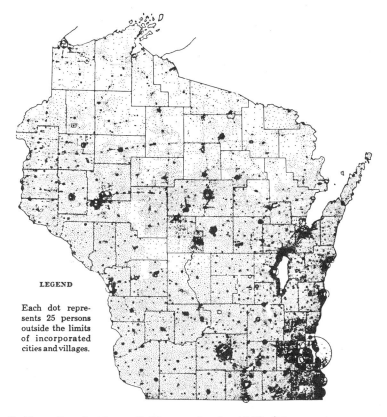

FIG. 3.11.   Population of Wisconsin in 1960 (Wisconsin Legislative Reference Bureau 1964).

them, and nationwide summaries are not compiled. However, most nations provide a brief summary of their livestock statistics (often outdated) to the United Nations, and this material is published annually in the Animal Health Yearbook.

Planning for the load of diagnostic samples, the amount of vaccine required, or the possible scale of endemnity payments would be difficult without accurate information about the agricultural use of land (Fig. 3.1), size of the region's livestock population, number of herds, and their location (Friend 1979; Worden 1979).

The success of disease-control and eradication programs is dependent upon access to all animals within the region for diagnosis, vaccination, or condemnation. Consequently, an accurate knowledge of the roadway and communication systems is essential. The experience of

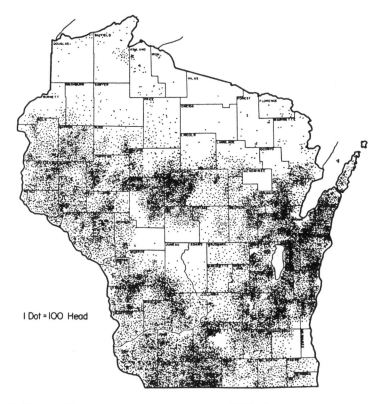

FIG. 3.12. Milk cows in Wisconsin in 1978 (Wisconsin
Agricultural Reporting Service 1980).

field diagnosticians who had to travel for as long as a
week by horseback to reach some of the more isolated
estancias in Tierra del Fuego (Argentine-United States
Joint Commission 1966) or the logistic problems encountered in parts of Mexico during the foot-and-mouth
disease campaign would cause any planner to hesitate.
Operations in such inaccessible regions can be carried
out successfully only with foreknowledge of the conditions that will be encountered. The experience during
the Mexican aftosa program indicates that plans must
make ample allowances for delays caused by weather and
terrain (Machado 1968).

The headquarters unit and supply depot should be
located in the regional network of roads and communication lines at a point that provides the best access to
the region and a good site for receiving and storing
goods obtained from outside. Since access must be

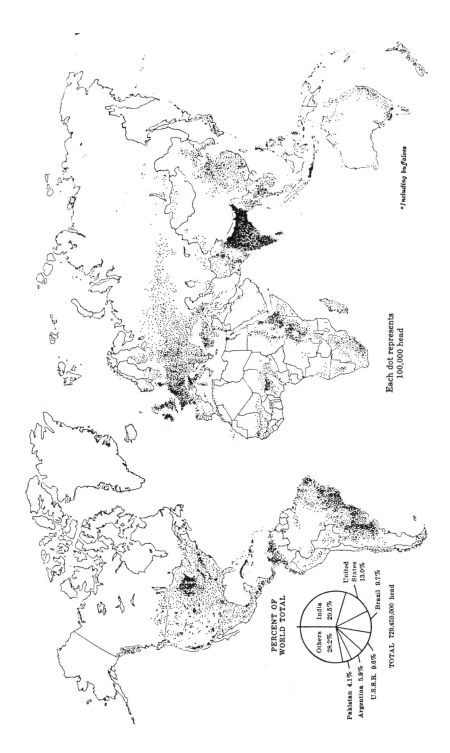

PERCENT OF
WORLD TOTAL

India
29.5%

United
States
13.0%

Brazil 9.7%

U.S.S.R. 8.6%

Argentina 5.9%

Pakistan 4.1%

Others
28.2%

TOTAL 729,459,000 head

Each dot represents
100,000 head

*Including buffaloes

FIG. 3.13. World cattle numbers, average 1957–1961 (Guidry 1964).

continuous throughout the year, meteorologic as well as geographic information is needed when logistic plans are made for regions plagued with heavy snows or prolonged wet seasons that restrict local travel on some roadways.

It is important for program planners to know that most of the regional information that is needed has been collected by some agency and is available if one knows where and how to obtain it. The specific information on the region, if properly used, will avoid costly errors and speed not only the development of the program but also its completion.

PEOPLE

Information Required

When we were discussing a set of disease-control problems with an older colleague, he commented, "Those are all people problems, not animal-disease problems." After reflection we realized he was right, but we did not know how to convince certain farmers and officials that our disease-control program should be implemented. This subject, management of people to control human disease, was the focus of a recent symposium of the Society for Study of Human Biology (Clegg and Garlick 1980).

The objectives of a program staff in their approach to the people of the region should be to (1) inform the community about the purpose of the program and its operations, and (2) open channels for the discussion of issues and negotiation of any conflicts that arise. It is important to include all segments of the affected population.

No government is powerful enough to implement or enforce a program that is not understood by the affected populace or respected by them. In almost all communities there are groups that seldom talk with each other. Occasionally this division is open and deep, and any semblance of alignment by the program staff with one of these groups will make it difficult or impossible to work with the other. It is unlikely that a meeting called in a facility "belonging" to one group will be attended by members of the other. Since this fractionation is less apparent to outsiders, the program staff may erroneously believe they have reached the community. Unfortunately, no one will inform them of their failure, and the expected cooperation will never be obtained.

Sources of Demographic and Cultural Information

Required information about the social organization of the region is not as well mapped and tabulated as information about animal populations (Wharton 1969). Nevertheless, a great deal can be learned rapidly from several accessible sources. General and agricultural censuses provide demographic information on the regional population with regard to geographic distribution and the size of certain cohorts (Fig. 3.11).

In all parts of the world farmers belong to one or more organizations that assist them in marketing their produce (marketing cooperatives), purchasing supplies of feeds and fuels (purchasing cooperatives), and improving their livestock (breeding associations). Any region may have one or more of each type of organization, each of which may differ in degree of militancy or passivity. Consequently, the membership of competing organizations may differ in attitudes and affluence. All organizations should be examined as possible avenues of communication since their leaders are usually willing to give program staff membership data and assist them in reaching members.

Social and religious organizations have a dominant role in the community in some regions and a minor one in others. In parts of Colombia the local Catholic priest has sometimes been the first to inform officials about disease outbreaks and has often helped them reach the farmers with disease-control information. Religious calendars determine the movement and slaughter of animals in certain countries, and religious practices significantly modify husbandry operations and options (Kahrs 1981; Sellers 1981). In some parts of Asia and Africa, a tribal chief is the individual through whom the farmers of the area are contacted. It is important for program officials to be aware of the customs in a particular region and follow the proper channels.

Farmers who keep themselves apart from any organization can often be reached in most countries through their children who take part in school vocational agricultural courses or in the counterpart of youth organizations such as 4-H and FFA (Future Farmers of America). In many countries agricultural extension meetings are held at the schools. Since it is a neutral site, many divergent groups can be assembled there under the auspices of the extension service or through the services of the local county agent.

In some regions sociologists and anthropologists have done community studies (Perez 1975) that map or analyze such things as community stability (in-and-out migrations), ethnic origins, rural organizations, attitudes toward innovation, and cultural practices (Dyson-Hudson and Dyson-Hudson 1969; Miller 1973; Saleh 1975). Cultural mores could include such epidemiologically important practices as drinking boiled instead of raw milk and making rennet rather than acid-fermented cheese. Sociological studies are published as theses, experiment-station bulletins (Kolb 1957; Marshall 1963), and articles in journals. A sociologist with training in rural communities can locate appropriate documents, interpret the observations, and conduct a special study when essential information is lacking. Although a few sociologists have looked at the special problems of introducing new measures for control of human diseases, the questions associated with the acceptance of animal-disease control measures are still largely unstudied (Horowitz 1979). Evaluation of the impact of an innovation on individuals as if the impact were independent of the setting in which it occurred is criticized by sociologists (Saint and Coward 1977).

Studies of rural people can be done while plans for disease control are being developed, as was shown in Colombia (Victoria-L. and Arevalo-A. 1970; Tellez-S. 1975). In that instance, a problem in communication was avoided when the study team learned that two groups of farmers (to whom a disease-control program for bananas was being directed) who spoke Spanish had immigrated into the region from different areas and used different words when referring to the parts of the banana plant and the practices used in its culture. Knowing this, the disease-control officials prepared the recommendations in two separate dialects.

The understanding of words is only part of the problem of communication. Acceptance or rejection of concepts is even more fundamental (Ruttan and Hayami 1973). It is very difficult for an individual who has been trained from childhood to accept scientific rationale to understand that some people may hold other beliefs (Imperato 1977). Scientific explanations of quarantine, depopulation, and disinfection are apt to be misunderstood by people who are convinced that disease is a punishment by spirits for wrongdoing (Cockburn 1964). Furthermore, in such a situation the control official faces an ethical problem. A scientific explanation of the methods not only attacks the beliefs of the people but also, if successful, subverts a culture. If the methods are explained in terms of local beliefs, disease control might occur without disturbing the culture, but the official may feel this approach is intellectually dishonest. The choice is difficult.

Even in a future-oriented society, it is not easy to argue that individuals should accept present privations for future good. In a society that is present- or past-oriented, such an argument is nonsensical. Innovations are considered by such people to be a threat to well-being and probably sinful as well.

The story is told of a government official who was attempting to convince the elders of an Indian village that water should be drawn from sanitary wells rather than from the polluted river and he had brought a microscope to prove his point. The chief elder counteracted this challenge of their beliefs by dashing the microscope to the floor. "Now where are your little animals?" he asked the sanitarian who had just shown him the swimming microorganisms.

Individuals who have been trained in such fields of epizootiology as veterinary medicine, entomology, bacteriology, and sanitary engineering rarely have sufficient background in anthropology, linguistics, religion, or communication to deal with human problems that may be encountered in animal-disease control programs. Help in identifying probable problem areas should be obtained from a trained expert in human relations when the disease control program is still in the planning stages, not after a problem endangers the whole program.

The benefits of understanding the cultural attitudes of a people is illustrated by the successful effort to eradicate hydatid worms from Iceland (Dungal 1957; Schwabe 1969). Since the population was completely literate and the long evenings were suited to reading, the program planners decided that any material published in the Icelandic tongue (even though Danish is also spoken) would be given attention. The life cycle of the hydatid worm and a system for its control was therefore published in Icelandic and every farm family became thoroughly acquainted with the reasons for control and the methods to be used. Eradication was soon accomplished with relatively little cost.

Historical Patterns

All communities undergo some change, and in many areas of the world change is rapid. The rural population changes by out-and-in migration. Insufficient replacements for children who move to the cities increases the median age of the community. Consequently, farms are either consolidated or abandoned. In southwestern Wisconsin several processes, some very slow and some rapid, can be observed in one county. In the past 100 years, the Irish who pioneered the hilly and rocky farms of the upper west Mounds district have been replaced by Norwegian immigrants. These farms are now being purchased by city dwellers for recreational land. South of this district a religious group, whose members practice simple living and natural farming, has purchased farms for its members. To the north, on the sands of the Wisconsin River basin, multimillion dollar corporation farms have appeared, bringing irrigation equipment and large machinery with them. The result is a very heterogeneous rural community where no single speaker exists and any proposal must be explained in light of the interests of each group.

In Sudan, as in most of the African Sahel, people displaced to the south by the years of drought of the early seventies were changed by the experience. Some returned to the north; others did not. In that entire area there has been increasing pressure by administrators to settle the indigenous nomadic herdsmen by offering them land and homes in return for loss of mobility. Unfortunately, the ecologic and social aspects of this change have been examined only superficially (Horowitz 1979).

The introduction of a new practice into plant agriculture can have unexpected results in animal agriculture. The development of high lysine corn and its introduction into the swine ration not only provided improved nutrients but also increased the fecundity of swine parasites. Consequently the need for anthelmintics was increased.

Almost universally, rural populations are skeptical of government programs that inevitability originate from urban centers. If the rural community has little voice in government affairs, the response can be hostile. There may also be ethnic differences, but an Irish official probably overstated it when she said, "Of course it works in England, they are more law-abiding people than are we Irish or for that matter you Americans."

AN EXAMPLE OF REGIONAL ASSESSMENT

As the result of a meeting between President Frondizi of Argentina and President Kennedy of the United States, a joint Argentine-United States Commission was created to study foot-and-mouth disease. The primary emphasis was to study the disease's effect on trade between the two nations.

One proposal studied by the commission was the

creation of a foot-and-mouth disease-free-zone on the island of Tierra del Fuego (Argentine-United States Joint Commission on Foot-and-Mouth Disease 1966). Consequently, an epizootiological survey was carried out on the island between January and April in 1963. The survey was conducted by Argentine and Chilean teams that used plans approved by the commission with technical advice from F. B. Leech, a British statistical consultant. The survey was designed to obtain data on the number of farms, kind and size of livestock populations, nature of land usage, size of pastures and flocks, significance of contact between animal species, swine feeding methods, kinds of animal movement, and size of animal slaughter. In addition, sera were collected from representative animals and examined for antibodies to the serotypes of foot-and-mouth disease prevalent in South America.

It is clear (Table 3.2) that the survey teams did

Table 3.2. Survey of Tierra del Fuego

	Argentine Side	Chilean Side
Number of farms (recorded or estimated)	61	400
Livestock populations		
Number of farms reporting	58	185
Sheep	668,611	684,118
Cattle	4,435	2,898
Swine	438	697
Number of farms with 1 species only	1	45
Land usage		
Number of farms reporting	58	179
Total area, ha	1,072,683	958,607
Number of pastures	906	971
% pastures less than 500 ha	47	61
% pastures over 2000 ha	17	4
Size of sheep flocks		
Number of farms reporting	24	134
Number of flocks	154	237
% flocks under 500	24	24
% flocks over 2000	53	37
Contact between sheep and swine	2/56[*]	25/108
Contact between sheep and cattle	38/57	101/134
Access of swine to garbage	14/29	33/66
Importation of sheep	22/48	124/185
Exhibition of sheep on mainland	6/48	0/154
Annual slaughter of sheep	166,988	6,550[+]

Source: Argentine-U.S. Joint Commission on Foot-and-Mouth Disease 1966.
[*]Number of farms reporting contact/total number of farms.
[+]Most sheep sent to mainland for slaughter—data not available.

not reach all livestock owners or obtain full information from them because (1) the maps were incomplete or
outdated (Fig. 3.14); (2) some owners lived in remote
mountainous areas and could be reached only after
several days of travel on horseback; and (3) traditionally, the owners were afraid any information divulged

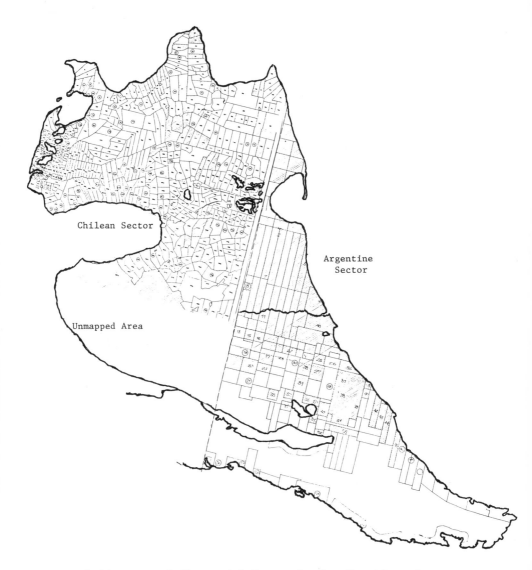

FIG. 3.14. Map of Tierra del Fuego showing location of
farms (adapted from Argentine-United States Joint Commission
on Foot-and-Mouth Disease 1966).

about their holdings might be used by government tax agents.

Nevertheless, the survey showed that the number, size, and management of farms were different on the Argentine and Chilean sides of the island. While the predominant husbandry was sheep production, a suffici- ent population of cattle and swine was found to be of epidemiological concern. Although no proven serologic reactors were found, foot-and-mouth disease was subse- quently introduced to the island by cattle from the mainland that were brought in to supply oil field workers with fresh beef. The disease was promptly eradicated.

REFERENCES

Anderson, R. K.; Berman, D. T.; Berry, W. T.; Hopkin, J. A.; and Wise, R. 1978. Report National Brucellosis Technical Commission. Anim. Plant Health Insp. Serv., USDA, Washington, D.C.

Anderson, S. G. 1952. Murray Valley encephalitis: Epidemiological aspects. *Med. J. Aust.* 1:97-100.

Animal Health Yearbook. 1978. Rome: FAO/WHO/OIE.

Argentine-United States Joint Commission on Foot-and- Mouth Disease. 1966. Studies on Foot-and-Mouth Disease. NAS-NRC Publ. 1343. Washington, D.C.

Audy, J. R. 1958. The localization of disease with special reference to the zoonoses. *Trans. R. Soc. Trop. Med. Hyg.* 52:308-328.

Bacon, P. J., and Macdonald, D. W. 1981. Habitat and the spread of rabies. *Nature* 289:634-635.

Birch, L. C. 1957. The role of weather in determining the distribution and abundance of animals. *Cold Spring Harbor Symp. Quant. Biol.* 22:203-215.

Clegg, E. J., and Garlick, J. P., eds. 1980. Disease and Urbanization. Symposia of the Society for the Study of Human Biology, vol. 20. Atlantic Highlands, N.J.: Humanities Press.

Cockburn, W. C. 1964. The implications of large-scale programmes for the control of infectious disease. Global Impacts of Applied Microbiology. New York: John Wiley & Sons, pp. 456-461.

Curtis, J. T. 1959. The Vegetation of Wisconsin. Madison, Wis: Univ. Wis. Press.

Darlington, P. J. 1957. Zoogeography: The Geograph- ical Distribution of Animals. New York: John Wiley & Sons.

Dungal, N. 1957. Eradication of hydated disease in Iceland. *N.Z. Med. J.* 56:213-222.

Dyson-Hudson, R., and Dyson-Hudson, N. 1969. Subsis- tence herding in Uganda. *Sci. Am.* 220(2):76-89.

Friend, R. E.   1979.   Animal production and economic data systems in Canada, Japan, Australia, and New Zealand.   In Proceedings of International Symposium on Animal Health and Disease Data Banks. Misc. Publ. 1381.   USDA, Washington, D.C., pp. 241-275.

Geological Survey.   1962.   Blue Mounds quadrangle, Wisconsin.   U.S. Dep. Interior.

Guidry, N. P.   1964.   A graphic summary of world agriculture.   Misc. Publ. 705.   USDA, Washington, D.C.

Hansen, W. R., and Yuill, T. M.   1976.   Role of wildlife hosts in the epizootiology of LaCrosse virus in Wisconsin.   In Wildlife Diseases, ed. L. A. Page.   New York: Plenum Press, pp. 453-463.

Hayes, R. O., and Hess, A. D.   1964.   Climatological conditions associated with outbreaks of eastern encephalitis.   Am. J. Trop. Med. Hyg. 13:851-858.

Hemmes, J. H.; Winkler, K. C.; and Kool, S. M.   1960. Virus survival as a seasonal factor in influenza and poliomyelitis.   Nature 188:430-431.

Hess, A. D., and Holden, P.   1958.   The natural history of the arthropod-borne encephalitides in the United States.   Ann. N.Y. Acad. Sci. 70:294-311.

Hine, R. L., ed.   1968.   Wildlife, people, and the land.   Publ. 621.   Dep. Nat. Resour., Madison, Wis.

Hope-Simpson, R. E.   1981.   The role of season in the epidemiology of influenza.   J. Hyg. Camb. 86:35-47.

Horowitz, M. M.   1979.   The sociology of pastoralism and African livestock projects.   Agency for International Development Program Evaluation Discussion Paper 6.   Bur. Program Policy Coord., AID, Washington, D.C.

Hyslop, N. St. G.   1974.   Effects of the environment on immunity to disease.   In International Livestock Environment Symposium Proceedings.   St. Joseph, Mich.: Am. Soc. Agric. Engrs., pp. 383-390.

Idso, S. B.; Jackson, R. D.; and Reginato, R. J.   1977. Remote-sensing of crop yields.   Science 196:19-25.

Imperato, P. J.   1977.   African Folk Medicine: Practices and Beliefs of the Bambara and other Peoples.   Baltimore: York Press.

International Livestock Environment Symposium Proceedings.   1974.   St. Joseph, Mich.: Am. Soc. Agric. Engrs.

Kahrs, R. F.   1981.   Virus diseases of cattle.   In Virus Diseases of Food Animals, vol. 1, ed. E. P. J. Gibbs.   London: Academic Press, pp. 137-155.

Knipling, E. F.   1960.   The eradication of the screwworm fly.   Sci. Am. 203(4):54-61.

Kolb, J. H. 1957. Neighborhood-family relations in rural society. Res. Bull. 201. Agric. Exp. Stn., Univ. Wis., Madison.

Levine, N. D. 1963. Weather, climate and bionomics of ruminant nematode larvae. In Advances in Veterinary Science, vol. 8, eds. C. A. Brandly and E. L. Jungherr. New York: Academic Press, pp. 215-261.

Machado, M. A., Jr. 1968. An Industry in Crisis: Mexican-United States Cooperation in the Control of Foot-and-Mouth Disease. Univ. Calif. Publ. in Hist., vol. 80. Berkeley and Los Angeles: Univ. Calif. Press.

Malaga-Cruz, H.; Lopez-Nieto, E.; and Wanderley, M. 1979. Caracterizacion de la poblacion animal. Pan Am. Foot-and-Mouth Dis. Cent., Rio de Janeiro, Brazil.

Marshall, D. G. 1963. Wisconsin's population: Changes and prospects, 1900-1963. Res. Bull. 241. Univ. Wis., Madison.

Marshall, I. D. 1959. The influence of ambient temperature on the course of myxomatosis in rabbits. J. Hyg. 57:484-497.

Mason, H. G., and Iltis, H. H. 1958. Preliminary reports of the flora of Wisconsin No. 42, Rosaceae I--rose family. Wis. Acad. Sci. Arts Lett. Trans. 47:65-94.

Miller, R. J. 1973. Cultural practices and disease control programs. In Animal Disease Eradication: Evaluating Programs. Proc. NAS Workshop, April 12-13, Univ. Wis. Ext., Madison, Wis., pp. 29-33.

Mohler, J. R. 1925. The California and Texas foot-and-mouth disease outbreaks. J. Am. Vet. Med. Assoc. 67:84-90.

National Oceanic and Atmospheric Administration. 1978. Wisconsin. Climatological Data 83(4):1-19.

Ollerenshaw, C. B., and Smith, L. P. 1969. Meteorological factors and forecasts of helminthic disease. Adv. Parasitol. 7:283-323.

Pan American Foot-and-Mouth Disease Center. 1979. Guidelines for compiling and recording information to characterize foot-and-mouth disease regionally in South America. Rio de Janeiro, Brazil.

Perez, F. 1975. Estudio socioeconomico de santander de quilichao. Boletin de Investigacion 15. Instituto Colombiano Agropecuario, Bogota, Colombia.

Richardson, R. H., ed. 1978. The Screwworm Problem: Evolution of Resistance to Biological Control. Austin, Tex.: Univ. Texas Press.

Rockford Map Publishers, Inc. 1971. Atlas and plat book: Iowa County, Wisconsin. Rockford, Ill.

Ruttan, V. W., and Hayami, Y. 1973. Technology transfer and agricultural development. *Tech. Cult.* 14:119-151.

Saint, W. S., and Coward, E. W., Jr. 1977. Agriculture and behavioral science: Emerging orientations. *Science* 197:733-737.

Saleh, A. A. 1975. Disincentives to agricultural production in developing countries: A policy survey. Foreign Agric., Mar. supplement. USDA, Washington, D.C.

Schnurrenberger, P. R.; Martin, R. J.; and Doby, P. B. 1965. Disease control through the study of population characteristics. *U.S. Livest. Sanit. Assoc. Proc.* 69:29-34.

Schwabe, C. W. 1969. Veterinary Medicine and Human Health, 2nd ed. Baltimore: Williams & Wilkens Co.

Seber, G. A. F. 1973. The Estimation of Animal Abundance and Related Parameters. London: Griffin.

Sellers, R. F. 1981. Factors affecting the geographical distribution and spread of virus diseases of food animals. In Virus Diseases of Food Animals, vol. 1, ed. E. P. J. Gibbs. London: Academic Press, pp. 19-29.

Siegel, H. S. 1974. Environmental stress and animal health: A discussion of the influence of environmental factors on the health of livestock and poultry. In International Livestock Environment Symposium Proceedings. St. Joseph, Mich.: Am. Soc. Agric. Engrs., pp. 14-20.

Smith, C. V. 1964. Some evidence for the windborne spread of fowl pest. *Meteorolog.* 93:257-263.

Smith, L. P., and Hugh-Jones, M. E. 1969. The weather factor in foot-and-mouth disease epidemics. *Nature* 223:712-715.

Soil Conservation Service. 1962. Soil survey of Iowa County, Wisconsin. Ser. 1958, no. 22, USDA and Univ. Wis., USGPO, Washington, D.C.

Tellez-S., J. 1975. La comunicacion en el oriente Antioqueno: Disponibilidad de medios. Boletin de Investigacion 34. Instituto Colombiano Agropecuario, Bogota, Colombia.

Temple, R. S., and Thomas, M. E. R. 1973. The Sahelian drought: A disaster for livestock populations. *World Anim. Rev.* 8:1-7.

Thaxton, P., and Siegel, H. S. 1970. Immunodepression in young chickens by high environmental temperature. *Poult. Sci.* 49:202-205.

Tromp, S. W. 1973. Meteorological changes and resistance to infection. Lancet, June 30, p. 1517.

Van Ness, G. B. 1971. Ecology of anthrax. *Science* 172:1303-1307.

Van Ness, G., and Stein, C. D. 1956. Soils of the United States favorable for anthrax. *J. Am. Vet. Med. Assoc.* 128:7-9.

Victoria-L., F., and Arevalo-A., M. 1970. Canales de comunicacion que usan los habilantes del proyecto de desarrollo rural del norte del cauca. Boletin de Investigacion 16. Instituto Colombiano Agropecuario, Bogota, Colombia.

Walker, J. W.; Pfow, C. J.; Newcomb, S. S.; Urban, W. D.; Nadler, H. E.; and Locke, L. N. 1969. Status of duck virus enteritis (duck plague) in the United States. *U.S. Anim. Health Assoc. Proc.* 73: 254-278.

Wang, J. Y., and Suomi, V. E. 1958. The phyto-climate of Wisconsin, 2. Temperature: Normals and hazards. Res. Rep. 2. Agric. Exp. Stn., Univ. Wis., Madison.

Watson, R. M. 1969. Aerial photographic methods in censuses of animals. *East African Agric. For. J.* 34:32-37 (special issue, July).

Wharton, C. R., Jr., ed. 1969. Subsistence Agriculture and Economic Development. Chicago: Aldine Publishing Co.

Wilson, W. O. 1974. Livestock environment research and needs for additional knowledge: Poultry. In International Livestock Environment Symposium Proceedings. St. Joseph, Mich.: Am. Soc. Agric. Engrs., pp. 422-424.

Wisconsin Agricultural Reporting Service. 1980. Wisconsin dairy facts. Wis. Dep. Agric., Trade, Consum. Prot., Madison, Wis.

Wisconsin Department of Public Instruction. 1962. Reading Wisconsin's landscape, 2nd ed. Madison, Wis.

Wisconsin Department of Transportation. 1980-1981. Official highway map of Wisconsin, Doc. Sales, Madison, Wis.

Wisconsin Legislative Reference Bureau. 1964. The Wisconsin Blue Book 1964. Madison, Wis: Dep. Adm. Doc. Sales Distrib., pp. 70-225.

Wisconsin Legislative Reference Bureau. 1973. The State of Wisconsin 1973 Blue Book. Madison, Wis: Dep. Adm. Doc. Sales Distrib.

Worden, G. 1979. Livestock data systems in the United States for economic analysis. In Proceedings of International Symposium on Animal Health and Disease Data Banks. Misc. Publ. 1381. Washington, D.C.: USDA, pp. 233-236.

4

Livestock Production Systems

EVOLUTION

While no farms are alike, in the sense that one can be used as an experimental control for another, there often are compelling reasons why epidemiologists and officials must allocate farms into such categories as tenancy, kind of livestock, size of herd, or type of management (Schnurrenberger et al. 1965).

Various systems of classifying livestock operations have been proposed (McDowell 1972). One system than brings all levels--simple and complex, ancient and modern--together and gives new insights is based on the view that livestock production is an evolutionary process in which the human race has gained increasing control over animals intended for use. In that evolution (Reed 1977), the harvester has taken over the determination of which animals will be mated, what they will eat, where and how they will live, and when they will die. Control over animals has been increased to the point that in some enterprises animals have become little more than production units in a factory assembly line.

Unfortunately, as the animal user has moved to fuller utilization and higher levels of control, the methods and structures developed to facilitate increased animal management have created new problems (Brander 1979) and new diseases (Strauch 1978).

Game Harvesting

The least control over animal utilization is possessed by the hunter. In the distant past all people depended upon wild animals for much of the pro-

tein in their diet; some people still do. When the
hunt failed, for whatever reason, the people starved.
Such a case occurred just a few years ago in the Northwest Territories of Canada when the caribou herd
changed its traditional migration route and the Indian
hunters were unable to find it. Hunting has always
been precarious because animal populations fluctuate in
response to weather and climatic change, and natural
scarcities are accentuated by competition between
hunters of different groups. The hunting group that
improves its skills and weapons has the advantage in
procuring game and stopping poachers.

Game is a renewable resource if the breeding
cohort is left undisturbed, but there is convincing
evidence that even 10,000 years ago successful hunting
bands' overkills resulted in the extinction of more
than a dozen species of large North American game
animals. The first human population explosion probably
occurred during such a period of improved hunting success and was followed by the first of recurring dark
ages. The hunter, then as now, was subjected to some
diseases of game animals, particularly predation-
dependent parasites, and hunting bands were subjected
to arthropodborne hematoprotozoan parasites and viruses
as well. While only a few bands of hunters still forage for game on land, animals of the sea are still
hunted, and some aquatic species are threatened with
extinction.

Nomadic Herding

The second level of animal utilization came with
the appearance of nomadic herders. Herding may have
evolved from keeping the young of a prey species as a
pet or deliberately capturing and rearing a sacred
animal for purposes of worship or magic. It is not
likely that the hunting chiefs sat down as game became
scarce and agreed on a way to maintain essential breeding stock. Nor is it probable that domestication of
livestock was undertaken as a way to feed people.
However it happened, the rearing of animals and the
planting of crops began over 10,000 years ago (Reed
1977) and probably brought about the second population
explosion and the beginning of civilization. Farming
and animal domestication also increased the motives for
human conflict and provided the means for its intensification when it occurred. During many early centuries, dynasties rose and fell as disciplined nomadic
herdsmen overran the villages and the cities of grain
producers. The nomad has been feared and romanticized
in legends and literature from that day to the present.

As a livestock producer, the nomad's first objective was to maintain a breeding herd and improve it by
culling (Horowitz 1979). In the necessary search for
pasture and water, the herd was moved north and south
following the seasons or up into the mountains and down
into the valleys, just as herds are still moved in
parts of Africa and Asia (Epstein 1971). While constant watch, as described in the Bible, usually protected the herd from predation, the nomad was forced to
share pastures with herds belonging to other groups
that also moved through the land. If the pastures were
overgrazed, the deterioration that followed was has-
tened in years of drought. Even today, the degradation
process is rarely recognized until it is too late.
Some degraded pastures became wastes and were lost
forever, and the diseases that were left behind on the
pastures and in the water holes affected the cattle
that followed. Even the powerful nomads, who often
terrified villagers, were powerless to control the
drought and disease that ravaged the herd on which
their life depended.

Sedentary Livestock Production

The third level of livestock production was
reached by the sedentary livestock producer. It is
unlikely that the nomads took this step because a
sedentary life is not possible in the arid lands
occupied by most nomadic people. Villagers in the more
humid areas presumably acquired a few animals and
expanded their herds when they learned how to irrigate
land and clear forests. Initially, livestock development was limited to regions where forage could be grown
all year. As the settlers learned how to gather and
store forage, livestock production moved into colder
climates. With control over forage production, the
emerging farmers were able to determine stocking rates
and nutrition of their animals as well as their breeding. While there was considerable segregation of
animals of one village from those of the next, the
movement of traders enabled cattle plagues to cross
entire continents more than a millennium ago. This
hazard, which still exists (Ellis and Hugh-Jones 1976),
was recognized in some ages and at some places. Bans
against transient animals entering pastures were enforced by guns both in Europe ages ago and in the central
United States before the arrival of the railroads.
Among the greatest legacies of the sedentary
herdsman was the development of all the standard breeds
of livestock (Neumann 1977) and the establishment of an
agroecosystem that could be sustained for centuries

(Trow-Smith 1957; Hodgson 1971; Hodgson 1977). However, the demands of a rapidly growing, urbanized population for more food at lower cost forced a change to intensive livestock production. The disincentives that rapidly decreased the role of nomadic and sedentary agriculture (Saleh 1975) in the production of food have not, and should not, eliminate these forms of agriculture because they remain the best agricultural options for some lands (Horowitz 1979).

Intensive Livestock Production

Intensive production arose in this century through a deliberate effort to alter the environment of the animal in order to prolong and accelerate production. Typical of the innovations that eventually changed the face of animal production was the discovery that artificial lighting of hen houses prolonged lay (Wilson 1966). The extended season necessitated the use of calcium and cod-liver oil to supplement the chickens' diet (Bird 1964). It also required closer confinement to reduce the cost per bird of better shelter and increased control over the environment. Inherent in these changes was an increase in the density and size of the animal herd or flock and a limitation of the functions performed in a given animal enterprise (specialization). Size and specialization were dictated by the economic limitations placed on the producer. Unit production costs had to be reduced so the producer could remain competitive while paying for the increased capitalization costs required for improvements. Many of the innovations were linked and had to be undertaken simultaneously or not at all. Furthermore, the farmer had to keep pace with neighbors, or the needed tools would no longer be available and the product would be difficult to market. Improvements in technology came first and most rapidly in the rearing of egg and meat birds, the least developed sectors of livestock production, and then spread to swine and later to dairy and beef. In all types of livestock the objective was increased productivity in terms of earlier maturity, faster growth, more uniform conformation, and greater production of milk, eggs, or number of offspring (Horsfall 1975). The results have been very impressive and have led many urbanites to expect that such increases in efficiency can continue indefinitely (Culver and Ericksen 1973).

Greater yield has been purchased at a cost that is still not clearly appreciated. The livestock producers, who previously did everything without assistance and asked only that consumers buy their product have lost their independence. Now, the genetic capability of the herd, the feedstuffs, the energy required to do work, and the capitalization required to buy improvements are supplied by others according to their design. Furthermore, the producer is faced with new problems (Andersen and Aalund 1975). Wastes from the herd may be too great to be used safely on the farm and must be applied or disposed of according to rules established by others. To achieve the desired productivity from both the land and the herd, the farmer must use chemicals whose short-term value is evident but whose long-term affects are unknown (Matyas 1978). The long-term effect is the crux of the quandary. The agroecosystem of good farmers of the past was stable and could endure for centuries, but today's farmer does not know whether the best of the intensive-producing farms can remain viable enterprises for even a century. Change is so rapid and continuous (Lewontin 1980) that there has been no time for long-term value assessment. However, it is known that the change in livestock production systems has resulted in the appearance of new diseases (Hanson 1957, 1974) and environmental problems.

INNOVATIVE LIVESTOCK PRODUCTION AND DISEASE CONTROL

Increased Herd Size

In the 30 years following World War I, poultry flocks were expanded from a few hundred birds to several thousand birds and finally to hundreds of thousands of birds (Table 4.1). Dairy herds doubled and tripled in size, and a few herds of over 10,000 animals appeared. Feedlot operations for beef cattle grew from several hundred cattle to over a hundred thousand cattle.

The size of today's herd is determined by who is handling it; a single operator aided by automatic equipment or a manager with a staff. The latter could be an individual entrepreneur (rancher), a corporation (large feedlot operation), or a cooperative (Israeli kibbutz). The minimum herd size is determined largely by effective utilization of the labor force and essential equipment. For instance, a current U.S. regulation that requires a producer of fluid milk to have a pipeline milker and refrigerated bulk tank dictates a minimum milking herd of 50 or more animals. Automated feeding equipment and standard housing demands that the minimum broiler house contain five to ten thousand

Table 4.1. Changes in Poultry Industry

Classification	1925	1950
Chicken	General purpose bird	Layerbirds or broiler birds
	Egg production less than 100 eggs	Egg production up to 300 eggs or more
	Broiler maturity, 18 wk	Broiler maturity, 9 wk
	Moulting-brooding uncontrolled	Moulting-brooding controlled
Breeding	Haphazard breeding	Hybrids produced through scientific breeding
	Genetic base unrestricted	Genetic base restricted to a few inbred lines
	On-farm hatching	Nation supplied by a few breeder-hatchers
Feeding	Feed raised on premise	Feed purchased, origin nationwide
	Diet of whole grains and scraps	Diet of formulated mash supplied in bulk
	Essential nutrients unknown	40 essential nutrients incorporated in diet
	Periodic feeding by hand	Automatic feeding equipment
	Drugs not used in feed	Drugs routinely added to feed
Management	Small flocks of 50-500	Large flocks of 50,000 to 500,000
	Free range or large yards	Confinement to houses or cages
	No environmental control	Controlled light and temperature
	Low density (1 to 5-10 sq ft)	High density (1 to 0.58 sq ft)
	Multigeneration operation	One-generation operation (all-in, all-out)
Diseases	Carrier-type diseases dominant	Crowd diseases dominant
	Vaccine use limited (1)	Vaccines widely used (6)
	Little veterinary interest	Significant veterinary interest
	Deficiency diseases common	Deficiency diseases rare
	Few diseases characterized	Many diseases characterized

Table 4.2. Analysis of Determinants of Swine Enzootic Pneumonia
    in Herds from a Danish Slaughterhouse

Factor/Category	Estimated Relative Risk
Herd Size	
1-399 pigs slaughtered per year	1.0
400-1,000+ pigs slaughtered per year	6.9
Replacement	
On-farm weaning	1.0
Purchase of weaners	7.3
(when adjusted for herd size)	(5.1)
Ventilation	
No-fan system	1.0
Fan system	3.0
(when adjusted for herd size,	(1.8)
not significant)	

Source: Willeberg 1979.

birds. The income received from such a broiler house
makes it necessary for the operator to have several
such units. The essential point is that labor, equipment, unit profit, and animal species determine the
size of a flock or herd (Wragg 1970). There is very
little flexibility, and individual preference has
little weight. However, herd size largely determines
the risk of disease with the risk increasing as herd
size increases (Table 4.2). Inflexibility in the
relationship of the determinates of herd size seldom
allows the owner to reduce risk by reducing herd size.

Specialization

The sedentary herdsman maintained the breeding
stock and sold surplus animals and livestock produce,
often doing part of the processing such as separating
cream from milk and making butter. Forage and grain
needed for the herd came from the farm. Many of the
improvements were undertaken without recourse to
credit. Few livestock producers in developed nations
can operate in this fashion today. The market demands
another type or quality of product, and the costs of
labor, taxes, and materials make it impossible to
follow old practices.
The dairy farmer has not only replaced the herd
bull with semen from a national breeding cooperative
but also may purchase an insemination and pregnancy
testing service. Because the herd is larger than one
individual can manage with hand labor, the farmer has
purchased tractors, forage-handling equipment, milking
machines, and a large range of automatic equipment. In
spite of the fact that most of the forage (green chop,

silage, and hay) is grown on the farm, feed supplements must be purchased from a dealer who may also grind the farmer's grain and blend it with the supplement. Milk is no longer delivered to the dairy by the farmer. Instead, once or twice a day a trucker pumps it from the refrigerated tank on the farm to the refrigerated truck and finally to the receiving tanks at the dairy. No processing of milk or meat is done on the farm. Veal calves and culled cows are butchered at an inspected establishment. The milk trucker, the inseminator, the veterinarian, and individuals servicing mechanical equipment visit the farm and herd regularly.

The large institutional dairy herds have gone even further. Replacement animals are purchased from a dealer who may have obtained them from a small breeder and reared them on contract. All feed is purchased, and all manure is removed from the premises. Both services may be contracted. Milking is done by crews who may have no other duties, and feeding and cleaning is handled by other laborers.

Poultry production has become even more institutionalized (Fig. 4.1). Most meat and layer birds are now specially selected hybrids. Production of chicks for sale to producers is controlled by international corporations who maintain grandparent stock by line breeding, grow out parental stock, and set up cross-breeding flocks. The eggs go to franchise hatcheries who deliver the chicks to producers through dealers (Coates et al. 1975). Rearing of broilers or production of layers may be done by individuals who contract to buy chicks and sell broilers or layers or by a corporation who hires a staff to operate broiler or layer facilities.

A long sequence of activities is required to produce a market egg or broiler, and no one person controls more than a segment of it. In fact, the producer may have the least input. The contract upon which the producer obtains credit from a bank, feed dealer, or poultry corporation usually spells out the management details--sometimes even the brand of feed and kind of drugs and vaccines that shall be used. Since these integrated enterprises span states and even nations, it is often difficult to get complete information on farm practices, and it may be impossible for local operators to institute changes. For example, the individual having the authority to make a change in vaccine may be a manager who sits at a desk 1,000 miles from the flocks. Is it any wonder that the evaluation of disease-control measures in such integrated enterprises becomes complex indeed (McCauley 1974; Parsons

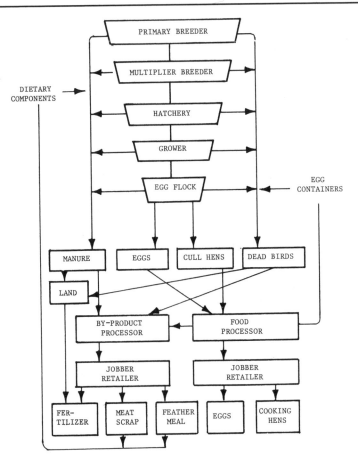

FIG. 4.1. Relationships of five production specialists of
the chicken-egg industry.

et al. 1976; Smith 1977; Stephens et al. 1979).
    The flow of materials and people within modern
livestock enterprises is not readily apparent to an
outsider (Dalton 1975), and the existence of irregularities is difficult to discern.   For example, an
error that introduces a poison, such as polybrominated
biphenyl, into a food supplement is undetectable until
after the product has been widely distributed and
has contaminated or killed animals on 1,000 farms
(Crossland 1979).   Similarly, a worthless vaccine can
compromise the immunity of a million animals and a
contaminated product can introduce disease into all
sections of the country.

Confinement

A hundred years ago confinement meant fences of rock, logs, or wire, and some of these barriers still keep animals in a pasture or pen. Under such circumstances, the space allocated to an animal was relatively large and often permitted the individual to not only feed on a variety of forages but also select a comfortable place out of the wind or sun and even away from irritating flies.

Today, confinement means a managed environment, often a structure in which the animal is on wire, slats, or a concrete floor. The space may be covered and insulated against heat and cold and screened against insects. Even the air may be heated or cooled and filtered (Chute and Stauffer 1962). These refinements reduce the space per animal, sometimes to the point where the animal is unable to turn around. The resulting increase in animal density usually leads to social stress and increased vulnerability to disease and infection (Muggenburg et al. 1967). The greater risk of loss from communicable disease has led some operators to change to specific pathogen-free breeding stock (Cooper 1970). Others have proposed area certification (Smith 1977).

Confinement of the animal's wastes may also be required. Older farmers, faced with accumulation of animal wastes in pens and stables, usually stored manure in piles next to the stables during inclement weather and during the appropriate season transported it to the fields and spread it as fertilizer. In many areas today, storage of animal wastes is restricted to approved containment structures. It may be removed from the stable or lot and spread daily or accumulated in sanitary pits, special ponds, or more elaborate liquid-manure storage and handling systems. The primary objective is to reduce pollution of surface or underground waters and the nuisance of odors and flies. Most of these systems save the nutrients needed by soils, but they add to production costs by increasing requirements for capital investment. Furthermore, they sometimes create special disease hazards. The stability of pathogens and parasites in manure that is handled in different ways has yet to be adequately documented. Sometimes the gases produced during fermentation of liquid wastes escape into areas used by animals and people and cause poisoning and even death.

All nutrients, including minor minerals and vitamins that were formerly sought out in pastures and on dung hills, must be delivered to the confined animal.

Table 4.3. Source of Protein in the Diet of Mink—An Example of
    Change Forced by Market Place Competition

Product	Period of Use	Problems Encountered
Horse meat	Primary source before 1965	Yellow fat disease (unsaturated fats) *Klebsiella* infections
Freshwater fish	1940-present	Contaminated by poly- chloronated biphenyl Thiaminase
Saltwater fish	1940-1977	Unknown
Fish meal	1960-1967	Dimethenitrosamine
Whale meat	1950-1968	Botulism Type C
Chicken by-products	1955-1977	Mycoplasmosis? Diethylstibesterol infertility
Beef by-products	Sporadic	*Klebisiella* infection *Pasteurella* infection
Fur seal meat	1962-present	Exposure to San Miguel sea lion disease
Downer and dead cattle	Sporadic	Black leg Anthrax Malignant edema
Pork products	1940-present	Pseudorabies Avian tuberculosis *Salmonella cholera-suis*
Sheep and goat products	Sporadic	Scrapie
Complete dry mink food, pelleted	1970-present	No known problems

Feed is dried or preserved in some other fashion; its
constituents are ground or pelleted for easier handling
and automated delivery; its components are formulated
to obtain a balance of known nutrients and fortified
with drugs to combat parasitism and infection or speed
growth. The result has been increased feed efficiency,
rapid weight gains, and sometimes reduced production
costs (Horsfall 1975). There (Table 4.3) have also
been unanticipated adverse effects (Lee 1952) as well
as concern over possible problems not yet encountered
(Mosier 1976). Concern for the welfare of confined
animals (Curtis 1980; Russell and Ainsworth 1981) has
led to regulatory action by some governments (Protection of Animals Act 1980).

Genetic Engineering

Until the last several decades, genetic improvement of animals was limited to age-old methods of
selecting and breeding animals of superior quality.
Then, first with chickens, and later with other

species, inbred lines were selected for certain genetic traits that could be appreciated only when they were crossed to produce hybrids with the desired qualities of both parent lines. The hybrid outdistanced animals selected by conventional systems because of the rapidity with which it could be designed to meet economic demands for early maturity, rapid growth, higher ratio of lean-to-fat meat, and other desired qualities (Taylor 1964).

The new technology (Ruttan 1973) required an intimate knowledge of genetics and was far too sophisticated for anyone but specialists. The source of much of the world's breeding stock was rapidly concentrated in the hands of a few entrepreneurs.

Genetic change in mammalian populations is slower than in avian populations because only the male is readily manipulated by the geneticists. This may be changed if it is possible to exploit the ovarian implantation technique in which ova from superior females fertilized *in vitro* by semen from superior males are implanted in grade females. This process will enable more rapid increase of high quality animals than is possible with conventional breeding.

Geneticists select qualities of commercial importance. The selection process that has been followed regarding the resistance of the animal to disease is by no means clear. Resistance to parasitic, bacterial, and viral diseases is genetically controlled, but controlling mechanisms are complex. The conflict between improved production and resistance to disease is illustrated by selection of milk cows for increased productivity and the associated increase in udder size without provision for adequate physical support for an increasingly heavy organ. The increased prevalence of mastitis can be related, in part, to structural failures that increase the probability of mechanical injury to the udder.

Selection for a genetic trait, such as increased milk production, is a lengthy process that is slowed if an additional trait, such as disease resistance, is added. Unfortunately, disease resistance is not a single genetic trait. Consequently, genetic selection for disease resistance is seldom practical as long as there are other options for controlling disease.

Two strategies have been tried to compensate for the increased infection vulnerability of animals that either are reared intensively without having been bred for increased resistance to disease or that may have suffered a decrease in their genetic resistance. One strategy is the development of specific-pathogen-free breeding stocks of chickens and swine for rearing in

clean environments (Betts et al. 1960). The second is
the development of animal housing that excludes common
pathogens. An example of the latter is the positive-
pressure air-filtered house for poultry (Drury et al.
1969).

Mechanization

The increase in herd size and the confinement of
increasing numbers of animals in less and less space
would not be possible without mechanization (Dexter
1977; Just et al. 1979). The initial stimulus for
mechanization was the increasing cost and unavailability of human labor as well as the low cost of
energy. The economic realities that forced the farmers
to increase their herd size also forced them to mecha-
nize in order to handle more animals. This use of
machines as hired hands gave the producers such new
abilities as thermostatic control of air and water
temperatures that insured safe storage of produce and
better cleaning of surfaces, and auger-fed delivery
from bulk tanks of feed mixed with the vitamins and
drugs necessary to improve growth rates and reduce
waste. Handling feed in bulk storage tanks brings such
secondary advantages as protection from rodent damage
and contamination, protection from spoilage (as may
occur in the storage of ensilage and grains under low
oxidation conditions) and reduced costs of bulk
delivery from a supplier.

We have become so accustomed to mechanization that
it is difficult to imagine a poultry industry without
scores of regulatory devices, but it can be done. For
centuries hen eggs have been artificially incubated in
Egypt in ovenlike chambers heated by fermenting manure
or burning straw. An operator, who detects increases
or decreases in temperature by feeling the warmth of an
egg held to his closed eyelid, keeps the chamber temperature within a degree of 38°C by opening and closing
apertures in the chamber wall.

Mechanization also permits intermittent or continuous removal of solid wastes. The resulting environmental control of pathogen buildup on surfaces and in
the air helps make close confinement of animals possible. Mechanical systems are also necessary for
cleaning surfaces by hosing, disinfecting with sprays,
forced-air movement, and air filtration.

STRUCTURAL MODEL

Individuals who grew up on livestock farms know
the seasonal events, how one thing follows another,

each in its due time. For these persons, the consequences of good and bad decisions as well as the inevitability of various events has become innate, and they
do not find it necessary to prepare a structural model
of the farm operation because the imprint is carried in
their minds. Preparation of a model is necessary, however, for those who need a picture of the operation in
order to (1) understand how disease-control measures
can be introduced and (2) predict the effect of selected measures on the operation and its profitability.
Construction of the basic operational diagram is
simple. Complexity arises as constraints are added,
and when the effect of variables and their economic
evaluation are considered, it becomes increasingly
difficult to proceed without the aid of a computer.

In a swine operation (Hubbard 1976), which can be
used as an example for any livestock operation, the sow
is the fundamental unit. The sequential events (Fig.
4.2) include the sow's prebreeding care, breeding,
gestation, and farrowing followed by weaning the litter
and its growth and finishing. Each event has a known
duration that predetermines the occupation of certain
quarters and the need for specific services. Prebreeding care lasts 4 weeks, breeding 3 weeks, and gestation 12 1/2 weeks. Weaning is done at 4 to 6 weeks,
and 21 to 28 weeks is usually allowed for growing and
finishing. The animal is usually moved to new quarters
during each period and it's diet is modified. At
appropriate times, treatments such as iron shots or
tail clipping are given and vaccines and anthelminthics
are administered. Timing of the treatment is very
important; earlier or later introduction might cause
complications or be less efficacious. At certain
times, the sow and offspring are more vulnerable to
stresses and require closer observation and more
supportive measures.

The system does not always run smoothly. The sow
or boar may be sterile, the sow may abort, or the
litter may sicken and die. When the cycle stops for
any of these reasons, the sow is either returned and
prepared for rebreeding or culled and sold for slaughter. Failure within the operation may involve only one
sow and her litter or part or all of the herd. If the
whole herd is affected, infectious disease or general
mismanagement is usually the cause. Although finishing
may be delayed by bad weather and poor feed, it may
also be delayed for market reasons to obtain a better
sale price.

In the past, only one breeding cycle was completed
per year. Farrowing was timed for weather favorable to
the piglets, and finishing was correlated to utiliza-

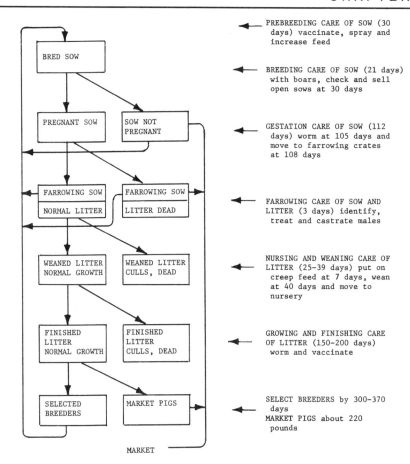

FIG. 4.2. Swine operation model (adapted from Bache and
Foster ca. 1976).

tion of the new grain crop. Currently, with housing
that protects young animals against adverse weather and
storage facilities that prevent rapid loss of feed to
rats or spoilage, most swine producers farrow twice a
year; some attempt continuous farrowing. While the
latter increases risk to airborne disease (Bohl 1970),
multiple farrowing gives better utilization of facilities and labor. However, its tight schedule is less
amenable to integration into a mixed farming
enterprise.

When a livestock operation is diagramed, each
event and its possible outcomes must be identified. A
sow, when bred, conceives and farrows, conceives and
aborts, or fails to conceive. The size of the litter

that is farrowed is normal (8-11), or less than normal because of reabsorption *in utero* or death at birth. When lactation is normal, an average-sized (6-8) litter is weaned; if lactation is abnormal, the piglets are runted or die.

Although each event can terminate in one of several ways, probabilities for the occurrence of any one of these terminations is known for the "average" herd. The termination of gestation may result in live births or no live births and will have a numerical value depending on the litter's size. Probable size is predictable. For some areas the probable size of the litter at birth is 10.0; at weaning it is 7.0. As the probable outcomes and numerical values are introduced into the diagram, it becomes possible by ordinary bookkeeping methods to determine the expected production of the operation (pounds of pigs to be sold) and predict quantitative values for such elements as pounds of feed, hours of labor, and number of days of use for farrowing pens or finishing barn. Further computation can show the change that an increase or decrease of one piglet in the size of the litter at weaning would have on overall production as well as the saving that an increase of 10 percent in feed efficiency (pounds of feed to pounds of weight gain) would have in total feed consumed. The impact of disease on the operation can be quantitated if the loss can be measured as mortality, decrease in feed efficiency, or by some other value. If the model has been transformed into computer language, the effect of various restraints on production as well as the effect of removing those restraints can be evaluated easily. This information can also be easily converted into monetary values so that the profit and loss of each intervention can be calculated.

With an understanding of the operation, researchers appreciate the need to develop control measures that cause the least disruption in the schedule, and control officials are better equipped to know best how to obtain the necessary cooperation and compliance from livestock producers.

ECONOMIC MODEL

A look at the monthly milk check or the sales receipts from a truckload of hogs or broilers is apt to give the observer a false idea about the profitability of a livestock operation. Operating expenses (feed and labor) as well as the return on money invested in the farm (interest or profit) must be examined (Trede and Boehlje 1976; Bache and Foster (ca. 1976). For exam-

ple, a successful swine breeder told a university class
visiting his operation, "I would have done better this
past year if I had put the money that I have tied up in
the farm into the bank to draw interest and then, had I
wanted to, I could have sold my own labor for going
rates." Such alternatives must be considered in any
appraisal of farm profitability.

The sow operation diagramed in Fig. 4.2, the
performance standards shown in Table 4.4, and the
estimates prepared by the Purdue University group for
an operation of 150 sows clearly illustrate the financial realities of the operation (Table 4.5). It is
assumed that the physical plant cost $163,000 (Table
4.6). In the first year of operation cash receipts
were only $4,752 (Table 4.7). Operating expenses of
$68,338 did not include overhead expenses. In the
second year cash receipts rose to $172,000 and opera-
ting expenses to $110,670, giving a balance of $61,330
before amortization and labor costs were deducted.
Succeeding years followed the same pattern as the
second year. In a real situation, the prices of items
produced and sold would vary and production standards
might not be achieved. While this would complicate the
calculations, it would not alter the central question:
"How much will be left for profit after the farmer pays
himself a salary and the amortization costs of $39,497
a year?" In this case, the farmer would be well into
the fifth year before the enterprise showed a profit
(Table 4.7). Although it takes time to pay off capital
costs, farming should not be the kind of operation that
an old and discouraged farmer had in mind, when he was
asked what he would do with a million dollars, "I would
just keep farming until it was all gone."

Economists would look at the swine operation in
terms of the value of the money invested (see discounting in chapter 12). They would point out that the
$163,000 required for capital could draw 9 percent
interest. Consequently, the present and future values

Table 4.4. Performance Standards: Farrow to Finish

Item	Standard
Conception rate	Gilts 80%, sows 90%
Live pigs farrowed/litter	10.0
Pigs weaned/litter	7.6
Mortality from weaning to market	1.5%
Gilts kept for replacement annually	84 for 150-sow operation
Rate of gain	220 lb at 6-7 mo
Feed conversion	400 lb feed/100 lb gain
Labor	4,200 hr for 150 sows

Source: Bache and Foster (ca. 1976).

Table 4.5. Cash Flow for 150-sow Operation, 1975

Item	
Cash receipts	
Market pigs, 2162	$161,716
Dry sows, 60	7,395
Non breeding gilts, 24	2,304
Boars, 6	585
	$172,000
Operating expenses (direct costs)	
Purchased feed	$ 38,000
Feed grain (cost of production)	59,190
Veterinary and medicine	1,500
Boar purchase	1,800
Marketing costs	4,080
Heating fuel	3,000
Electricity	600
Truck and tractor care	1,000
Miscellaneous (bedding, etc.)	1,500
	$110,670
Overhead expenses	
Investment (amortization)	$ 24,797
Labor (4,200 hours at	
$3.50 per hour)	14,700
	$ 39,497
Total expenses	$150,167
Net return	$ 21,833

Source: Bache and Foster (ca. 1976).

Table 4.6. Facility Investment for 150-Sow Operation

Facilities by types of use	Cost
Farrowing (50 sows)	$ 55,000
Nursery (400 pigs)	15,000
Finishing	52,700
Breeding (58 females)	3,660
Gestation (116 females)	19,140
Supporting equipment	17,500
(feed center, manure handling, etc.)	
	$163,000*

Source: Bache and Foster (ca. 1976).
*Depreciation: 15 years on buildings ($71,340) and 8 years on equipment ($91,660).

of the sum are different. In 10 years, unless the
$163,000 was worth $209,700 or had provided an increase
of $146,700, the investor would have lost money even
though the original $163,000 was still there. This
future value of an investment must be considered and

Table 4.7.   Economic Appraisal of 150-Sow Operation

Year	Cash Receipts	Operational Expenses	Overhead Expenses	Balance
1	$ 4,752	$ 68,338	$ 7,350	$-70,936
2	172,000	110,670	39,497*	-49,103
3	172,000	110,670	39,497	-27,270
4	172,000	110,670	39,497	- 5,437
5	172,000	110,670	39,497	16,396
6	172,000	100,670	39,497	38,229
7	172,000	110,670	39,497	60,062
8	172,000	110,670	39,497	81,895
9	172,000	110,670	39,497	103,728
10	172,000	110,670	39,497	125,561

Source: Bache and Foster (ca. 1976).
*Overhead: Labor ($14,700) and amoratization ($24,797).

discounted in terms of present money. If the $163,000
had not appreciated in the 10-year period, its worth,
based on a 9 percent discounting rate, would be only
$85,900 today.

ECONOMIC FACTORS AND DISEASE CONTROL

This brief excursion into the economic problems of
the individual farmer has two purposes: (1) to prepare
for an examination of regional economic problems in
chapter 12 when a proposed disease-control program is
evaluated, and (2) to give a better understanding of
the farmer's perspective when disease occurs and
disease-control options must be considered.
It should be evident that the farmer must be concerned with uncertainty as well as losses. Losses
obviously cut income but both decreased income and
uncertainty limit the options. Although introduction
of control can stop losses and increase the income,
control comes with its own price tag based on the use
of veterinary services, drugs, vaccines, and labor. In
some instances, it may also require either a minor
capital investment (dipping vat) or a major one
(positive-pressure air-filtration house). McDowell
(1972) concluded that it takes more than a 25 percent
projected increase in production with a probability of
attainment of over 90 percent to attract the interest
of conservative livestock operators. Furthermore, even
among individuals who are classed as early adapters of
technology, a projected production increase of 10 percent with a 90 percent probability must be assured for
the improvement or program to be accepted. In some
instances, particularly when neighbors adopt a certain

practice, a farmer may have to choose between making the improvement or ceasing operation. An older farmer is more likely to make the latter decision than a young farmer. In almost all instances, farmers faced with such choices want as much information as possible from sources they trust (Kleibenstein et al. 1976) as well as time to consider the situation without interference. Few individuals, particularly farmers, can be expected to make quick decisions on matters that affect their future income and solvency. If pressured to make a quick decision, they may reject the proposal offhand.

REFERENCES

Andersen, H. and Aalund, O. 1975. Intensive animal production in Denmark: Some environmental aspects. *Agric. Environ.* 2:65-73.

Bache, D. H., and Foster, J. R. Ca. 1976. Pork production systems with business analyses. Pork Industry Handbook PIH-15. Coop. Ext. Serv., Purdue Univ., West Lafayette, Ind.

Betts, A. O.; Lamont, P. H.; and Littlewort, M. C. G. 1960. The production by hysterectomy of pathogen-free, colostrum-deprived pigs and the foundation of a minimal-disease herd. *Vet. Rec.* 72:461-468.

Bird, H. R. 1964. The changing environment of the chicken. In Newcastle Disease Virus: An Evolving Pathogen, ed. R. P. Hanson. Madison, Wis.: Univ. Wis. Press, pp. 35-46.

Bohl, E. H. 1970. Transmissible gastroenteritis. In Diseases of Swine, 3rd ed, ed. H. W. Dunne. Ames, Ia.: Iowa State Univ. Press. pp. 171-173.

Brander, G. C. 1979. The relevance of human and animal health considerations in veterinary education. In Veterinary Epidemiology and Economics. Int. Symp. Vet. Epidemiol. Econ. Proc. 2:319-325. Canberra: Aust. Gov. Publ. Ser.

Chute, H. L., and Stauffer, D. R. 1962. Specific pathogen free poultry flocks in Maine. Agric. Exp. Stn. Rep. 106. Univ. Maine.

Coates, W. S.; Rosenwald, A. S.; and Swanson, M. H. 1975. Replacing your laying stock. Leaflet 2786. Coop. Ext., Univ. Calif., Davis.

Cooper, D. M. 1970. Poultry: Principles of disease control. I. Production of specified pathogen-free stock by management-environment control. *Vet. Rec.* 86:388-396.

Crossland, J. 1979. Fallout from the disaster: Polybrominated biphenyls. *Environment* 21(7):6-14.

Culver, D. W., and Ericksen, M. H. 1973. American
     agriculture: Its capacity to produce. The Farm
     Index, USDA, Washington, D.C., Dec.
Curtis, S. E. 1980. Animal welfare concerns in modern
     pork production: An animal scientist's analysis.
     U.S. Anim. Health Assoc. Proc. 84:27-46.
Dalton, G. E., ed. 1975. Study of Agricultural
     Systems. London: Appl. Sci. Publ. Ltd.
Dexter, K. 1977. Press notice: The impact of tech-
     nology on the political economy of agriculture,
     March 25, Ministry Agric., Fish., Food, London.
Drury, L. N.; Patterson, W. C.; and Beard, C. W.
     1969. Ventilating poultry houses with filtered
     air under positive pressure to prevent airborne
     diseases. *Poult. Sci.* 48:1640-1646.
Ellis, P. R., and Hugh-Jones, M. E. 1976. Disease as
     a limiting factor to beef production in developing
     countries. In Beef Cattle Production in Develop-
     ing Countries, ed. A. J. Smith. Edinburgh: Univ.
     Edinburgh, pp. 105-116.
Epstein, H. 1971. The Origin of the Domestic Animals
     of Africa, vol. 1. New York: Africana Publ.
     Corp.
Hanson, R. P. 1957. Origin of hog cholera. *J. Am.
     Vet. Med. Assoc.* 131:211-218.
———. 1974. The reemergence of Newcastle disease.
     In Advances in Veterinary Science and Comparative
     Medicine, vol. 18, eds. C. A. Brandly and E. L.
     Jungherr. New York: Academic Press, pp. 213-229.
Hodgson, H. J., ed. 1977. Potential of the world's
     forages for ruminant animal production. Winrock
     Int. Livest. Res. Train. Cent., Petit Jean
     Mountain, Morrilton, Ark.
Hodgson, R. E. 1971. Place of animals in world agri-
     culture. *J. Dairy Sci.* 54:442-447.
Horowitz, M. M. 1979. The sociology of pastoralism
     and African livestock projects. Agency for Inter-
     national Development Program Evaluation Discussion
     Paper 6. Bur. Program Policy Coord., AID,
     Washington, D.C.
Horsfall, J. G., chairman. 1975. Agricultural Produc-
     tion Efficiency. Washington, D.C.: NAS.
Hubbard, D. D., ed. 1976. Guidelines for uniform
     swine improvement programs. Ext. Serv. Program
     Aid 1157. USDA, Washington, D.C.
Just, R. E.; Schmitz, A.; and Zilberman, D. 1979.
     Technological change in agriculture. *Science* 206:
     1277-1280.
Kliebenstein, J. B.; Kesler, R. P.; and Rottmann, L. F.
     1976. Factors affecting the production decisions

of hog farmers. *J. Am. Soc. Farm Managers Rural Appraisers* 40(2):69-71.

Lee, A. M. 1952. Our newer knowledge of bovine hyperkeratosis. *U.S. Livest. Sanit. Assoc. Proc.* 56: 175-194.

Lewontin, R. C. 1980. Economics down on the farm. *Nature* 287:661-662.

McCauley, E. H. 1974. The contribution of veterinary service to the dairy enterprise income of Minnesota farmers: Production function analysis. *J. Am. Vet. Med. Assoc.* 165:1094-1098.

McDowell, R. E, 1972. <u>Improvement of Livestock Production in Warm Climates</u>. San Francisco: W. H. Freeman and Company.

Matyas, Z. 1978. New animal husbandry techniques and health risks for the human population. In <u>Natural History of Newly Emerging and Re-emerging Viral Zoonoses</u>. Munich Symp. Microbiol. Proc. 3:37-55. Munich: WHO Collaborating Centre for Collection and Evaluation of Data on Comparative Virology.

Mosier, J. 1976. Report of the subcommittee on effects or lack of effects to the public health from use of antibiotics in animal feeds. *U.S. Anim. Health Assoc. Proc.* 80:307-314.

Muggenburg, B. A.; Kowalczyk, T.; Hoekstra, W. G.; and Grummer, R. H. 1967. Effect of certain management variables on the incidence and severity of gastric lesions in swine. *Vet. Med.* 62:1090-1094.

Neumann, A. L. 1977. <u>Beef Cattle</u>, 7th ed. New York: John Wiley & Sons.

Parsons, J. H.; Davies, A. J.; and Stevens, A. J. 1976. Report on the joint exercise in animal health and productivity. Minist. Agric., Fish., Food, Middlesex, UK.

Protection of Animals Act 1980. 1981. Victoria Gov. Gazette, No. 16, Melbourne.

Reed, C. A., ed. 1977. <u>Origins of Agriculture</u>. The Hauge, Paris: Mouton Publ.

Russell, J., and Ainsworth, E. 1981. What farmers should know about animal welfare. *Farm Journal*, Oct., pp. 21-23.

Ruttan, V. W. 1973. Induced technical and institutional change and the future of agriculture. Agric. Dev. Counc., Inc., New York, Dec.

Saleh, A. A. 1975. Disincentives to agricultural production in developing countries: A policy survey. Foreign Agric. Mar. supplement, USDA, Washington, D.C.

Schnurrenberger, P. R.; Martin, R. J.; and Doby, P. B. 1965. Disease control through the study of population characteristics. *U.S. Livest. Sanit. Assoc. Proc.* 69:29-34.

Smith, P. L. 1977. A poultry flock health certification program in a VVND quarantine area: A proposal. *U.S. Anim. Health Assoc. Proc.* 81:345-352.

Stephens, A. J.; Esslemont, R. J.; and Ellis, P. R. 1979. The evolution of a health and productivity monitoring system for dairy herds in the UK. In Veterinary Epidemiology and Economics. Int. Symp. Vet. Epidemiol. Econ. Proc. 2:53-58. Canberra: Aust. Gov. Publ. Serv.

Strauch, D. 1978. Indications for a possible role of viruses as a health risk for the human population arising from new animal husbandry techniques. In Natural History of Newly Emerging and Re-emerging Viral Zoonoses. Munich Symp. Microbiol. Proc. 3:56-63. Munich: WHO Collaborating Centre for Collection and Evaluation of Data on Comparative Virology.

Taylor, L. W. 1964. The chicken as an evolving host. In Newcastle Disease Virus: An Evolving Pathogen, ed. R. P. Hanson. Madison, Wis.: Univ. Wis. Press, pp. 23-34.

Trede, L. D., and Boehlje, M. D. 1976. An economic and financial evaluation of swine production systems. *J. Am. Soc. Farm Managers Rural Appraisers* 40(2):5-9.

Trow-Smith, R. 1957. A History of British Livestock Husbandry to 1700. London: Routledge and Kegan Paul.

Willeberg, P. 1979. The analysis and interpretation of epidemiological data. In Veterinary Epidemiology and Economics. Int. Symp. Vet. Epidemiol. Econ. Proc. 2:185-198. Canberra: Aust. Gov. Publ. Serv.

Wilson, W. O. 1966. Poultry production. *Sci. Am.* 215(1):56-64.

Wragg, S. R. 1970. The economics of intensive livestock production. *Vet. Rec.* 86:33-37.

5

Livestock Marketing and Disease Control

MARKETING AND THE CONSUMER

It has been known for years that the commercial movements of infected animals (Mease 1817) and animal products containing infectious agents (Aulaqi 1979) are the primary way many livestock diseases are spread (Fig. 5.1). The entry of disease onto the clean property of a buyer can be prevented to only a limited extent because a buyer needs technical assistance to ascertain whether the animal purchased is free from disease. In addition, the buyer cannot avoid the losses from misrepresentation of the animal's soundness without the availability of legal recourse based on established legislation.

Livestock

Certification that animals purchased are free of disabling disease is dependent upon the activities of government agencies that conduct tests and provide assurance that the animal is as it has been represented (chapter 10). Animals moving in market channels (Fig. 5.2) are either going (1) from one farm to another as young stock, replacement stock, or breeders; or (2) to slaughter (Dowell and Bjorka 1941). Infected animals going to slaughter are not likely to spread as much disease as infected animals that are being moved from one farm to another. The latter will continue to live and shed disease agents (Miller et al. 1979). Disease-control authorities recognize this reduced risk and apply less stringent regulations to animals going to slaughter. Regulations become increasingly stringent

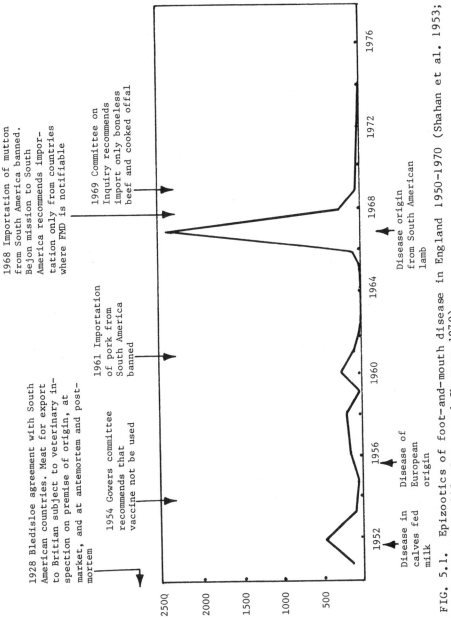

FIG. 5.1. Epizootics of foot-and-mouth disease in England 1950-1970 (Shahan et al. 1953; Northumberland 1968; Swann and Sharman 1979).

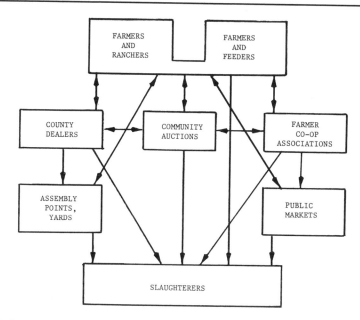

FIG. 5.2. Commercial channels for market cattle (adapted from Dowell and Bjorka 1941).

for animals being moved (1) from one farms to another, (2) from one political jurisdiction to another, or (3) from one country to another (Hejl 1974). Certain kinds of animals cannot be moved between some nations because of embargoes. Embargoes and temporary moratoria on movement of animals or animal products have far-reaching economic effects that must be considered by disease-control officials before they implement bans on movement (Sundquist et al. 1979). If breeders are unable to import live animals because of legal prohibition, they may try to import frozen semen and a new product of recent technology, frozen ova. Although importing these products is probably less risky than importing breeding animals, the nature of the risk has not yet been fully evaluated.

Livestock Products

Since most animal products such as meat, milk, and eggs, are intended for human consumption, they are subject to inspection for wholesomeness. These products may also be fed to animals, for example, milk or milk replacers to calves and meat scraps in garbage to swine (Wright 1943; Hall 1952; Hugh-Jones 1976). Animal dis-

eases such as hog cholera and foot-and-mouth disease
may be spread when animal products intended for human
consumption are fed to livestock (Henderson and
Brooksby 1948; Dawson 1970; Hedger and Dawson 1970).
Consequently, regulations covering food products are
directed to both human and animal health and importation of meat and cheese may be barred even though the
product meets the requirements for wholesomeness as a
human food (Griffiths 1972; Hejl 1976).

Some animal products are not intended for human or
animal consumption but are used in the manufacture of a
variety of products such as hides for leather, milk
solids for casein, and organs for production of enzymes
and hormones. These products are also controlled to
prevent accidental or deliberate diversion to animal
feed. Since processing usually removes or destroys
animal pathogens (Glencross 1972) the concern over
diversion pertains to the raw material before it enters
the manufacturing process. Workers may also be endangered during the manufacturing process, as illustrated
by woolsorter's disease (Brachmann et al. 1966). When
the hazard is believed to be high, movement of the
material is banned. In instances of lesser risk, movement is regulated to provide safeguards.

Certain animal products, such as meat meal, meat
scraps, feather meal, and bone meal, are destined to be
fed to animals after processing. The raw materials
include animal offal and condemmed animal parts from
packing and processing houses, discarded eggs from
packinghouses and hatcheries, and dead and downer animals from farms. When properly heat-processed in a
well-run rendering plant, the end product is safe
(Tittiger 1971). To insure safety, regulations are
directed at two critical aspects of the operation:
(1) the heating period and the temperature used, and
(2) the care taken to avoid recontaminaton of the
sterilized product after it comes out of the cooker
(Hess et al. 1970). Processed products of this type
can go into feeds of almost every species of livestock
and poultry. In spite of such precautions, numerous
instances of disease transmission are known (Morehouse
and Wedman 1961). A notorious example was the distribution of anthrax-contaminated bone meal to hundreds of
midwestern farms in 1952 (Stein and Stoner 1953). The
bone meal had been heat processed in Europe from raw
material obtained in Africa, but it was recontaminated
by transport in a ship that had held the raw material
but had not been decontaminated. Fresh-frozen animal
products of diverse origin, such as freshwater fish,
seal, chicken heads, and pig spleens, are fed to mink

and sometimes other carnivores that require a high protein diet. Diseases and poisonings that have been transmitted to mink (Table 4.3), can be transmitted to swine and poultry that gain access to mink yards and scavenge in areas where mink food is spilled (Madin 1981). A few such occurrences illustrate the complexity of determining the ultimate consumer.

The production of biologics may also contribute to the spread of disease. A notorious instance was the importation of seed virus by an American company producing human smallpox vaccine. When vaccine production was initiated by inoculating the seed of bovine origin into calves in the company facilities, the foot-and-mouth disease virus that contaminated the inoculum induced overt disease that spread into adjacent herds and infected thousands of animals before it was eradicated. Today, many vaccines are produced in cell cultures that require for their maintenance two animal products, trypsin and fetal calf serum. Both products can be and have been contaminated with animal pathogens, and it is difficult, if not impossible, to eliminate the contaminating agents without reducing the quality of the two products. Production of biologics depends, primarily, on safety tests designed to detect certain known pathogens. However, it is possible that some exotic viruses that damage only the fetus would not be detected by standard tests and could be widely disseminated before their presence was revealed.

Forages and other plant products may also be contaminated with materials of animal origin and have served as fomites for disease agents (Moosbrugger 1957).

Although the process is usually of marginal profitability, animal wastes are sometimes compacted, dried, and sold in bags as fertilizer. Shipping, in some instances, involves movement from one political jurisdiction to another. Survival of pathogens is dependent upon the process of preparation and drying. Although it is known that certain parasites can remain active for months in droppings on pasture and certain viruses persist for months in pond water (Berg 1967), no one has made a realistic assessment of the risks involved in the commerce of animal fertilizer.

MARKET CHANNELS AND TRANSPORT

Mechanics

At one time most animals moved to market on foot along the caravan routes of Asia and the cattle trails

of America.   Until   recently   cattle   in   South   America
moved to market this way and in scattered communities
throughout   the   world   this   method   is   still   used.
Wastage is high when the animals are slowly driven to
their destination, since the trip may take many weeks
and they must forage for food in areas where it may be
scanty.
    In the United States about one hundred years ago,
cattle drovers were replaced by cattle cars moving on
rails.   These, in turn, have been replaced in the last
30 years by cattle trucks moving on highways.   Around
the world today, most animals are moved by railroad
cars, trucks, ships, and barges (Houthuis 1957).   However, air freight is important in the international
shipment of breeding stock and the transport of certain
animal products (Blood 1947).   Over the years, the most
fundamental change in transport has been the decrease
in time in transit.   What once took weeks now takes a
couple of days or a few hours.   Animals are spared
wastage of flesh and exposure to disease.   On the other
hand, animals that are incubating a disease can now
arrive at their destination and be accepted as apparently normal.   In earlier days they would have developed the disease and died or recovered before arrival.
The freedom of Australia, New Zealand, and the Americas
from many of the animal plagues of the Old World can be
attributed, primarily, to the culling effect of the
long ocean voyage on sailing ships (Pierce 1975).   The
second change brought about by improved transportation
is the greater accessibility of distant markets to producers who otherwise would be forced to sell locally or
not at all.

Diversion and Illicit Movement

    Now as in the past, animals (Fig. 5.2) and animal
products (Figs. 5.3 and 5.4) are seldom sold directly
by the producer to the ultimate consumer.   One or more
intermediaries, such as dealers, jobbers, exporters,
importers, wholesalers, and retailers, are usually
involved (Roy et al. 1966).   The intermediate operator,
because of inadequate records and questionable handling
practices, inevitably complicates the job of disease-
control officials who wish to trace the origin of
diseased animals (Figs. 5.5, 5.6 and 5.7) or products
(Christenberry 1979).   In order to meet the demands of
one or more buyers, jobbers often assemble animals from
many producers, temporarily holding them on property
they own or arranging for someone else to hold them.
For example, exporters of wild birds buy trapped birds
from collectors and hold them in treatment stations

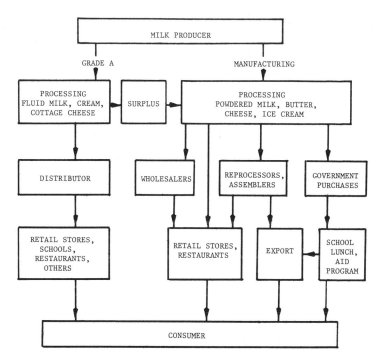

FIG. 5.3. Marketing channels for milk (adapted from Mortenson 1977).

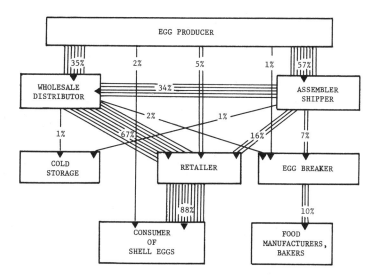

FIG. 5.4. Marketing channels for eggs: Volume in percentages (adapted from Mortenson 1977).

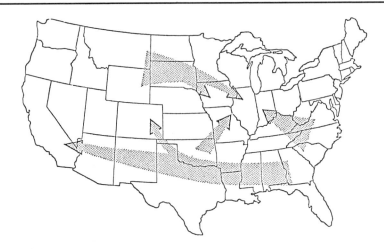

FIG. 5.5. Major directional movements of feeder cattle in
the United States (Anderson et al. 1978).

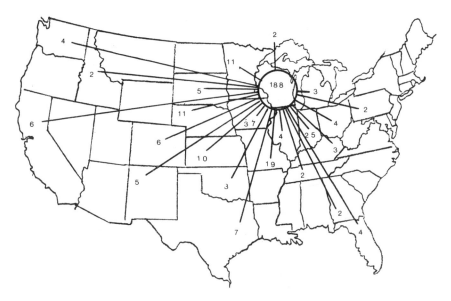

FIG. 5.6. Directional movements: Shipments of dairy cattle
and calves out of Wisconsin in 1979.   Numbers in thousands
(Wisconsin Agricultural Reporting Service 1980).

until an importer in another country obtains the
license necessary to authorize shipment. This assembly
of domestic or wild animals (Lennette and Emmons 1972)
for or during shipment provides an opportunity for
transmission of disease from infected animals to other

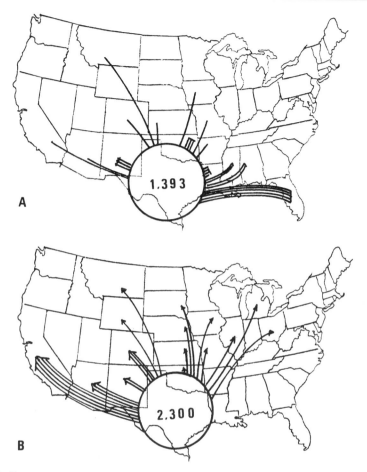

FIG. 5.7. Directional movement: Shipments of nonfed cattle into and out of Texas 1962. Numbers in thousands: A, in-shipments; B, out-shipments (Anderson et al. 1978).

susceptibles including people. The stressful events of assembly and shipment also depress the resistance of many animals and create such disease problems as shipping fever of cattle (a disease of complex etiology to which several viruses and bacteria contribute) (Sinha and Abinanti 1962) and airsacculitis of poultry (another disease of complex etiology to which mycoplasma, other bacteria, and sometimes viruses contribute). Temporary (and unrecorded) contact sometimes occurs when animals encounter one another as they are loaded or unloaded from river and coastal ships or when

crated fowl in different shipments share a baggage room
for several hours. For example, animals that were
being shipped on a tramp steamer to a European zoo from
an African nation free of rinderpest were infected with
the virus en route by diseased animals as they were on-
and off-loaded in ports of call (Boldrini 1954).
Disease transmission may also be caused by use of
products designated as animal feed for manufacturing;
for example, the diversion of dried milk originally
intended for the manufacture of casein, to the production of calf replacer (Acree 1976).

The most serious problems facing disease-control
authorities are: (1) illegal movement of livestock
within the country, and (2) smuggling of animals and
animal products into the country (Matulich 1972;
Courtenay and Robins 1975; Hanson 1975). The size of
the problem is difficult to assess. No country is free
of illegal movement, but its amount varies from border
to border and season to season. Smuggling has been
estimated to equal or surpass the legal trade between
some countries. High price differentials, high tariffs, severe restrictions, or complete bans on legal
movement favor illicit trade. In some countries, particularly where the pay of custom officials is low,
bribery facilitates the movement of legally restricted
animals. In other countries, animals are smuggled
across the border at unguarded points, and animal products are sometimes hidden in a legal shipment (Inskipp
(ca. 1975). Unquestionably, the illicit movement of
animals and animal products is the greatest threat to
the control or prevention of exotic disease. Exotic
Newcastle disease has been repeatedly introduced into
the United States in this way (Lancaster 1963; Hanson
1972, 1974), and African swine fever has entered
Europe, South America, and the Caribbean in contraband
goods.

DYNAMICS OF MARKET GEOGRAPHY

Production and Consumer Areas

Land that can produce an abundance of animal feed,
and is not being preempted for other uses, usually becomes an area of animal surplus that exports animals or
their products to areas that need animal protein (May
1959; Schertz 1979). The transportation cost of feed
usually keeps the livestock producer near or on the
land where feed is produced (Newberg 1963). Two other
important factors that contribute to the clustering of

producers are (1) the development of processing facilities, and (2) the costs of transporting the animal to
the processing plant and the product to the consumer
(McCoy 1972; McDowell 1972). Establishment or aban-
donment of processing facilities is dependent on an
adequate supply of animals, availability of labor at
competitive prices, and the erection and maintenance of
modern facilities. Animal production is stimulated in
areas close to a processing plant but suppressed in
areas further away, primarily because of the increased
costs of transportation.

Facilitators and Restrictors of Market Flow

     Disease-control officials are primarily concerned
with (1) the direction of flow of animals (Figs. 5.5,
5.6, and 5.7) and animal products, and (2) the regional
intensification of animal populations (Malphrus et al.
1968; Gustafson and Van Arsdell 1970; Schertz 1979).
Diseases tend to move out of exporting areas and into
importing areas (Ward 1972; Pan American Foot-and-Mouth
Disease Center 1981). For over 20 years, vesicular
exanthema remained a problem unique to California, primarily because that state imported rather than exported
swine (Madin 1981). Once the disease was accidently
introduced into the exporting area of the Midwest, it
rapidly spread into almost every state in the nation.
Regional changes that result in the development of new
exporting areas and the alteration of directional flow
should be watched closely by epidemiologists. Year by
year over the past several hundred years, the U.S.
swine industry has moved westward from a center on the
eastern seaboard to one that is now west of the Mississippi River. This movement followed the development of
lands more favorable for feed grain production. In the
last several decades, beef cattle production has rapidly developed in the Gulf coast area because of the
availability of year-round pastures (Anderson et al.
1978). The duck industry, once centered on Long Island
(Leibovitz 1978), has all but abandoned that location
for one in the Midwest and in addition has changed from
many producers of moderate size to two giant corporations. The speed of these changes may be as slow as
the western movement of the swine industry, which took
several hundred years, or as rapid as the transplanta-
tion of the duck industry, which took less than a
decade.
     While livestock production and processing responds
primarily to market incentives, development may be modified by community-imposed restraints, such as taxes,

trade agreements, and land zoning. For instance, high tariffs can restrict or stop the legal movement of animal products between countries. Such barriers exist in most parts of the world, largely for the purpose of protecting local producers. Movement of livestock and livestock products can also be temporarily stopped by a local or regional quarantine aimed at control of a new disease. Such a measure has tremendous economic impact and should be taken only when absolutely necessary (Sundquist et al. 1979).

Within a nation, participation of all producers may be restricted by producer-consumer agreements that have evolved with government approval to insure the delivery of a certain quantity and quality of a product, such as fluid milk (Schomisch 1967). In the case of milk, the producer-consumer agreement resulted in the development of milk sheds (Fig. 5.8), discrete regions from which milk is supplied to metropolitan areas. The milk shed for large cities, such as Chicago, may consist of areas in two or more states and encompass all communities within the region.

Animal production is usually prohibited by zoning in areas close to cities or recreational areas where livestock and humans do not coexist well because of air or water pollution.

LIVESTOCK MARKET CYCLES

An examination of the agricultural census record of the past 150 years reveals that cattle populations have risen and fallen in cycles of about 11 years (Fig. 5.9) (Anderson et al). This fluctuation is directly associated with the rising and falling prices of cattle and the resulting price of meat. Since sucessive decreases in cattle population have not been as great as the preceding decrease, the overall effect, when charted on a graph, looks like a back-tilted stairstep. The cattle population has increased more or less in line with that of the human population. Although the reality of the cattle cycle is not questioned, the reason for it can only be deduced.

When the market is bullish, cattle prices rise. Cattle producers increase the size of their herds, and new cattle operations are started. As the cycle and the population build, more and more cattle go to market. Eventually the market becomes saturated. The market then becomes bearish and cattle prices fall. Producers respond by reducing their breeding programs. Continuing low prices cause the failure of some marginal operations and prevent potential producers from

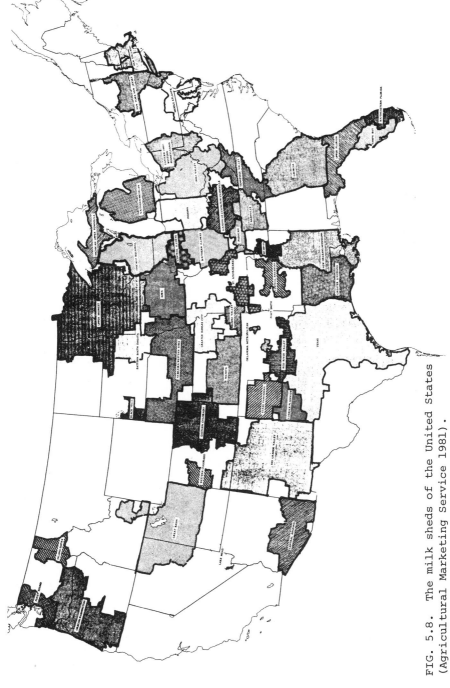

FIG. 5.8. The milk sheds of the United States (Agricultural Marketing Service 1981).

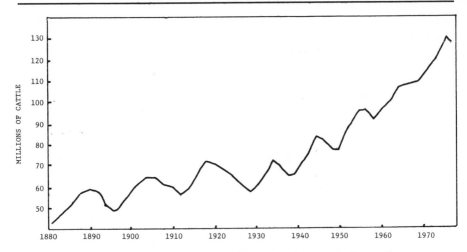

FIG. 5.9.   Cattle cycle 1880 to 1976 based on cattle and
calves on farms on January 1 (Anderson et al. 1978).

getting started.   As the cycle deepens and the national
herd becomes smaller, fewer cattle move to market.
When the flow to market reaches a certain low point,
scarcity causes the price to start up.   This does not
result in an immediate increase in the market supply,
however, because the breeding herds have been reduced
and must be rebuilt.   In fact, the supply may be decreased even further because the producers will retain,
not sell, all animals of breeding potential.

The cycle appears to arise out of a conflict between the short-term responses of the market and the
long-term responses of the breeder.   The latter is
restricted by the fecundity and reproductive cycle of
the cow as well as the growth rate of the calf.

The cattle cycle can be intensified by climatic
conditions, such as drought and severe winters that
restrict reproduction and increase mortality or mild
weather and abundant rains that facilitate reproduction
and growth.   Adverse weather can also cause major
eddies within the cattle cycle by accelerating or
slowing the cycle's effect in one region and not in
another.   For example, adverse weather may necessitate
a major movement of cattle to a region of more favorable weather for feeding and breeding purposes.   Any
major interregional movement of this nature can be
expected to increase problems of disease surveillance
and disease control.   Rising prices may also have an
effect on disease control.   For example, animals that
were not vaccinated for brucellosis because they were

intended for slaughter will be susceptible to that
disease if, in a period of rising prices, they are
retained and converted to breeders.

In general, disease surveillance based on marketed
cattle gives an accurate picture of disease in the
population when the national herd is large and the cull
rate is large. A less accurate picture is obtained
when the herd is low and the cull rate is low.

Cycles of varying length occur in all livestock
populations and are probably caused by the cascading
effect of one event upon another as well as the delays
inherent in animal biology that prevent the producer
from responding to the precipitating event.

REFERENCES

Acree, J. A. 1976. Importation of casein from foot-
    and-mouth countries. Advis. Comm. Foreign Anim.
    Dis. Sec. Agric., USDA, Hyattsville, Md. Mar. 30.
Agricultural Marketing Service. 1981. Federal milk
    order market statistics for September 1980. Fed.
    Milk Order Stat. 249. USDA, Washington, D.C.
Anderson, R. K.; Berman, D. T.; Berry, W. T.; Hopkin,
    J. A.; and Wise, R. 1978. Report National
    Brucellosis Technical Commission. Anim. Plant
    Health Insp. Serv., USDA, Washington, D.C.
Aulaqi, N. A. 1979. Movement of milk in the United
    States and its implications in the spread and
    control of foot-and-mouth disease. In A Study of
    the Potential Economic Impact of Foot-and-Mouth
    Disease in the United States, eds. E. H. McCauley,
    N. A. Aulaqi, J. C. New, Jr., W. B. Sundquist, and
    W. M. Miller. Tech. Rep. 10. Washington, D.C.:
    USGPO, pp. 169-184.
Berg, G., ed. 1967. Transmission of Viruses by the
    Water Route. New York: Interscience Publ.
Blood, B. D. 1947. Veterinary sanitary problems of
    air transport. J. Am. Vet. Med. Assoc. 110:1-8.
Boldrini, G. 1954. Un episodio di peste bovina su una
    nave del Lloyd triestino. Veterinaria Italiana
    Collana Di Mongrafie, supplement to Veterinaria
    Italiana 5:1182.
Brachmann, P. S.; Kaufmann, A. F.; and Dalldorf, F. G.
    1966. Industrial inhalation anthrax. Bacteriol.
    Rev. 30:646-657.
Christenberry, C. C. 1979. Traceback. Paper read at
    Conf. Concepts Tech. Control Erad. Anim. Dis.,
    Sept. 10-14, Auburn, Ala.
Courtenay, W. R., Jr., and Robins, C. R. 1975. Exotic
    organisms. Bioscience 25:700-701.

Dawson, P. S. 1970. The involvement of milk in the spread of foot-and-mouth disease: An epidemiological study. *Vet. Rec.* 87:543-548.

Dowell, A. A., and Bjorka, K. 1941. <u>Livestock Marketing</u>. New York: McGraw-Hill Book Co., Inc.

Glencross, E. J. G. 1972. Pancreatin as a source of hospital-acquired Salmonellosis. *Br. Med. J.* 2:376-378.

Griffiths, R. B. 1972. Disease-free zones and beef export. *World Anim. Rev.* 1:19-22.

Gustafson, R. A., and Van Arsdell, R. N. 1970. Cattle feeding in the United States. Agric. Econ. Rep. 186. USDA, Washington, D.C.

Hall, O. 1952. Garbage feeding control in Canada. *U.S. Livest. Sanit. Assoc. Proc.* 56:209-216.

Hanson, R. P. 1972. Worldwide spread of viscerotropic Newcastle disease. *U.S. Anim. Health Assoc. Proc.* 76:276-279.

————. 1974. The reemergence of Newcastle disease. In <u>Advances in Veterinary Science and Comparative Medicine</u>, vol. 18, eds. C. A. Brandly and E. L. Jungherr. New York: Academic Press, pp. 213-229.

————. 1975. Exotic organisms. *Bioscience* 25:700-701.

Hedger, R. S., and Dawson, P. S. 1970. Foot-and-mouth disease virus in milk: An epidemiological study. *Vet. Rec.* 87:186-188, 213.

Hejl, J. M. 1974. Fleming Key animal import center. *Fed. Regist.* 39(42), FR Doc. 74-4875.

————. 1976. Importation of meat and meat products from countries infected with certain animal diseases; clarification and relief of restrictions; importation of test samples. Anim. Plant Health Insp. Serv., USDA, Washington, D.C., Apr. 9.

Henderson, W. M., and Brooksby, J. B. 1948. The survival of foot-and-mouth disease virus in meat and offal. *J. Hyg.* 46:394-402.

Hess, G. W.; Moulthorp, J. I.; and Norton, H. R. 1970. New decontamination efforts and techniques of elimination of Salmonella from animal protein rendering plants. *J. Am. Vet. Med. Assoc.* 157:1975-1980.

Houthuis, M. J. J. 1957. Transport, ante-mortem care, and inspection of animals intended for slaughter. Agric. Studies 34. FAO, UN, Rome, pp. 111-122.

Hugh-Jones, M. E. 1976. A simulation spatial model of the spread of foot-and-mouth disease through the primary movement of milk. *J. Hyg. Camb.* 77:1-9.

Inskipp, T. P. Ca. 1975. All heaven in a rage: A study of importation of wild birds into the United Kingdom. The Royal Society for the Protection of Birds. The Lodge Sandy, Bedfordshire, England.

Lancaster, J. E. 1963. Newcastle disease: Modes of spread, parts 1, 2. *Vet. Bull.* 33:221-226, 279-285.

Leibovitz, L. 1978. Duck plague (duck virus enteritis). In Diseases of Poultry, 7th ed., eds. M. S. Hofstad, B. W. Calnek, C. F. Helmboldt, W. M. Reid, and H. W. Yonder, Jr. Ames, Ia.: Iowa State Univ. Press, pp. 621-632.

Lennette, E. H., and Emmons, R. W. 1972. Health problems associated with transport and use of non-domesticated animals: An overview. Sci. Publ. 235. Pan Am. Health Organ.

McCoy, J. H. 1972. Livestock and Meat Marketing. Westport, Conn.: The AVI Publ. Co., Inc.

McDowell, R. E. 1972. Improvement of Livestock Production in Warm Climates. San Francisco: W. H. Freeman and Company.

Madin, S. H. 1981. Vesicular exanthema. In Diseases of Swine, 5th ed., eds. A. D. Leman, R. D. Glock, W. L. Mengeling, R. H. C. Penny, E. Scholl, and B. Straw. Ames, Ia.: Iowa State Univ. Press, pp. 302-309.

Malphrus, L. D.; Liu, C. Y.; and Freund, R. J. 1968. Cattle and calf movement in the south. South. Coop. Ser. Bull. 134.

Matulich, W. 1972. Newcastle disease eradication task force exotic birds. *West. Poult. Dis. Conf. Proc.* 21:64-65.

May, J. M. 1959. The geography of milk. *J. Milk Food Technol.* 22:137-141.

Mease, J. 1817. The case of the North Carolina cattle. Memoirs of the Phil. Soc. Promot. Agric., Philadelphia.

Miller, W. M.; Aulaqi, N. A.; and Willard, C. J. 1979. Animal movement and disease spread: Pilot study. In A Study of the Potential Economic Impact of Foot-and-Mouth Disease in the United States, eds. E. H. McCauley, N. A. Aulaqi, J. C. New, Jr., W. B. Sundquist, and W. M. Miller. Tech. Rep. 9. Washington, D.C.: USGPO.

Moosbrugger, G. A. 1957. The dissemination of foot-and-mouth disease by agricultural produce. Proc. Symp. Vesicular Dis., Plum Island Anim. Dis. Lab., Agric. Res. Serv. 45-1, USDA, pp. 61-73.

Morehouse, L. G., and Wedman, E. E. 1961. Salmonella

and other disease-producing organisms in animal by-products: A survey. *J. Am. Vet. Med. Assoc.* 139:989-995.

Mortenson, W. P. 1977. Modern Marketing of Farm Products, 3rd ed. Danville, Ill.: Interstate Printers and Publ., Inc.

Newberg, R. 1963. Livestock marketing: North Central Region. II. Channels through which livestock move from farm to final destination. Res. Bull. 932. Ohio Agric. Ext. Stn., Wooster, Ohio.

Northumberland, Duke of. 1968. Report of the Committee of Inquiry on Foot-and-Mouth Disease 1968, part 1, Cmnd. 3999; part 2, Cmnd. 4225. London: Her Majesty's Stationery Off.

Pan American Foot-and-Mouth Disease Center. 1981. Report of the director to the scientific advisory committee. Rio de Janeiro, Brazil, pp 34-38.

Pierce, A. E. 1975. An historical review of animal movement, exotic disease, and quarantine in New Zealand and Australia. *N.Z. Vet. J.* 23:125-136.

Roy, E. P.; Moore, J. R.; and Walsh, R. G., eds. 1966. The broiler chicken industry. In Market Structure of the Agricultural Industries. Ames, Ia.: Iowa State Univ. Press, pp. 68-100.

Schertz, L. P. 1979. Another Revolution in U.S. Farming? Washington, D.C.: USGPO.

Schomisch, T. P. 1967. Wisconsin brucellosis campaign. M.S. thesis, Univ. Wis., Madison.

Shahan, M. S., chairman; Clower, T. B.; Hay, J. R.; Howe, I. G.; Kord, C. E.; Mulhern, F. J.; Traum, J.; and Baker, J. A. 1953. Report of the committee on vesicular diseases. *U.S. Livest. Sanit. Assoc. Proc.* 57:361-365.

Sinha, S. K., and Abinanti, F. R. 1962. Shipping fever of cattle. In Advances in Veterinary Science, vol. 7, eds. C. A. Brandly and E. L. Jungherr. New York: Academic Press, pp. 225-271.

Stein, D. C., and Stoner, M. G. 1953. Anthrax outbreaks in livestock during 1952. *Vet. Med.* 48:257-262.

Sundquist, W. B.; McCauley, E. H.; and Zanussi, D. 1979. Economic impact of moratoria on the movement of animals and animal products in the U.S. Staff Paper P79-31. Dep. Agric. Appl. Econ., Univ. Minn., St. Paul, Minn.

Swann, A. I., and Sharman, R. S. 1979. History of disease control and eradication in Great Britain, North America, and Mexico. Paper read at Conf. Concepts Tech. Control Erad. Anim. Dis., Sept. 10-14, Auburn, Ala.

Tittiger, F. 1971. Studies on the contamination of products produced by rendering plants. *Can. J. Comp. Med.* 35:167–173.

Ward, M. F. 1972. The relationship of marketing and economics to an animal disease control and eradication program. CENTO Seminar on the Control and Eradication of Viral Diseases in the CENTO region, June 12–17. Cent. Treaty Organ., Istanbul, pp. 147–149.

Wisconsin Agricultural Reporting Service. 1980. Wisconsin agricultural statistics. Wis. Dep. Agric., Trade, Consum. Prot., Madison, Wis.

Wright, W. H. 1943. Public health problems concerned in the disposal of garbage by feeding it to swine. *Am. J. Public Health* 33:208–220.

6

Legal Foundations

Regional disease-control programs place general welfare above the rights of individuals. Controls that interfere with individual freedom or cause loss of private property must be imposed in accordance with the law (Les Benedict 1970) and be subject to review. Furthermore, persons suffering losses, as a result of governmental action, must be given compensation.

ROOTS OF REGULATION

The development of law relating to disease control goes back almost one thousand years. In the first century A.D., Columella advocated animal quarantines to control disease (Schwabe 1969). However, the actual practice of quarantine was not instituted until 1374 when the Republic of Venice prevented plague-exposed travelers from mingling with its residents. Following the lead of several European countries, the United States established port-of-entry quarantine stations for livestock in 1890 (Hendershott 1965; Diamant 1978). All nations now impose some animal quarantine measures (Cockrill 1963; Watson and Brown 1981), largely enacted to prevent disease importation (Fig. 5.1). Compensation for losses of condemned animals goes back over 250 years. At that time Thomas Bates described compensation for diseased cattle, which were buried to comply with governmental decree, in a paper entitled, "A brief account of the contagious disease which raged among the milch cows near London in the year 1714 and methods that were taken for suppressing it" (Bates 1714). The owners of these English cattle received approximately 6,278 pounds for 5,418 cows and 439 calves that were valued at 32,508 pounds. Compulsory inspection of premises and commercial products as well as require- ments for licenses and permits to carry out specific activities have a somewhat shorter history.

SOURCE OF LEGAL AUTHORITY

Step-by-step the government has extended its right not only to regulate the commerce of animals and animal products but also to establish minimum requirements for the production and processing of animal and human foods (Abrahamson 1962; Hannah and Storm 1974). Many of these measures were devised to prevent the dissemina- tion of disease (Tables 6.1 and 6.2); others were intended to prevent fraud. Regulatory officials are usually responsible for the initial legal action re- quired to stop disease. However, this initiative can be shifted to the buyer if the community and its judic- ial system accept the concept of liability for off-site costs of disease. Authority for each action of the government resides in a law written by a legislative body and signed by the chief executive (Animal Plant Health Inspection Service 1976). The actual rules and the procedures for applying the rules lie in regula- tions prepared by responsible agencies (Meat and Poultry Inspection Service 1977). Laws and regulations can be challenged by citizens, reinterpreted by legal officers, and sometimes overturned by the courts.

Writing Laws and Regulations

The immediate impetus for a law is based on the testimony of citizens and officials in a legislative hearing where the case for and against legal code revi- sions is argued. The hearing may be instigated by administrators (Anderson 1966) or called in response to citizen pressure, the lobbying of special groups, a revised legal interpretation of a previous law, or the determination that a previous law is unconstitutional.

The new law is drafted by the legal staff of a legislator or legislative committee and subsequently is placed on the legislative agenda (Office of Federal Register 1975). The text is published in an official government record (Animal Plant Health Inspection Service 1973, 1975). A public hearing may be held, and the proposed legislation may be subjected to floor debate and amendments. If passed by the originating legislative chamber, it is sent to the other chamber (most governments have a bicameral legislative system) where it is placed on the agenda. Again hearings may

Table 6.1. Animal Plagues and Legislation for the Control of Animal Diseases in the United Kingdom

Year	Plagues and Actions	Year	Legislation
1714	Rinderpest introduced and eradicated in 4 mo.	1714	George I authorized eradication and paid for it from the Civil List.
1745	Rinderpest introduced and continued to spread.	1746	Order in Council authorized quarantine and eradication but action was not effective.
1759	Rinderpest eliminated after 14 yr.	1753	Problem of rinderpest discussed in Parliament.
1769	Rinderpest introduced and promptly eradicated.	1770	Order in Council authorized eradication measures for rinderpest and banned importation of foreign cattle.
1840	Foot-and-mouth disease, pleuropneumonia, and sheep pox introduced and allowed to spread.	1840	Demands of growing urban population for more meat resulted in relaxation of Order in Council of 1770 and resumption of importation.
1854	Widespread epidemic of rinderpest on Continent.	1847	Act passed in Council to empower queen to prohibit importation of livestock or admit livestock only after quarantine.
		1848	Act passed to regulate movement of livestock, poultry, and meat within UK.
1863	Concept of contagion was discredited by many physicians and veterinarians.	1857	Order in Council of 1847 that prohibited importation of livestock was revoked because of adverse opinions.
		1864	Order in Council to prohibit importation of livestock failed to pass.
1865	Rinderpest introduced in May and initially allowed to spread.	1865	Order in Council enforced notification of cattle plague and founded Veterinary Department.
1866	Rinderpest eradicated in September.	1866	Cattle Disease Prevention Act enforced.
1867	Rinderpest reintroduced and eradicated.	1869	Contagious Diseases (Animals) Act passed permanently authorizing quarantine and eradication measures.
1872	Rinderpest reintroduced and eradicated.		

1875	First shipment of refrigerated beef arrived from U.S.
1877	Rinderpest reintroduced and eradicated.
1878	Contagious Diseases (Animals) Act revised (still serves as basis of animal quarantine and eradication measures).
1884	Act passed to prohibit importation of livestock and livestock products from countries having contagious diseases.
1887	Board of Agriculture established and Veterinary Department included.
1894	Diseases of Animals Act revised to include comprehensive legislation.
1917	Veterinary Diagnostic and Research Laboratory established at Weybridge.

Source: Francis 1948; Swann and Sharman 1979.

Table 6.2. Animal Plagues and Legislation for the Control of Animal Diseases in the United States

Year	Plagues and Actions	Year	Legislation
1843	Pleuropneumonia introduced on Long Island and spread within 15 yr to all of northeastern U.S.	1859	Massachusetts legislature authorized eradication of pleuropneumonia and appropriated $1 million for the effort. Eradication accomplished in 1865.
1870	Foot-and-mouth disease introduced into New England but did not persist.		
1872	Influenza of horses interrupted transport of people and goods in urban East.		
1875	First shipment of refrigerated beef sent from U.S. to England.		
1879	England bans importation of live cattle from U.S. because of pleuropneumonia.		
1883	Germany bans U.S. pork as trichnia infected.	1884	Bureau of Animal Industry established. Reporting of animal disease initiated. Movement of diseased animals restricted.
1887	Effective action taken to eradicate pleuropneumonia.	1887	Authority given to purchase and destroy cattle infected with or exposed to pleuropneumonia.
		1890	Importation of diseased animals prohibited. Quarantine required for imported livestock and inspection of exports. Operation of stockyards regulated.
1902	Foot-and-mouth disease introduced and eradicated.	1903	Secretary of Agriculture authorized to make regulations needed to prevent dissemination of disease.
		1905	Quarantine of any state or territory authorized if needed.
1906	Tuberculin testing of cattle initiated.	1906	Transit of livestock regulated.

1908 Foot-and-mouth disease reintroduced and eradicated.

1913 The act of 1906 applied to railroads.

1914 Foot-and-mouth disease appeared in Michigan, spread through the midwest and was eradicated at great cost and effort.

1917 Tuberculosis found to be widespread in dairy cattle. Eradication program initiated.

1918 Swine flu appeared in Midwest simultaneously with human flu pandemic.

1920 Movement of reactor (TB) cattle to slaughter authorized.

1924 Foot-and-mouth disease introduced on West Coast and eradicated after spreading to deer.

1928 Live poultry included with livestock in all previous acts (1884, 1903, 1905) regulating diseased animals.

1929 Foot-and-mouth disease reappeared on West Coast and eradicated.

1930 Importation of livestock and unprocessed meat from countries with foot-and-mouth disease or rinderpest prohibited.

1932 Foot-and-mouth disease appeared and eradicated.

1934 National brucellosis eradication program initiated as a cattle reduction program.

1935 Pullorum control program established.

1937 Epizootic of equine encephalomyelitis killed thousands of horses.

1939 With the exception of nine countries, U.S. certified as modified bovine tuberculosis free.

1946 Foot-and-mouth disease introduced and spread rapidly through central Mexico. A joint U.S.-Mexican commission established. Disease not eradicated until 1954.

1946 Authorized inspection and certification of agricultural products.

Table 6.2 *continued*

Year	Plagues and Actions	Year	Legislation
		1947	Cooperation authorized with Mexico to eradicate foot-and-mouth disease or rinderpest introduced into that country. Funding appropriated.
		1948	Federal animal health laboratories established.
1952	Scrapie reintroduced into U.S. and eradication program begun.	1953	Special measures for eradication of scrapie and blue tongue authorized.
1954	Sterile male procedure for eradication of screwworm demonstrated on Island of Curacao.	1956	Authorized payment of claims for contaminated materials destroyed.
1959	Screwworm eradicated from southeastern U.S.	1961	Eradication of hog cholera authorized.
		1962	Broad powers given to Secretary of Agriculture to control and eradicate any communicable disease of livestock and poultry. Interference with disease control officials executing their powers made a federal crime. Authorized establishment of extraordinary emergency.
1971	Exotic Newcastle disease introduced into California and eradicated after a 2-yr effort at a cost of $56 million.	1972	Indemnities for loss of income from animals destroyed authorized for the first time.
		1972	Joint Mexican-U.S. Commission for screwworm eradication established.

Source: Shope 1958; Hendershott 1965; Hourrigan 1968; Vet. Serv. (ca. 1971a; ca. 1971b); Animal Plant Health Inspection Service 1978; Swann and Sharman 1979.

be held with the possibility of further debate and amendments. If passed, any changes must be resolved in a committee of the joint chambers before the proposed legislation goes to the chief executive for signature or veto. The new law usually becomes effective immediately upon receiving the executive's signature. A citizen who has been injured unjustly by the law may contest its applications or legality all the way through the courts to the Supreme Court (Walker 1974; United States Court of Appeals 1975; Bazelon 1981). The law may also be repealed by subsequent legislative action.

Regulations are administrative rules that define the way in which laws are implemented. Some are implied in the original legislation. Many more are written to show application of the law to new situations or enable an agency to carry out the responsibilities it has been given.

In the U.S. Department of Agriculture, the program or regulatory staff of the Animal Plant Health Inspection Service (APHIS) drafts the proposed regulation and submits it to review by other units in the department, other appropriate agencies, and the office of the general council. The concept for the regulation may have arisen within the technical staff of the agency or been suggested by professional or lay organizations acting informally as advisory groups (Fig. 6.1). The subsequent approved draft is given a preamble explaining its purpose and published in the *Federal Register*. Forty-five days are given for public review. Comments submitted in writing along with explanation are attached to the text of the regulation, and if the agency is satisfied, it is again published in the *Federal Register*.

The regulation is now official and can be challenged only in federal court for one or more of five reasons: (1) lack of legal authority, (2) inconsistency, (3) discrimination, (4) vagueness of language, or (5) factual errors. If the challenge is sustained, the regulation is invalidated; if not, it remains in effect.

Subordinate units of government, such as states, provinces, territories, or smaller municipalities, may also develop laws, regulations, and ordinances relating to the control of animal disease (U.S. District Court 1978). Such rulings are subordinate to federal or national law except where jurisdiction has been given to the local government. For example, interstate commerce, regardless of its origination point, is regulated by federal control, but commerce that moves only within the state or municipality is controlled by local

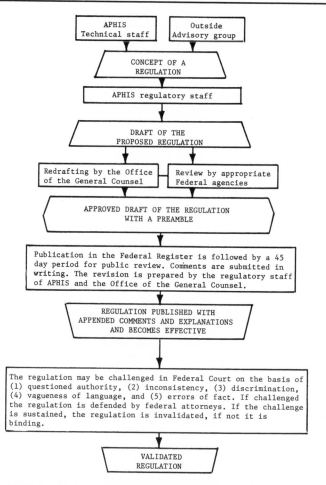

FIG. 6.1. Development of a federal regulation.

jurisdiction. The process used by subordinate government units in developing laws and regulations is similar to that of the federal government (Wisconsin
Legislative Reference Bureau 1979).

GOVERNMENTAL ACTIONS

Embargo

Embargo is a governmental action that forbids the
entry of animals or animal products from another
government or territory. According to the Act of

August 30, 1890, the President of the United States was
authorized "to suspend the importation of all or any
class of animals for a limited time, whenever he was of
the opinion that such an action was necessary for the
protection of animals of the United States against
infectious or contagious diseases."

Quarantine

Quarantine is an action that places a defined
area under the direct supervision of authorities
(Matovinovic 1969) who have the responsibility of bar-
ring the movement of any animals or animal products out
of the area (Food and Agriculture Organization 1956;
Conn 1967). This is spelled out in the Act of March 3,
1905, that authorized the Secretary of Agriculture "to
quarantine any state or territory . . . or any portion
. . . when he should determine that cattle or other
livestock [defined as including live poultry in the Act
of February 7, 1928] in such state or territory . . .
were affected with any contagious, infectious or communicable disease." The Act of 1905 also prohibited
transportation of livestock to and from quarantine
areas except as approved by the Secretary.

Inspections

Inspection is an action in which government agents
enter a premise where animals are reared or assembled
for slaughter for the purpose of conducting physical
examinations, taking temperatures, drawing blood, or
administering diagnostic reagents (Organization for
European Economic Co-operation 1959). Inspection also
includes any laboratory tests that are conducted with
the materials obtained, such as blood or fecal specimens, and may include the introduction of sentinel
animals for the purpose of detecting disease carriers.
The first authorization for inspections was given to
the U.S. Secretary of Agriculture in 1890, and this
power was subsequently expanded and clarified. For
instance, in 1926 the Supreme Court affirmed that the
secretary had the authority to direct agents of the
department to supervise inspection of animals suspected
or known to have infectious or communicable diseases.
The procedures for obtaining a diagnosis and the criteria used are defined in the regulations for program
(or scheduled) diseases. Organizations such as the
U.S. Animal Health Association have played a major role
in the establishment of these procedures and criteria
(Pickard 1952; Peacock 1972; Baker 1973; Mussman 1973).
In Europe such groups as the European Foot-and-Mouth

Commission and the animal-disease section of the Common
Market Commission have played a similar role. The
established criteria have been challenged in courts on
numerous occasions but have usually stood the
challenge.

Condemnation

Condemnation is a governmental action that author-
izes agents to destroy all the animals in a herd that
has been diagnosed as being (1) infected with a specified, highly communicable disease; or (2) contaminated
with substances that would be of danger to people
(Pickard 1952; *Federal Register* 1978; Hannah 1981). In
1977, APHIS attempted to condemn contacts (birds that
showed no indication of disease after leaving a flock
that was subsequently condemned) in an effort to control spread of virulent Newcastle disease. This action
was abandoned when the legality of the action was
questioned.

Indemnification

Indemnification is a governmental action that pays
owners for animals that are destroyed in disease control and eradication programs (*Journal American Veterinary Medical Association* 1976; Aulaqi and Sundquist
1979). An Act of May 3, 1956, extended the coverage to
include claims for materials (such as feedstuffs) destroyed because the materials were exposed to disease.
In 1972 payment was authorized for income that was lost
because animals were destroyed. For example, if a
flock of chickens must be destroyed, the owner would be
paid for the income that would have come from egg sales
during the period required to replace the flock.

Approval or Grading

Establishment of grading standards enable the
government inspector to reject or downgrade a product.
By this authority the government can enforce sanitary
standards for the production and processing of animal
and human food as well as control the marketing of
drugs and vaccines used in food animals (Peacock 1972;
Journal American Veterinary Medical Association 1979).

Permits

Interstate and international movement of animals
and products depends upon the issuance of permits to
import, export, or transport. Permits also authorize

individuals to establish only those businesses, erect only those structures, or transport only those goods that are in compliance with the regulations that limit these actions. Zoning and pollution abatement is accomplished largely by the restriction of permits for construction (Hannah 1974, 1976; Laitos 1975).

Licenses

The production of biologicals and pharmacological substances as well as the sale and administration of biologicals and pharmacologically active substances is controlled by licensing firms and individuals. To obtain a license, applicants must appear before an examining board or reviewing agency and demonstrate their understanding of approved practices (Whitaker 1974; Hannah 1979). The license is conditional upon conformity to approved practices (Humphrey 1961).

Research

This action enables the government to establish research laboratories and to support research in approved institutions (Rothschild 1971).

Specified Programs

The authorization and funding of a control program for a specific disease enable the authorities to carry out any measures necessary to eliminate it (Sharman and Walker 1973).

PENALTIES FOR NONCOMPLIANCE

Physical actions taken to prevent government agents from carrying out regulations and attempts to conceal information and defraud can be punished in the courts by imprisonment, fines, confiscation of property, or suspension or revocation of licenses and permits.

The complex regulatory structures that attempt to anticipate and prohibit antisocial acts could be simplified if the community would accept the concept of liability of individuals for off-site cost of their actions. However, the use of litigation to recover costs of the loss of a herd from disease introduced by a purchased animal despite its warranty, would not serve to control disease unless the legal process was so sure, adequate, and rapid that it would deter the sale of diseased animals. Nevertheless, the concept of using legal mechanisms to control disease in the private sector should be studied.

Some of the individuals who have responsibility for controlling animal diseases as well as most of the individuals who do the research and develop the concepts that underlie disease control have difficulty in separating the spheres of natural laws and human laws. Unfortunately, regulations that reflect the state of the art at the time they were written are difficult to modify as new scientific information becomes available. As a result, regulations still exist that knowledgeable people know are harmful or self-defeating. The rigidity that exists in the regulatory process of all governments makes the process of changing regulations laborious and time-consuming. Meanwhile, the regulation continues to be enforced. Furthermore, some changes must be accomplished step-by-step over an extended period because an immediate action that is scientifically desirable is economically or socially unacceptable. These limitations must be understood by biologists, epidemiologists, and regulatory officials because no government has ever had enough police to enforce any law that is against the wishes of an overwhelming majority of its people. Conversely, the wishes of the majority of the people have never been able to change government regulations quickly.

REFERENCES

Abrahamson, S. S. 1962. Law and the Wisconsin dairy industry: Quality control of dairy products, 1838-1929. S.J.D. thesis, Law School, Univ. Wis., Madison.

Anderson, R. J. 1966. The federal committee on pest control. Scientific Aspects of Pest Control. NAS-NRC. Publ. 1402. Washington, D.C., pp. 367-374.

Animal Plant Health Inspection Service. 1973. Proposed rules: Viruses, serums, toxins, and analogous products. *Fed. Regist.* 38(112): 15450-15456.

————. 1975. Proposed rules: Viruses, serums, toxins, and analogous products. *Fed. Regist.* 40(49): 11587-11590.

————. 1976. Regulations: Title 9--Animals and animal products (interstate transportation). Code of *Fed. Regist.* Amend. 76-2 through 76-106 beginning with *Fed. Regist.* 41 FR.766, Jan 5, and ending with *Fed. Regist.* 41 FR.52433.

————. 1978. Eradication of exotic Newcastle disease

in southern California, 1971-74. APHIS 91-34. USDA, Hyattsville, Md.

Aulaqi, N. A., and Sundquist, W. B. 1979. Indemnification under animal disease control programs with special emphasis on foot-and-mouth disease. In A Study of the Potential Economic Impact of Foot-and-Mouth Disease in the United States, eds. E. H. McCauley, N. A. Aulaqi, J. C. New, Jr., W. B. Sundquist, and W. M. Miller. Tech. Rep. 12. Washington, D.C.: USGPO, pp. 201-241.

Baker, E. D. 1973. Report of the committee on meat and poultry hygiene. U.S. Anim. Health Assoc. Proc. 77:138-140.

Bates, T. 1714. A brief account of the contagious disease which raged among the milch cows near London in the year 1714 and the methods that were taken for suppressing it. Philos. Trans. R. Soc. London.

Bazelon, D. L. 1981. The judiciary: What role in health improvement? Science 211:792-793.

Cockrill, W. R. 1963. The changing status of animal quarantine. Br. Vet. J. 119:338-349.

Conn, E. 1967. Organization and regulations for quarantine establishments set up in northern Ireland for the sanitary control of importations and exportations of animals and products of animal origin. Bull. Off. Int. Epizoot. 68:331-337.

Diamant, G. 1978. Regulatory veterinary medicine: And they blew a horn in Judea. J. Am. Vet. Med. Assoc. 172:45-54.

Federal Register. 1978. Animals destroyed because of scrapie. 43(180):41,183-41,184.

Food and Agriculture Organization. 1956. Report of the meeting on the appraisal of quarantine regulations for the importation and exportation of livestock, Feb. 13-17. Paris.

Francis, J. 1948. The contributions that quarantine, sanitary measures and eradication can make to preventive medicine. Vet. Rec. 60:361-367.

Hannah, H. W. 1974. Livestock waste disposal regulations: The veterinarian's position. J. Am. Vet. Med. Assoc. 164:32-33.

————. 1976. Some nuances of noise and smoke. J. Am. Vet. Med. Assoc. 169:1298-1299.

————. 1979. Professional licensing under siege. J. Am. Vet. Med. Assoc. 175:1162.

————. 1981. Drug residues: Who is liable? Anim. Nutr. Health, Jan.-Feb., pp. 6, 10-11.

Hannah, H. W., and Storm, D. F. 1974. Law for the Veterinarian and Livestock Owner, 3rd ed.

Danville, Ill.:   Interstate Printers and Publ.,
     Inc.
Hendershott, R. A. 1965. The history of regulatory
     veterinary medicine in the United States. *U.S.
     Livest. Sanit. Assoc. Proc.* 69:1-6.
Hourrigan, J. L. 1968. General historical notes on
     regulatory   veterinary   medicine   and   certain
     diseases of interest to regulatory veterinarians.
     Anim. Plant Health Insp. Serv., USDA, Hyattsville,
     Md., Oct. 21.
Humphrey, H. H., chairman. 1961. Veterinary Medical
     Science and Human Health. Committee on Government
     Operations, United States Senate. Washington,
     D.C.: USGPO.
Journal of the American Veterinary Medical Association.
     1976.   Legislation   for   compensation   of   hog
     cholera. 169:286.
————. 1979. Economics of antibiotics in feed. 174:
     235, 238.
Laitos, J. G. 1975. A legal-economic history of air
     pollution controls in Wisconsin. S.J.D. thesis,
     Law School, Univ. Wis., Madison.
Les Benedict, M. 1970. Contagion and the consti-
     tution: Quarantine agitation from 1859 to 1866.
     J. Hist. Med. 25:177-193.
Matovinovic, J. 1969. A short history of quarantine.
     Univ. Mich. Med. Cent. J. 35:224-228.
Meat and Poultry Inspection Service. 1977. Issuances
     of the meat and poultry inspection program. Anim.
     Plant Health Insp. Serv., USDA, Hyattsville, Md.,
     Feb. 18, pp. 79-143.
Mussman, H. C. 1973. The changing face of meat and
     poultry inspection.   J. Am. Vet. Med. Assoc.
     163:1061-1064.
Office of Federal Register. 1975. Document drafting
     handbook.   Natl. Arch. Rec. Serv., Washington,
     D.C.
Organization for European Economic Co-operation. 1959.
     Livestock diseases and the organization of veteri-
     nary services in Europe.   Documentation in Food
     and Agriculture, 1959 Ser. 5.
Peacock, G. V. 1972. Regulatory activities in veteri-
     nary biologics.   *U.S. Anim. Health Assoc. Proc.*
     76:53-57.
Pickard, J. R. 1952. Tuberculosis condemnations.
     U.S. Livest. Sanit. Assoc. Proc. 56:144-148.
Rothschild, Lord. 1971. Framework for government
     research and development.   Cmnd. 4814. Her
     Majesty's Stationery Off., London.
Schwabe, C. W. 1969. Veterinary Medicine and Human

Health, 2nd ed. Baltimore, Md.: Williams & Wilkins Co.

Sharman, E. C., and Walker, J. W. 1973. Regulatory aspects of velogenic viscerotropic Newcastle disease. *J. Am. Vet. Med. Assoc.* 163:1089-1093.

Shope, R. E. 1958. Swine influenza (flu, hog flu, swine flu). In Diseases of Swine, 1st ed., ed. H. W. Dunne. Ames, Ia.: Iowa State College Press, pp. 81-98.

Swann, A. I., and Sharman, R. S. 1979. History of disease control and eradication in Great Britain, North America, and Mexico. Paper read at Conf. Concepts Tech. Control Erad. Anim. Dis., Sept. 10-14, Auburn, Ala.

United States Court of Appeals. 1975. B. R. Slocum dba Animal World v. United States of America and Earl Butz. Fifth Circuit, no. 75-1242, June 16.

United States District Court for the District of Maryland. 1978. United States of America et al. v. Maryland - National Capital Park and Planning Commission et al., no. 78-934-Y, Nov. 6.

Veterinary Services. Ca. 1971a. Chronology of the development of regulatory control of animal health and animal food products in the United States. Anim. Plant Health Insp. Serv., USDA, Hyattsville, Md.

————. Ca. 1971b. Legal authorities under which Veterinary Services, APHIS, carries out its functions. Anim. Plant Health Insp. Serv., USDA, Hyattsville, Md.

Walker, J. W. 1974. Statement of reasons. U.S. District Court for the Southern District of Florida, Miami, Fla., Dec. 5.

Watson, W. A., and Brown, A. C. L. 1981. Legislation and control of virus diseases. In Virus Diseases of Food Animals, vol. 1, ed. E. P. J. Gibbs. London: Academic Press, pp. 265-306.

Whitaker, A. H. 1974. A history of federal pesticide regulation in the United States to 1947. Ph.D. diss., Emory Univ., Atlanta, Ga.

Wisconsin Legislative Reference Bureau. 1979. The State of Wisconsin 1979-1980 Blue Book. Madison, Wis.: Dep. Adm. Doc. Sales Distrib.

7

Related Institutions

INTERINSTITUTIONAL RELATIONSHIPS

An organization created to control disease or carry out any other innovative action, even if it is dependent on some existing agency, has an existence and identity of its own and must relate not only to its parent but also to all of the other organizations that exist within its working area. This is not a simple matter, and conflicts may arise that will threaten the organization's mission and survival.

The new organization is considered in relationship with (1) the parent agency, (2) the oversight and legislative bodies, (3) other federal agencies, (4) local governmental units, and (5) foreign government institutions.

PARENTAL AGENCY

An illustrious parent cannot insure the success of an offspring, but a parent with a bad record can give the offspring a serious handicap. The record of the parental agency similarly reflects upon its offshoot. If a new organization is associated with a parental agency whose officials are distrusted by the public, the new organization will have difficulty in getting established. A legislative body may assign a new program to an agency with a good record even if that agency is less congruent with the new organization than another agency is. A good record is based not only on accomplishments but also on success in public relations. Such a record is seldom achieved without a staff that uses imagination in planning, recruits effectively, and runs a fiscally responsible operation. All these characteristics are important in planning and establishing a new organization. This is particularly true in recruiting the staff and securing support for the program. Public belief in the veracity of officials develops slowly as actions verify promises that have been made. However, such belief is seldom generalized appreciably.

Ideally, the charge given a disease-control task force should fall clearly within the mission and competency of the parental agency. Eradication of an animal disease is obviously part of the responsibility of a department of agriculture and rural development (Figs. 7.1, 7.2 and 7.3). As an alternative, the new program could be assigned to a department of human health and welfare, but it would be less appropriate there and administrative problems would probably occur. For example, the Pan American Foot-and-Mouth Disease Center and its program for control of livestock diseases was established within the Pan American Health Organization, which is concerned primarily with human health. This action led to recurrent demands for justification. Consequently, a significant amount of the Center's staff time has been diverted to (1) showing how the animal-disease control effort is related to the agency mission and (2) finding ways to adapt the human health organization's methods to fit the special needs of an animal-disease-research laboratory (Seoane and Palacios 1967; Pan American Foot-and-Mouth Disease Center 1977).

While the new organization may eventually develop independent capabilities in a wide range of activities, initially it is dependent upon the parental agency for many administrative services, staff training, and specialized services such as those provided by a diagnostic laboratory. The long-standing experience of the permanent agency make it logical for the new organization, particularly an animal-disease task force, to seek fiscal advice and communication support from the older institution. Unless the new program is to be of long duration or very extensive, laboratory services are best provided by contract. This is especially true if research is needed to solve problems encountered in field operations. Sometimes the staff of a task force is tempted to turn its attention away from its primary assignment when it appears that answers to challenging problems could be obtained with a modest amount of research. For example, during the Newcastle disease eradication program in California, the director, with the support of the scientific advisory committee, repeatedly discouraged such diversion of staff time

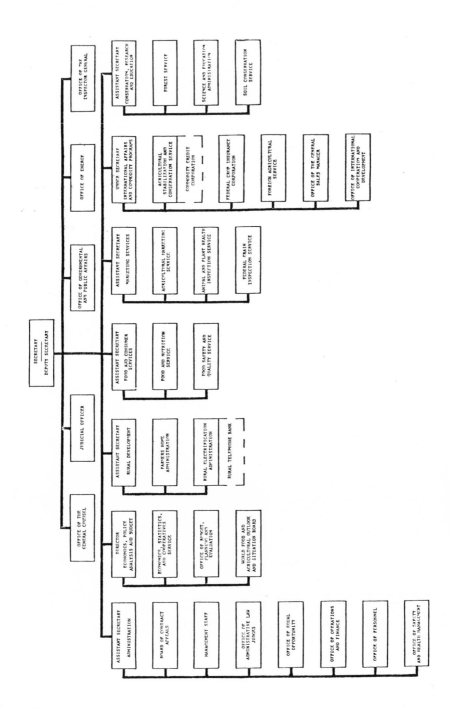

FIG. 7.1. Organization of a department of agriculture: United States in 1978.

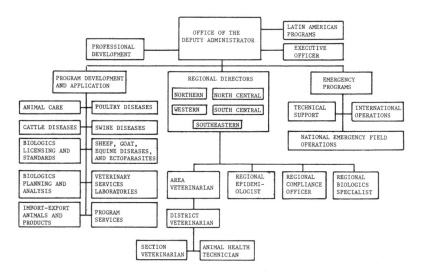

FIG. 7.2. Organization of an animal disease-control agency (Animal Plant Health Inspection Service in 1978).

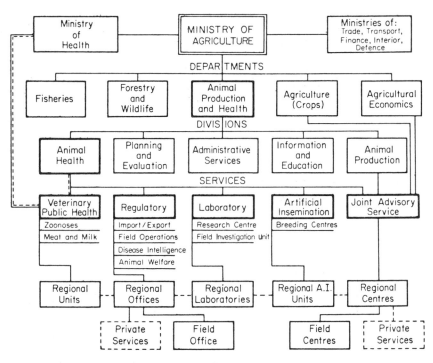

FIG. 7.3. Organization of a hypothetical animal service: European tradition (Reprinted by permission of Ellis 1974).

because the primary program activities would have been disrupted. Once the problem is identified, contract personnel should be brought in to conduct whatever study is needed to solve the problem, but only if support for such a study can be justified within the mission and programing units of the parent agency (Agricultural Research Service 1976).

OVERSIGHT AGENCIES

When reporting to superiors in the parental agency, the task force director and staff are dealing with administrators who have a general background even if they lack specific knowledge of the technical problems that must be surmounted. Only minimal explanatory information needs to be provided to make a request comprehensible. However, working with oversight personnel in the budget bureau and legislative bodies may be more difficult because they have different backgrounds. For this reason, progress reports and budget explanations should be presented in a way that is comprehensible by the government analyst as well as the person on the street (McGregor 1973). This is difficult for most technical people who are used to a shorthand terminology that is intelligible only within their cadre. Moreover, a speaker that is defending the program before a legislative committee may be subjected to some hostile interrogation, even when the program objectives have been lauded and its complexities have been presented briefly and clearly (Agency for International Development 1975). In such a situation, the speaker must remain patient, and have an adequate command of the facts.

Since, the executive branch operates all line agencies and keeps them under surveillance through a budget office (the Office of Management and Budget in the United States), it can direct an agency to (1) initiate programs that are compatible with the agency's mission and do not exceed the funding provided, or (2) discontinue any program. If an agency proposes new programs or increased funding for ongoing programs, the proposals must be approved by the budget office before they are presented to the legislative branch. These requirements permit the political officials within the executive branch, who change as administrations change, to exercise considerable control over the technical staffs of the agencies. If the officials lack knowledgeable advisors (Leopold 1976), the changes may be unfortunate.

The legislative branch has the power to (1) auth-

orize and appropriate funds for the executive agencies'
new and ongoing programs; (2) review ongoing programs
when it desires (Humphrey 1961; Agency for International Development 1975; Bentley and Long 1976) and, if
not satisfied, stop the program or remove its funding;
(3) ask an agency to plan a new program; (4) authorize
and fund a new program without the parent agency's participation in planning; (5) authorize or direct reorga-
nization of agencies; (6) combine, eliminate, or create
new agencies; and (7) redefine an agency's mission.

International agencies and financial institutions
conduct a similar evaluation of proposals and also
subject them to review (World Bank 1977).

SISTER AGENCIES

Executive branch agencies created to carry out
different missions discover that certain of their
activities inevitably overlap those of sister agencies
(Fig. 7.4) and the extent of this overlap may increase
as they are assigned added duties by the legislative
branch of government. In the United States the Department of Agriculture has the primary responsibility for
control of animal diseases, but it must cooperate with
customs and immigration officials in the Department of
Commerce when controlling the international movement of
diseased animals and animal products. Similarly, when
attempting eradication of a disease that infects wildlife, the Department of Agriculture must cooperate with
the Department of Interior, which has jurisdiction over
all migratory animals and controls wildlife on federal
lands (Animal Plant Health Inspection Service 1975;
Friend 1976). When using insecticides to control
vectors or when disposing of diseased animals, the
Department of Agriculture must cooperate with the
Environmental Protection Agency, which is responsible
for monitoring pollution.

Although some social decorum and a semblance of a
peck order exists among agencies, jurisdiction is
seldom clear-cut. If at all possible, disagreements
between agencies should be worked out prior to actual
confrontation because the procedures for resolving conflicts are slow. Arbitration at high administrative
levels and in the courts is time-consuming and may subject certain actions to uncertainties that would para-
lyze a control program. If resolution of a conflict
should require legislative action, the long delay could
have drastic effects on the program. The best course
is to anticipate areas of conflict, insofar as possi-

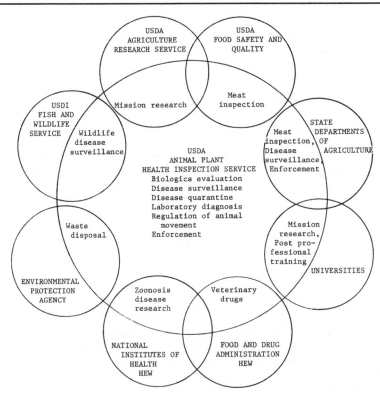

FIG. 7.4. U.S. agencies and institutions that had over-
lapping jurisdictions in animal disease control in 1980.

ble, and use committees and liaison agents to work out
solutions. Standard procedures have been developed for
some problem areas, such as the preparation and assessment of environmental impact statements (Mendenhall
1976). Any proposed program is outlined, critical
areas identified, and alternative procedures suggested
for reducing the impact. The statement is reviewed by
the concerned agencies and a course of action is
approved after discussion of the pros and cons.
        Apart from matters already identified as impact
categories, there are many areas of possible conflict.
Dialogue between the government units must be initiated
within a structure that obligates the participants to
meet regularly and frequently to identify such areas
and seek solutions before a confrontation develops
(Animal Protein Conservation Work Group ca. 1974). It
is important (1) for communications to begin before
tensions are created that inhibit dialogue, (2) for the

participants to be familiar with both the technical and administrative activities of their units, and (3) for the participants to have access to their top level administrators.

LOCAL ORGANIZATIONS

The greatest difference between local organizations and national agencies is the greater role of citizen participation in deliberations at the local level (Lagerroos 1977). Consequently, more individuals must be told the story and the ensuing discussion may not result in decisions as firm as those of a national agency.

A procedure used in the Wisconsin brucellosis program illustrates one method of securing democratic cooperation between local bodies and eradication officials (Schomisch 1967). Two control options, Plans A and B were offered. In Plan A farmers voted to put the towns (townships) into a compulsory eradication program. Plan B was a voluntary program. Peer pressure was sufficient to put most of the towns into Plan A. The legislature decreed that all towns in the county would be put into the program when three-fourths of the towns in a county had voted for it. Similarly, when three-fourths of the counties had elected the program, it would become compulsory for the entire state. Consequently, pockets of resistance were forced into the program by their peers and not by the task force officials.

The jurisdiction of national, state, and local organizations is based on law and precedent (Fig. 7.5). Nevertheless, procedures for consultation, negotiation, and arbitration should be in place in case new situations arise that require negotiation.

INTERNATIONAL INSTITUTIONS

Disease organisms do not recognize either internal jurisdictions or international boundaries (World Health Organization 1962; Fiennes 1964; Saulmon 1971; Arce 1979). A program to control a specific disease, even within a relatively small district, can involve a measure of international cooperation if that district is on an international border or special technical assistance is needed (Machado 1969).

All nations adhere to certain international trading agreements and usually have bilateral and multilateral treaties concerning the reporting of highly

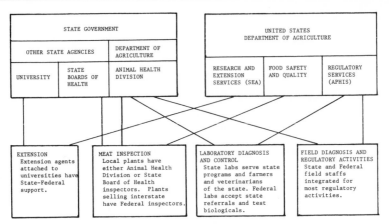

FIG. 7.5. Interrelationships of state and federal disease-control activities in the United States in 1978.

communicable diseases of livestock and the placing of restrictions on movement of animals (Cockrill 1965). In the case of animals to be exported, restrictions include disease-free certifications based on physical examination and certain other tests. Sometimes, agreements exist that require participating nations to assist each other in the event of a disease emergency or provide technical assistance and training (Argentine-U.S. Joint Commission on Foot-and-Mouth Disease 1964; Machado 1968; Agreement between the Ministry of Agriculture of Colombia and the USDA 1973; Kelley 1973; Lancaster 1976).

When no prior agreement exists between the nation needing aid and the nation wishing to offer aid, international agencies, such as the Food and Agriculture Organization of the United Nations (Gibbs 1981) or the Interamerican Institute for Agricultural Sciences of the Organization of American States, will administer emergency aid programs (Murnane 1980). While assistance to other countries may be given for humanitarian reasons, self-interest usually plays an important role.

The development of effective relationships with foreign governments requires a two-way flow of information and open discussion of future plans (Soles 1972; National Research Council 1977). Both administrative and technical staffs must be involved in talks that take place. For instance, if a joint disease-control effort is being considered, an international body should be created before the program is initiated and the responsibility of both governments to this body clearly defined (Machado 1968).

CONFLICT RESOLUTION

Conflicts between agencies arise because of philosophical or political differences, disagreement over social and economic priorities, and jurisdictional rivalries.

The judiciary is empowered to interpret legislation when its meaning is questioned and to resolve conflicts created by jurisdictional ambiguities. The judiciary may also rule that a legislative act or an executive order is not authorized by the constitution and therefore is invalid.

The legal advisors of the federal agency that is developing an action program have the responsibility to identify such legally defined relationships as the creation of coordinating commissions, appointment of liaison officers, preparation of impact statements, and the holding of special hearings. The language of the agency's regulations must make the meaning clear. It may be necessary to define word usage where misinterpretation is possible or even rewrite the regulations if they are in conflict with those of other agencies. Conflicts that cannot be avoided by planning should be identified at the earliest opportunity so that a negotiated resolution can be obtained before the conflict jeopardizes field actions.

Nelkin (1979) argues that controversy is sometimes essential to the resolution of problems that arise if a technical procedure is not socially acceptable to a segment of the population. For example, local resistance in California to the Newcastle disease eradication program was focused on a technical procedure, involving the sentinel bird, that was used to detect inapparent carriers of the virus in commercial flocks. The healthy and fully susceptible sentinel chicken, housed in a cage and placed in a flock with suspected carriers, became diseased and died in 5 to 7 days, dramatically demonstrating the danger that such flocks posed for healthy flocks. An order obtained in the state court stopped the program temporarily, but declaration by the United States Secretary of Agriculture of "a state of extraordinary emergency" took jurisdiction away from the state courts, and the detection program was resumed. Since the resulting delay of several weeks occurred at a critical time, epidemiologists believe that period of unchecked spread increased the cost of the program by several million dollars (Animal Plant Health Inspection Service 1978). Delays incurred while waiting court resolution of such conflicts may carry a high price. Consequently, standing commissions, special conferences, and liaison agents are

often employed by nations to avoid or resolve conflicts
(Fogedby 1956; COSALFA 1973; European Commission 1974).
    Civil conflict is near the surface in many devel-
oping countries and sometimes erupts in open civil war.
The resulting disruptions in government services and
their effect on proposed disease-control or eradication
programs must be seriously considered when deciding
whether to attempt a program in a country where civil
war is possible. If the decision is made to go ahead,
the only disease-control strategies that should be used
are those that can tolerate temporary suspensions of
effort without losing all the ground that has been
gained (Lawrence et al. 1980).

REFERENCES

Agency for International Development. 1975. AID in an
    interdependent world. Office of Public Affairs,
    Washington, D.C.
Agreement between the Ministry of Agriculture of the
    government of Colombia and the Department of Agri-
    culture of the government of the United States of
    America. 1973. USDA, Washington, D.C., Aug. 18.
Agricultural Research Service. 1976. Management and
    planning system. USDA, Washington, D.C.
Animal Plant Health Inspection Service. 1975. Memor-
    andum of understanding between Department of
    Agriculture and Department of Interior. USDA,
    Washington, D.C.
————————. 1978. Eradication of exotic Newcastle disease
    in southern California, 1971-74. APHIS 91-34.
    USDA, Hyattsville, Md.
Animal Protein Conservation Work Group. Ca. 1974.
    Animal protein conservation report. Anim. Plant
    Health Insp. Serv., USDA, Hyattsville, Md.
Arce, A. A. 1979. History of animal control and
    disease eradication in Latin America. Paper read
    at Conf. Concepts Tech. Control Erad. Anim. Dis.,
    Sept. 10-14, Auburn, Ala.
Argentine-United States Joint Commission on Foot-and-
    Mouth Disease. 1964. Documentation of Argentine,
    United States, and Pan American Foot-and-Mouth
    Disease Center reports on foot-and-mouth disease,
    1961-1964. NAS-NRC, Washington, D.C.
Bentley, O. G., and Long, R. W. 1976. Brief comments
    about interim report: Special oversight review of
    agricultural research and development. Agricultu-
    ral Research Policy Advisory Committee. Secretary
    of Agriculture, Washington, D.C.
Cockrill, W. R. 1965. IV. The principles and applica-

tion of international disease control. *Vet. Rec.* 77:1438-1448.

COSALFA. 1973. First special meeting of the South American commission for the control of foot-and-mouth disease, July 20-21, Bogota, Colombia. Pan Am. Health Organ., Washington, D.C.

Ellis, P. 1974. The development of animal health services. *Agric. Adm.* 1:199-219.

European Commission for the Control of Foot-and-Mouth Disease. 1974. Report of the meeting of the research group, Apr. 1-2, FAO, UN, Rome.

Fiennes, R. N. T. W. 1964. Animal disease and quarantine regulations: The dangers of disease transmission from wild animals in captivity to human beings or domestic stock. *Bull. Epizoot. Dis. Africa* 12:93-96.

Fogedby, E. 1956. European commission for the control of foot-and-mouth disease. Proc. Symp. Vesicular Dis., Sept. 27-28, Plum Island Anim. Dis. Lab., Agric. Res. Serv. 45-1, USDA.

Friend, M. 1976. Brucellosis eradication in wildlife. Fish Wildl. Serv., U.S. Dep. Interior, Washington, D.C.

Gibbs, E. P. J., ed. 1981. Virus Diseases of Food Animals, vol. 1. London: Academic Press, pp. 31-42, 317-330.

Humphrey, H. H., chairman. 1961. Veterinary Medical Science and Human Health. Committee on Government Operations, United States Senate. Washington, D.C.: USGPO.

Kelley, O. J. 1973. Agency for International Development. *U.S. Anim. Health Assoc. Proc.* 77:210-215.

Lagerroos, D. 1977. Your role in the act: A citizens guide to the Wisconsin Environmental Policy Act. Off. State Plann. Energy, Madison, Wis.

Lancaster, J. E. 1976. International cooperation and Newcastle disease surveillance. *West. Poult. Dis. Conf. Proc.* 25:27-30.

Lawrence, J. A.; Foggin, C. M.; and Norval, R. A. I. 1980. The effects of war on the control of diseases of livestock in Rhodesia (Zimbabwe). *Vet. Rec.* 107:82-85.

Leopold, A. C. 1976. Letter to Chairman, Board of Agriculture and Renewable Resources, NRC, Sept. 1, University of Nebraska.

McGregor, R. C. 1973. Government criteria for evaluating competing programs. Animal disease eradication: Evaluation programs. Proc. NAS Workshop, Apr. 12-13, Univ. Wis. Ext., Madison, Wis.

Machado, M. A., Jr. 1968. An Industry in Crisis:

Mexican-United States Cooperation in the Control of Foot-and-Mouth Disease. Univ. Calif. Publ. in Hist., vol. 80. Berkeley and Los Angeles: Univ. Calif. Press.

————. 1969. Aftosa: A Historical Survey of Foot-and-Mouth Disease and Inter-American Relations. Albany, N.Y.: State Univ. New York Press.

Mendenhall, W. S., Jr. 1976. Darien Gap Highway: Final environmental impact statement, Panama-Colombia. U.S. Dep. Transp., Fed. Highw. Adm., Washington, D.C.

Murnane, T. G. 1980. The role of the Interamerican Institute for Agricultural Sciences in animal health programs in Latin America and Caribbean countries. *U.S. Anim. Health Assoc. Proc.* 84:17-22.

National Research Council. 1977. Supporting Papers: World Food and Nutrition Study, vol. 5. Washington, D.C.: NAS.

Nelkin, D., ed. 1979. Controversy: Politics of Technical Decisions. Beverly Hills, Calif.: Sage Publ.

Pan American Foot-and-Mouth Disease Center. 1977. Report to the director by the scientific advisory committee. Rio de Janeiro, Brazil.

Saulmon, E. E. 1971. International aspects of animal disease control. *U.S. Anim. Health Assoc. Proc.* 75:10-13.

Schomisch, T. P. 1967. Wisconsin brucellosis campaign. M.S. thesis, Univ. Wis., Madison.

Seoane, E., and Palacios, C. 1967. Report on foot-and-mouth disease, present and future problems on the American continent, and the importance of the Pan American Foot-and-Mouth Disease Center. Pan Am. Health Organ., Washington, D.C.

Soles, R. E. 1972. Pan American Highway: Running a dream through a swamp. *Nation* 214:233-236.

World Bank. 1977. Basic issues emerging from the Bank's experience with animal health project loans. Washington, D.C.

World Health Organization. 1962. International quarantine. *WHO Chron.* 16:48-50.

8

Ongoing Research Programs

JUSTIFICATION

Nature of Research

Research is a methodology for not only finding answers to questions and solutions to problems but also defending those findings with some confidence (Beveridge 1957). Research has given us an understanding of the spread and development of disease as well as the feasibility of the interventions that arrest it.

From the point of view of individuals who are charged with control of disease there are two kinds of research (Mitchell 1956): (1) preparatory studies in which investigators learn enough about the significance of the problem and the nature of the disease process to initiate control, and (2) concurrent studies undertaken to solve problems that become apparent after control of the disease has begun (McDaniel 1976). This is clearly an operational classification. The division of research into basic and applied is also operational because, in this distinction as in the former one, the categorization concerns the use of the research findings and says nothing about the nature of the research itself (McElroy 1977).

The nature of research lies in what is asked and how it is asked. This question distinguishes fundamental from trivial research. One may amass a great deal of evidence for the association of two events on the assumption that it supports a hypothesis. Yet the association may have nothing to do with the hypothesis if the question was improperly asked and the testing was not rigorous. In such a case, the answer is trivial. Although the public, when paying for the benefits

155

of research, does not need to be concerned about the various classifications, it should be aware of the distinction between good research, which is characterized by careful planning, sound methodology, and critical analysis, and poor research, which lacks one or all of these characteristics.

Establishment of Objectives

The public has the right to ask what research is required in order to develop and carry out animal disease-control programs. The research should (1) establish the basis of a strategy for control, (2) develop methods to be used in intervention, (3) develop a basis for improving methods of control, and (4) develop a basis for reassessing strategy.

The proponents of research (National Program Staff 1976) do not agree on who (user, administrator, or producer) should select the research objectives (Cooke 1981) or how the responsibility for completion should be shared (Fig. 8.1). Pasteur was not faced with this controversy. As a research scientist (producer), he sat down with the brewer or farmer who had a problem (the user) and together they established the nature of the question that needed to be asked. No administrators were there to keep them apart. Today, with the growth of government bureaucracy, research laboratories are established as entities with their own mission, and disease-control task forces and programs are formed independently (Humphrey 1961; Braye et al. 1976). Not

	TECHNOLOGY, PROGRAM, PERFORMANCE	SUBJECTS	BENEFIT-COST, POLICY, RESOURCES	
PROGRAM STAFF SCIENTISTS	ALTERNATIVES, REVIEW, EVALUATION, WORKSHOP	FUNCTIONS	FORECAST, ANALYSIS, UTILIZATION, EFFICIENCY ASSESSMENT	LINE ADMINISTRATORS, ANALYSTS, ECONOMISTS
	SCIENCE, METHODS, REFERENCES, MANUSCRIPTS	INTERESTS	RESULTS, EQUIPMENT, FACILITIES, FUNDING	

FIG. 8.1. Distribution of functions and interests between line and staff (adapted from Purchase and Cotton 1978).

only are these functions under different directors, but the directors themselves are under several administrative levels that must be penetrated before the responsible individual is reached. The separation of units caused by the growing bureaucracy results in ever increasing communication problems. Experience has shown that direct and close communication between user and producer without the intervention of an administrative filter (1) provides a deeper insight into the problem, (2) stimulates innovative thinking, and (3) reduces the interval between problem recognition and solution development. Continuous and serious effort, illustrated by special intragency study groups (Animal Protein Conservation Work Group ca. 1974), is required to restore communication that has been inhibited or destroyed by the separation caused by institutional growth. The U.S. Animal Health Association and the U.S. Department of Agriculture established a committee in 1982 to investigate charges that federal research laboratories were not responsive to national needs. The preliminary findings reported by the committee were failure of communication between user of research and producer of research rather than unresponsiveness.

An administrative approach known as a matrix organization (Mee 1973), which was used initially in the development of the aerospace program to shorten communication lines and maintain accountability, has been adopted by the research planning staff of the U.S. Department of Agriculture (Purchase and Cotton 1978). Individuals from line units are assigned to a research project with defined objectives. The members of this multidisciplinary project group pursue the research objectives with the support of their individual line units. When the investigation is completed, the individuals are reassigned or returned to their original units. All the persons sharing a research objective communicate directly rather than through administrative channels. This approach permits greater innovation and more rapid progress. Although matrix organization is very appropriate for the administration of applied research, its usefulness in fundamental research has not been established (Anderson 1974).

ENVIRONMENT FOR RESEARCH

Throughout the world, departments of agriculture have established laboratories to conduct research on the broad or narrow problems that must be understood to control animal diseases. Some of these laboratories

have an excellent record of productivity (National
Research Council 1972). Regardless of their record,
they are praised or criticized (Hightower 1973; Division of Vector Biology and Control 1976) in ways that
give knowledgeable people, both within and outside the
laboratories, little confidence in the assessments made
by politicians and public media.

Three characteristics should be examined when
determining a laboratory's productivity: (1) institutional structure, (2) physical facilities, and (3) tra-
ditions (Mayer and Mayer 1974; Blume 1980). Decision
makers who consider these characteristics are hoped to
be better prepared to judge research institutions.

Institutional Structure

The mission of the laboratory should be clearly
defined and, when changed circumstances make it desirable, redefined (Rothschild 1971, 1972; Bentley and
Long 1976). A medical research laboratory that was
established in a remote community with a unique disease
problem illustrates this point. During its first few
decades, the laboratory staff was very productive and
built a good foundation for an understanding of the
nature, epidemiology, and control of the disease they
were investigating. However, when the original mission
was completed, no new assignment was given, the staff
was not integrated into other institutions, and the
laboratory was allowed to drift. Although a few individuals developed good but unrelated research projects,
the laboratory clearly was not functioning efficiently.
Such a situation can be prevented by an ongoing assessment of research objectives and institutional assignments (Fig. 8.2).

Once an institution is established and the staff
is selected (Grover and Wallace 1979), it must be given
a certain degree of autonomy to develop and carry on a
coherent program. Furthermore, it should neither be
subjected to such arbitrary pressures as dismissal of
half of its staff because of a government budget emergency nor a change in assignment because certain political groups wish to push a pet idea. Such a problem
was described in 1714 by John Bates who was chairman of
a commission appointed by the British crown to develop
a control program for rinderpest, which had invaded
England from the continent. Bates complained of being
sidetracked repeatedly from his studies by requests
from members of the royal retinue to investigate new
magical cures they had heard about. The time Bates
used in researching and refuting these cures could have

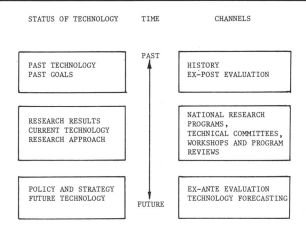

FIG. 8.2. Channels through which the program-planning staff functions (adapted from Purchase and Cotton 1978).

been used more effectively on the original assignment.

Researchable ideas are generated by investigators in the course of laboratory studies and by people confronted with disease problems in the field. Ideas from the field can be translated into laboratory experiments if research and field personnel have the opportunity to communicate and visit. The foot-and-mouth disease research program at Pirbright in England (Animal Virus Research Institute 1974) and the Plum Island Animal Disease Research Center in New York (Shahan 1956; Callis 1971; Agricultural Research Service 1982) have both benefited by sending some of their staff into the field and by having guest investigators from the field come to their institutions for periods of research. The innovative ideas that develop in these interchanges can be incorporated into the projected research program. This is particularly true when the staff participates with the director in planning. There must, however, be flexibility to take new directions and grow or regroup. Ad hoc internal review of research areas, an approach that has been under trial at Plum Island Animal Disease Center for several years, has some promise. Individuals who volunteer for this intensive review bring to it experience gained in other areas of research (Bachrach et al. 1976). External reviewers have also been used at both federal and private institutions (Advisory Committee on Foreign Animal and Poultry Diseases 1978; Pan American Foot-and-Mouth Disease Center 1979). The best results were obtained when the area under review was relatively narrow and

enough time was allocated to permit an in-depth
examination with ample opportunity for individual
interchange.

Within the institution, lagging investigators must
be stimulated and productivity rewarded. The special
chemistry that sometimes develops between individuals
stimulates them to greater productivity. For example,
one director, with tongue in cheek, pointed out a
middle-aged male investigator whose productivity had
lagged until he was given the assistance of a very
able, young, female professional. Perhaps the chemistry was male chauvinism, but the competition stimulated
both persons to work hard. In other instances associates may inhibit one another. The director must try
to find the place where each individual will be most
productive.

Some means of rewarding productivity must be provided; it can take the form of advancement, increase in
salary, opportunity to travel to meetings, or opportunity for study.

Physical Facility

Site. Any group charged with selecting the site for an
animal disease laboratory should consider five things:
(1) availability, at a reasonable cost of sufficient
land to provide room for the proposed structure and
pssible expansion; (2) on site availability of all
utilities including water, sewer, electricity, and an
assured source of power; (3) proximity to a community
having attractive, reasonably priced housing for
employees and cultural and recreational resources; (4)
access to good surface and air transportation; and (5)
reasonable access to library facilities and consultative groups. The need for sufficient land is self-
evident. A casual attitude toward the availability of
utilities has created serious problems, particularly in
developing countries. For example, a multimillion
dollar animal disease laboratory has been standing idle
in South America for five years for lack of water and
sewer. In other instances some electrical equipment in
laboratories in developing countries is nonfunctional
much of the time because electrical service is unde-
pendable. Problems in developed nations sometimes
arise in recruiting qualified researchers if housing
and living costs are too high and the educational and
cultural resources that professional people want for
their families are not available. Good air and surface
access are needed for efficient administration, diagno-

stic laboratories, laboratories engaged in training programs, and laboratories that must maintain sophisticated equipment. The problem of access to supplemental library services and consultative experts in related fields has been used with some justification as an excuse for poor productivity. Proximity to another research center or a major university, which permits an individual researcher to spend a morning in a library or nearby laboratory, gives that particular laboratory a recruiting edge over another facility where the individual must apply for permission and money to travel and spend several days in the effort. Most investigators simply will not go to such lengths to find an answer. Consequently, the research atmosphere is impoverished.

Design. The most important aspects of the design of a laboratory are laboratory safety (Center for Disease Control 1974) and the reduction of any adverse impact that laboratory activities may have on the area's environment (Fig. 8.3). Research involving animal pathogens has long been considered potentially hazardous to the health of livestock in the region and, sometimes, to the health of the researchers themselves. Radioisotopes now in widespread use in biological laboratories require many of the same precautions in handling that are needed for infectious agents. The use of a single barrier to confine hazardous infectious material is not enough (Wedum et al. 1972). Three barriers--spatial, mechanical, and procedural--must be utilized.

It is generally accepted that a laboratory dealing with highly communicable livestock diseases should be separated from local susceptible livestock by a reasonable distance. In some countries this is accomplished by siting the laboratory on an island. The late Richard Shope suggested to the author that locating such a laboratory in a metropolitan area had merit as the separation from livestock would be equally sure. In several European countries, a distance of a kilometer or less is interposed between the laboratory and livestock operations. The law in the United States and Australia states that laboratories where foreign animal diseases are studied must be situated on land separated by water, on an island or peninsula, from animal populations.

The primary safety effort, however, is a mechanical one of confining pathogens within units in the laboratory by use of air filtration and air locks and by the processing of sewage and solid wastes (Callis and Cottral 1968). The effectiveness of isolation

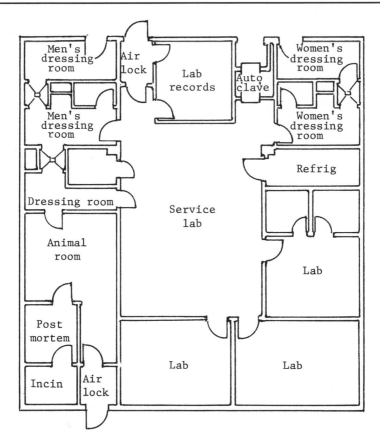

FIG. 8.3. National Animal Disease Laboratory module, United
States Department of Agriculture.

engineering, however, is dependent upon the absolute
adherence of the staff to operational procedures that
are established to confine the pathogen (Office of
Biosafety 1974). In a laboratory operating at a high
level of security, the investigator enters through a
change room and shower suite where street clothing is
removed and laboratory clothing donned. At the end of
the day the individual showers before dressing in
street clothes. Any notebooks taken along must be
passed through a gas sterilizer. All air from the unit
passes through absolute filters or an incinerator, and
all fluid and solid wastes are treated with heat or
incinerated. Engineering of such a laboratory must
give attention to such details as air leakage through
electrical ducting and the availability of backup electricity during power failures. Within the laboratory

the flow of work should be carefully structured so that hazardous operations take place in glove boxes or laminar flow chambers. Color coding and the identification of all materials is essential.

The well-being of both people and laboratory animals must be given careful attention (Institute of Laboratory Animal Resources 1965). The housing and care of laboratory animals requires careful planning of the facilities and strict adherence to standard procedures (Runkle and McMaster 1964).

Research is characterized by innovation and change. Facilities rapidly become obsolete unless they are designed to permit structural and layout changes that keep up with the research. While it is impossible to foresee the future, short-term changes in which emphasis is increased in certain phases of work can be anticipated. Additional space or reallocation is an inevitable need in every laboratory. This problem may be solved by using modular rooms that can be easily shifted from one activity to another to facilitate rapid expansion or changes of activity. A second strategy for change is to place essential utilities in runs that are always accessible for the attachment of new outlets at low cost and without major disruption. Some older laboratories are still functioning well because these two strategies were used and the space was provided for construction of new wings or placement of new accessory structures.

Traditions

Research productivity is basically determined by something that is much less tangible than the physical plant and operational funding. An iconoclastic university scientist, who had served some time as an administrator, maintained that there is an inverse relationship between bricks and mortar and scientific ideas. Although this belief can be questioned, there seems to be little evidence of a positive relationship. Research accomplishments depend upon the composition of the staff and its training, dedication, and motivation (Fig. 8.4).

The staff and administrators at institutions that are world renowned for their record of scientific productivity have, when pressed, identified four procedures and concepts they felt were important in making their institutions outstanding.

High standards. Most important is the establishment of high standards by which the work and an individual is measured. In these institutions work is reviewed by

BASIC DRIVES	PRIMARY MOTIVES	DERIVED MOTIVES	EXAMPLES OF SELF-ACTUALIZATION
BIOLOGICAL	PSYCHOLOGICAL ↑ ↓ SOCIAL	SECURITY	Have job stability
		OPPORTUNITY	Be promoted and grow in abilities
		PARTICIPATION	Have a voice in job affairs
		RECOGNITION	Be appreciated and know that you count
		ECONOMIC	Have a decent standard of living
		ACCOMPLISHMENT	Feel that you are doing some-thing worthwhile
		COMMUNICATION	Know what is going on
		POWER	Have a chance to gain ascendency over others
		CONFORMITY	Be part of the team
		INDEPENDENCE	Satisfy personal freedom

FIG. 8.4. Motivating factors (adapted from Scott 1967).

knowledgeable peers and papers are published in refereed journals that are internationally recognized
(Garfield 1979). The staff understands that their
individual ability to meet the high standards of their
particular laboratory will determine the degree of
respect it will receive in the scientific world
(Shepherd and Brown 1956).

Morale. Morale within the institution is based on the
administrators' ability to serve the research community
that they head, represent it effectively to the funding
agencies, higher authorities, and the public, and protect the right of individual researchers to get a hearing for their ideas and receive recognition for their
contributions (Guba 1958).

Creative atmosphere. A creative atmosphere is dependent upon the provision of frequent opportunities for
informal interaction among investigators as well as
spontaneous discussion and sharing of ideas in the
lunchroom, at coffee breaks, and in seminars. Communication of developing ideas is essential for insights
that result in innovation, but it must be spontaneous
rather than rigorously structured (Newman 1958). In
addition, opportunities must be created for users and

researchers to interact, either by bringing users to the laboratory to discuss problems or sending investigators to the field to see the problem firsthand. Furthermore, investigators need to meet with peers at national or international meetings on a regular basis. All of these interactions have a measurable effect on research productivity, but their relative significance differs from one investigator to another (Goodfield 1977).

Sabbaticals and fellowships. Interaction of longer duration is needed to bring about institutional changes. Sabbaticals for staff and fellowships for visitors provide two mechanisms. An early director of the Rockefeller Institute has been quoted as telling his staff scientists, "I want you to take a leave for three months. Whether you go to another laboratory or lay on the beach doesn't matter to me, but I believe that unless you periodically change your environment you will lose the creativity and productivity that I expect from you." This viewpoint is shared, in part, by directors of many institutions who usually expect their staff to spend the sabbatical period in another laboratory and give an accounting on return. The reverse action is the acceptance of visiting investigators and fellows into the laboratory. Ideas are introduced by these exchanges, and systems of operation are questioned. New ideas brought back from sabbaticals and introduced by visiting investigators and fellows keep institutions alive and functioning.

PRIORITIES

The criteria and process used in establishing research priorities are of central importance to the legislative branch of government, which funds research, and the public, who are the eventual beneficiaries. The public believes that general welfare should override benefits to a few or the cultivation of selfish interests, and they hold that critical problems should be given priority over trivial problems (Mayer and Mayer 1974; Arndt and Ruttan 1975; Whitaker and Wennergren 1976). More and more the public is giving voice to the idea that such decisions should not be entirely deferred to the scientific community.

Criteria

Almost all research proposals are now subjected to review before funding is made available. Two criteria that are applied in the review involve only the scientific community; the third involves the public as well: (1) determination of scientific merit, (2) evidence of capability (Cole et al. 1977), and (3) mission relevance (Committee on Science and Technology 1975; Purchase and Cotton 1978).

Scientific merit, although readily understood by scientific practitioners, is not easily explained to the public. It examines the proposed research process, which the investigator should have clearly stated in the proposal. The hypothesis is the fundamental consideration. What is the idea to be tested? Is the experimental design logical? Have tools been developed to test the hypothesis? Is the investigator aware of similar developments in the field to prevent overlap and repetitive effort?

Evidence of capability is also considered during the review. Does the investigator have the physical facilities, the tools, and the training required to undertake the proposed investigation? Has this been documented carefully?

Mission relevance is yet another consideration. Will the investigation provide, either in the short or the long run, solutions to the problems that fall within the mission of the agency and laboratory as established by legislative action? This review of relevance not only restrains certain lines of research and encourages others but also gives the public a voice through legislative authorization in setting research priorities.

Review

The means by which these three criteria are applied to a proposal is important (Fig. 8.5). Reviews of grants and contracts often employ a two-step procedure that to a limited extent has been used for internal allocation of research funds within large research institutions. The first step involves the review of the research proposal by peers (who have no vested interest in the proposal) for its scientific merit and the research capability of the investigator. This may be conducted in a meeting in which a critique is presented followed by defense and discussion. A written appraisal and a numerical priority rating based on the consensus of the conferees is given to both the investigator and the administrator (Cole et al. 1977).

The second step is an administrative review that weighs the mission relevance of the proposal and its priority in relationship to other proposals. Ad hoc

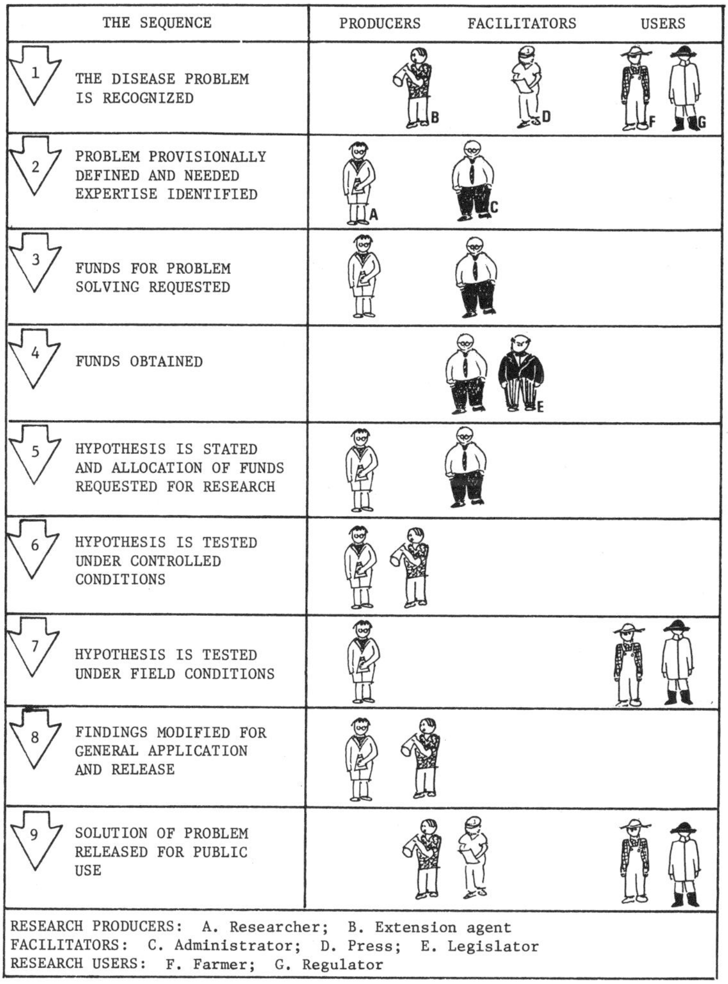

THE SEQUENCE	PRODUCERS	FACILITATORS	USERS
1. THE DISEASE PROBLEM IS RECOGNIZED	B	D	F G
2. PROBLEM PROVISIONALLY DEFINED AND NEEDED EXPERTISE IDENTIFIED	A	C	
3. FUNDS FOR PROBLEM SOLVING REQUESTED			
4. FUNDS OBTAINED		E	
5. HYPOTHESIS IS STATED AND ALLOCATION OF FUNDS REQUESTED FOR RESEARCH			
6. HYPOTHESIS IS TESTED UNDER CONTROLLED CONDITIONS			
7. HYPOTHESIS IS TESTED UNDER FIELD CONDITIONS			
8. FINDINGS MODIFIED FOR GENERAL APPLICATION AND RELEASE			
9. SOLUTION OF PROBLEM RELEASED FOR PUBLIC USE			

RESEARCH PRODUCERS: A. Researcher; B. Extension agent
FACILITATORS: C. Administrator; D. Press; E. Legislator
RESEARCH USERS: F. Farmer; G. Regulator

FIG. 8.5. Solving animal disease problems.

representatives of the public sector sometimes sit with the administrators and participate in this review.

Funding

Support for research is obtained by either competitive funding of grants or contracts to public or private institutions or administrative determination of support for proposals generated by sections and laboratories within an agency (Bentley and Long 1976). A two-step review can be used in both instances, although in some agencies the decision as to whether a project is to be undertaken is made by administrators who have little experience in evaluating research and who seek little assistance in making their decision.

Some government agencies use both external grants and contracts and internally administered funds. A good argument can be made for using both sources because the combination provides flexibility in expanding and reducing programs and avoids the ascendency of fixed beliefs. For example, Russia lost years of research effort in the plant field when Lysenko, who did not believe in Mendelian genetics, gained control of research funding and cut off all support for plant breeding methods that contradicted his ideas. As a result, other sciences were also adversely affected (Gorham et al. 1975). On a much smaller scale, individuals with strong beliefs have prevented the exploration of certain ideas in laboratories that they dominated. If a nation or field of science is dependent upon an institution under such domination, progress can be seriously hampered. Much of the innovation in industry comes from small companies where new ideas are allowed to prove their worth. The advantages of having several sources of funds when structuring research institutions or supporting research are clear from the records of research contributions in almost every field of scientific endeavor (National Research Council 1972, 1977). Unfortunately, competition for grant support does have its price. The time researchers spend in developing grantsmanship expertise is time taken away from research (Leopold 1979).

THE RESEARCH PROCESS

Diversity is needed in structuring research institutions because of the complex process by which a new idea develops and moves into a practical application. Some researchers distinguish four steps in the process: (1) hypothesis, (2) synthesis, (3) application, and (4) transfer. Problems arise when administrators try to separate hypothesis and snythesis, which are generally considered to be fundamental research, from application and transfer, which are considered to be applied research. There is a widespread belief that the fundamental research is more rigorous and prestigous. In reality, the same care and high standards are required in all steps of the process. The last two steps are most easily understood by administrators of disease-control programs, and who consider them to be of greatest importance. Operationally, directors of control programs must handle the problems that arise and account for funds that are wasted when the standard of research conducted in the field falls short of what is expected in the laboratory. A new test for a disease reactor that resulted from an insight into an immunological process seldom provides a technology that works well when first taken out to the field. The additional research that may solve the problem of its field application may also lead to a more fundamental understanding of the immunological process. Certainly, establishing that the test is dependable requires a thorough knowledge of immunology and skill at experimental research. While the transfer of a laboratory test such as detection of carriers from one disease to another, or applying the test to another species may seem simple and immensely practical, it is seldom something that can be done by personnel whose only experience is routine testing. Instead, for the field application to be practical, it must undergo rigorous testing by experimentalists with thorough knowledge of the specialty. Bushland (1978) illustrated this process in his description of the problems that arose in Florida and Texas as the screwworm eradication program proceeded. These problems involved not only the genetic differences between the fly populations in the laboratory and the field (Richardson et al. 1982) but also procedures for effective dispersal and understanding of the behavior of the fly (Beal ca. 1980). The program's success depended upon correct problem diagnosis and solution.

A new approach that identifies misconceptions in hypotheses uses available information to build a model. The model reveals missing information and (since a model is, simply speaking, a budget) imbalances in the budget. For example, the use of a model revealed that transmission of virus from chipmunk to chipmunk by mosquitoes and from one mosquito generation to the next transovarially were not sufficient to maintain LaCrosse encephalitis virus in a woodlot. Yet this endemic virus is maintained year after year throughout its range. Investigators were then led to discover venereal transmission in mosquitoes that contributes to virus perpetuation and oral transmission to foxes preying upon chipmunks that spread the virus between woodlots.

ACCOUNTABILITY

Both the scientific community and the public are concerned with the accountability of scientists.

Persons involved in research have overriding ethical
and moral obligations to make all findings available to
other scientists and the general public. Both the content of the results and the manner in which it is presented provide the basis on which the investigator will
be judged. Scientific judgment is based on the quality
and quantity of published research, but public judgment
is based on the individual's scientific standing and
the proven or potential application of the research.
Judgment of the public will determine, in large part,
the investigator's continued access to research facilities and funds. The scientist's affiliated institution
is judged on the productivity and renown of its staff.

Most research results require months or years of
hard work. If the results are to be relevant to current needs, the problem must have been anticipated and
ample time allowed for completion of the research. If
the investigator either fails to have the solution when
it is needed or obtains it before it is needed, the
relevance of the research is doubted and the investigator's motivation is questioned.

Many of society's competing special interest
groups demand that science attend to their needs first.

Table 8.1. Evaluation of Marek's Disease Vaccine and Comparison
      of Adoption Times

Cost of vaccine development		Ten-Year Total ($ million)
Public sector research	1965–1974	17.1
Private sector research	1965–1974	15.0
		32.1

Benefits of vaccine development	Annual Savings ($ million)
Reduced leukosis broiler condemnations	27.3
Reduced associated broiler condemnations	6.3
Reduced broiler mortality	5.6
Reduced broiler breeder mortality	5.0
Reduced egg-type chicken mortality	15.4
Reduced condemnation of egg-type chickens	0.1
Improved feed utilization	3.2
Increased egg production	105.5
	168.4

Years required for adoption (95% acceptance)		
Vaccine for Marek's disease	1971–1973	2
Mechanical harvesting of grapes	1968–1971	3
Hybrid corn, Iowa	1933–1940	7
Monogerm sugar beet seed	1956–1965	9
Hybrid sorghum	1955–1970	15
Hybrid corn, United States	1933–1969	36

Source: Adapted from Purchase and Schultz 1979.

As expected, the most articulate gain the most attention (Hightower 1973; Wade 1973). The resulting unrea-
sonable demands on scientists and research laboratories
may obscure inadequacies of planning and organization
as well as occasional evidences of bad judgment and
possible malfeasance (Smith 1979). Research accomplishments are usually warmly welcomed but their social
and economic value is uncommonly measured. The history
of research regarding its relevance to defined needs
merits documentation. Cole et al. (1962) documented
the value of hog cholera research, and Purchase documented lymphoid leukosis research (1976) and Marek's
disease research (1977) (Table 8.1), but many more
quantitative evaluations of the value of research
should be made (Weisbrod 1971; American Veterinary
Medical Association 1974; Horsfall 1975; Evenson et al.
1979).

REFERENCES

Advisory Committee on Foreign Animal and Poultry
    Diseases to the Secretary of Agriculture. 1978.
    Minutes of joint meeting with the consultants to
    the Plum Island Animal Disease Center, June 27-28,
    USDA, Washington, D.C.
Agricultural Research Service. 1982. The Plum Island
    Animal Disease Center. USDA, Washington, D.C.
American Veterinary Medical Association Council on
    Research. 1974. Justifications for veterinary
    animal health research. *Am. J. Vet. Res.*
    35:875-887.
Anderson, N. G. 1974. Science and management tech-
    niques. *Science* 183:726-727.
Animal Protein Conservation Work Group. Ca. 1974.
    Animal protein conservation report. Anim. Plant
    Health Insp. Serv., USDA, Hyattsville, Md.
Animal Virus Research Institute. 1974. The Animal
    Virus Research Institute: 1924-1974. Pirbright,
    UK.
Arndt, T. M., and Ruttan, V. W. 1975. Resource allo-
    cation and productivity in national and interna-
    tional agricultural research. Agric. Dev. Counc.,
    Inc., New York.
Bachrach, H. L.; Campbell, C. H.; Dardiri, A. H.; Hyde,
    J. L.; McKercher, P. D.; and McVicar, J. W. 1976.
    In-depth review foot-and-mouth disease research.
    Plum Island Anim. Dis. Cent., Greenport, N.Y.
Bates, T. 1714. A brief account of the contagious
    disease which raged among the milch cows near

London in the year 1714 and the methods that were taken for suppressing it. *Philos. Trans. R. Soc. London.*

Beal, V. C., Jr. Ca. 1980. The interaction of the environment with heredity in the eradication of the screwworm fly and the relationship of field observations to the strain versus species question. Anim. Plant Health Insp. Serv., USDA, Hyattsville, Md.

Bentley, O. G., and Long, R. W. 1976. Brief comments about interim report: Special oversight review of agricultural research and development. Agricultural Research Policy Advisory Committee. Secretary of Agriculture, Washington, D.C.

Beveridge, W. I. B. 1957. The Art of Scientific Investigation. New York: W. W. Norton and Co., Inc.

Blume, S. S. 1980. A managerial view of research: A review of Scientific Productivity, ed. F. M. Andrews. *Science* 207:48-49.

Braye, E. T.; Moulton, W.; O'Berry, P.; Schwabe, C. W.; and Pritchard, W. R. 1976. Report of the committee on animal health, National Research Council World Food and Nutrition study. NAS, Washington, D.C.

Bushland, R. C. 1978. Eradication and suppression of the screwworm fly by the sterile male technique, ed. Comm. Jt. US/USSR Acad. Study Fundam. Sci. Policy. NAS, Washington, D.C.

Callis, J. J. 1971. Plum Island Laboratory: Its role in foreign animal disease research. *Agric. Sci. Rev.* 9(3):1-13.

Callis, J. J., and Cottral, G. E. 1968. Methods for containment of animal pathogens at the Plum Island Animal Disease Laboratory. In Methods in Virology, vol. 4, eds. K. Maramorsch and H. Koprowski. New York: Academic Press, pp. 465-480.

Center for Disease Control. 1974. Laboratory safety at the Center for Disease Control. U.S. Dep. Health Educ. Welfare Publ. CDC 75-8118, Atlanta, Ga.

Cole, C. G.; Henley, R. R.; Dale, C. N.; Mott, L. O.; Torrey, J. P.; and Zinober, M. R. 1962. History of hog cholera research in the U.S. department of agriculture, 1884-1960. Agric. Inf. Bull. 241. USGPO, Washington, D.C.

Cole, S.; Rubin, L.; and Cole, J. R. 1977. Peer review and the support of science. *Sci. Am.* 237(4): 34-41.

Committee on Science and Technology. 1975. Agricul-

tural research and development: Special oversight
hearings of the U.S. House of Representatives.
USGPO, Washington, D.C.

Cooke, G. W., ed. 1981. Agricultural Research, 1931-
1981: A History of the Agricultural Research
Council and a Review of Developments in Agricultural Research During the Last Fifty Years.
London: Agricultural Research Council.

Division of Vector Biology and Control. 1976. WHO-
supported collaborative research projects in
India: The facts. *WHO Chron.* 30:131-139.

Evenson, R. E.; Waggoner, P. E.; and Ruttan, V. W.
1979. Economic benefits from research: An example from Agriculture. *Science* 205:1101-1107.

Garfield, E. 1979. Controversies over opiate receptor
research typify problems facing awards committees.
Curr. Contents No. 20, pp. 5-18.

Goodfield, J. 1977. Humanity in science: A perspective and a plea. *Science* 198:580-585.

Gorham, J.; Graves, J.; Lambert, G.; Shille, V.; and
Twiehaus, M. 1975. U.S. Veterinary Scientist
team visit to USSR, May 15-June 13, 1975. USDA,
Washington, D.C.

Grover, F., and Wallace, P. 1979. Laboratory Organization and Management. Butterworths: Sevenoaks,
UK.

Guba, E. G. 1958. Morale and satisfaction: a study in
past-future time perspective. *Adm. Sci. Q.* 3:195-
209.

Hightower, J. 1973. Hard Tomatoes, Hard Times: A
Report of the Agribusiness Accountability Project
on the Failure of America's Land Grant College
Complex. Cambridge: Schenkman Publ. Co.

Horsfall, J. G., chairman. 1975. Agricultural Production Efficiency. Washington, D.C.: NAS.

Humphrey, H. H., chairman. 1961. Veterinary Medical
Science and Human Health. Committee on Government
Operations, United States Senate. Washington,
D.C.: USGPO.

Institute of Laboratory Animal Resources. 1965. Guide
for laboratory animal facilities and care. U.S.
Dep. Health Educ. Welfare, USGPO, Washington, D.C.

Leopold, A. C. 1979. The burden of competitive
grants. *Science* 203:607.

McDaniel, H. A. 1976. Laboratory support for emergency programs. *U.S. Anim. Health Assoc. Proc.*
80:319-323.

McElroy, W. D. 1977. The global age: Roles of basic
and applied research. *Science* 196:267-270.

Mayer, A., and Mayer, J. 1974. Agriculture, the

island empire. *J. Am. Acad. Arts Sci.*, Summer, pp. 83-95.

Mee, J. F. 1973. Matrix organization. In The Encyclopedia of Management, ed. C. Heyel. New York: Van Nostrand Reinhold Company, pp. 560-562.

Mitchell, C. A. 1956. Coordination of research and regulatory functions. Proc. Symp. Vesicular Dis., Sept. 27, 28, Plum Island Anim. Dis. Lab., Agric. Res. Serv. 45-1, USDA.

National Program Staff. 1976. Diagnosis and control of foreign animal diseases: Development of improved methods for the diagnosis and control of foot-and-mouth disease and other foreign animal diseases. Natl. Res. Program 20460, Agric. Res. Serv., USDA, Washington, D.C.

National Research Council. 1972. Report of the committee on research advisory to the U.S. Department of Agriculture. NAS, Washington, D.C.

————. 1977. Brucellosis Research: An Evaluation. Washington, D.C.: NAS.

Newman, J. R. 1958. Book review: Reason and Chance in Scientific Discovery by R. Taton. *Sci. Am.* 198(4):141-148.

Office of Biosafety. 1974. Laboratory safety at the Center for Disease Control. I. Administrative aspects. II. Preventive aspects. U.S. Dep. Health Educ. Welfare Publ. CDC 75-8118.

Pan American Foot-and-Mouth Disease Center. 1979. Report to the director by the scientific advisory committee. Rio de Janeiro, Brazil.

Purchase, H. G. 1976. An evaluation of research on lymphoid leukosis and Marek's disease. *West. Poult. Dis. Conf. Proc.* 25:2.

————. 1977. The etiology and control of Marek's disease of chickens and the economic impact of a successful research program. In Virology in Agriculture. Montclair, N.J.: Allanheld, Osmun & Co., Inc., pp. 63-81.

Purchase, H. G., and Cotton, C. C. 1978. Providing integration in a highly differentiated research organization: The role of a program staff. *IEEE Trans. Eng. Manage.* EM-25(3):68-71.

Purchase, H. G., and Schultz, E. F. 1979. The economics of Marek's disease control in the United States. *World's Poult. Sci. J.* 34(4):198-204.

Richardson, R. H.; Ellison, J. R.; and Averhoff, W. W. 1982. Autocidal control of screwworms in North America. *Science* 215:361-370.

Rothschild, Lord. 1971. Framework for government

research and development. Cmnd. 4814. Her Majesty's Stationery Off., London.

————. 1972. Framework for government research and development. Cmnd. 5046. Her Majesty's Stationery Off., London.

Runkle, R. S., and McMaster, W. W., Jr. 1964. Laboratory animal housing, parts 1, 2. *J. Am. Inst. Archit.* 41(3):55-58, 41(4):77-80.

Scott, W. G. 1967. Organization Theory: A Behavioral Analysis for Management. Homewood, Ill.: Richard D. Irwin, Inc.

Shahan, M. S. 1956. Animal disease research at Plum Island. Proc. Symp. Vesicular Dis., Sept. 27, 28, Plum Island Anim. Dis. Lab., Agric. Res. Serv. 45-1, USDA.

Shepherd, C., and Brown, P. 1956. Status, prestige and esteem in a research organization. *Adm. Sci. Q.* 1:340-360.

Smith, R. J. 1979. NCI bioassays yield a trail of blunders. *Science* 204:1287-1292.

Wade, N. 1973. Agriculture: Social sciences oppressed and poverty stricken. *Science* 110:719-722.

Wedum, A. G.; Barkley, W. E.; and Hellman, A. 1972. Handling of infectious agents. *J. Am. Vet. Med. Assoc.* 161:1557-1567.

Weisbrod, B. A. 1971. Costs and benefits of medical research: A case study of poliomyelitis. *J. Polit. Econ.* 79:527-544.

Whitaker, M. D., and Wennergren, E. B. 1976. U.S. universities and the world food problem. *Science* 194:497-500.

9

Ongoing Training Programs

PERSONNEL REQUIREMENTS

In most developed countries the supply of trained
people is sufficient to carry out large emergency programs and ongoing disease-control activities if the
personnel requirements are defined, needed people identified, and a suitable system of recruitment developed
(McLaughlin et al. 1976; Chrysler 1977). This is not
true in most developing countries because the supply of
trained people is inadequate to carry out even elemen-
tary services (Table 9.1) (Arambulo et al. 1976).
Control of animal disease is dependent upon an
organized effort carried out by a corps of professionally trained people. The great variety of tasks in-

Table 9.1. Populations

	Developed Nations		Less-Developed Nations	
		United		
Classification	USA	Kingdom	Colombia	Nigeria
Cattle	171,185,000	19,975,000	30,969,000	10,957,000
Horses, mules	8,974,000	140,000	1,607,000	978,000
Sheep, goats	18,145,000	28,095,000	2,892,000	30,913,000
Pigs	63,898,000	8,979,000	1,544,000	898,000
All livestock	262,202,000	57,189,000	37,012,000	43,746,000
Veterinarians	30,000	5,963	219	189
Human population	209,000,000	56,000,000	23,000,000	58,000,000
Population ratios				
Humans/vet	6,966	9,391	105,023	306,878
Cattle/vet	5,706	3,349	141,410	57,973
Livestock/vet	8,740	9,590	169,005	231,460

Source: *Animal Health Yearbook* 1974.

volved and the complex decisions that must be made challenge both the skills and knowledge of any inter- disciplinary team. Neither the veterinarians (Morey et al. 1976) who make up the largest component of the team nor members of any other profession have the breadth of training needed for some of the administra- tive posts or the specialization required for some of the technical posts. Even though the additional train- ing and experience can be acquired through the happen- stance of service in a series of different positions, the needs of an institution for experts and leaders is too important to depend upon chance (Baker and Perlman 1967). Planning to provide opportunities for training and experience needed to qualify individuals for leadership and counsel is essential (Bailey 1978).

VETERINARY EDUCATION

Education of veterinarians is dependent upon standards established by licensing bodies in each country and the response of schools to those standards (Cockrill 1964; Joint Committee on Veterinary Education 1975) although other forces may exist (Miller 1979). In all countries a veterinary school candidate must have completed secondary school satisfactorily and, in some countries, the equivalent of two or three years of college work as well. The pre-veterinary curriculum is usually science-oriented and little attention is given to the arts and humanities. The narrowness of the pro- fessional curriculum does not prepare the students for administrative responsibilities, and this deficiency concerns many leaders in both veterinary and human medicine (Goodfield 1977).

The professional curriculum covers a three- or four-year period and is divided between science and technical courses. The extent of clinical training varies. In better schools it is given in the third and fourth year and makes up most of the fourth year. The time demands of required courses are so restrictive that the students do not have the option of specializa- tion (Lyle 1969; Blackmore and Harris 1979; Leech 1979; Thrusfield 1979) or exposure to broadening cultural influences (Howe 1979).

Postprofessional training, if it is taken, follows three tracks. The student may (1) take a graduate de- gree emphasizing research in microbiology, physiology, public health, or some other academic discipline (Schwabe 1969; Sadler 1975); (2) undertake independent or supervised study, usually during university resi- dency, toward passing the examination of a specialty board such as pathology; and (3) take several years of internship in a clinical facility to gain specialization in a field such as small animal surgery.

The three tracks are designed to train the personnel for research institutes, veterinary schools, hospitals, and some positions in government and industry. Unfortunately, such education not only fails to meet the important needs of other institutions who employ veterinarians in administrative positions (Humphrey 1961; Swann 1975), but also fails to provide individuals with the sensitivity and breath of knowledge needed to work effectively in community or international programs. Multinational corporations and international agencies are finding that a lack of training in linguistic skills, while a matter of concern, is less critical than unadaptability and narrowness of attitude. Although no course of training can change inflexible individuals, certain education methods can broaden the outlook of most individuals and enable them to adjust to rapidly changing situations.

IN-SERVICE TRAINING PROGRAMS

When government and industry are faced with the problem of preparing staff for new tasks, in-service training programs should be designed for carefully selected and unselected participants (Fig. 9.1). These

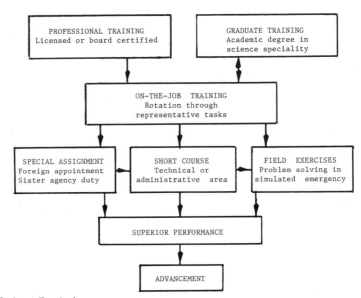

FIG. 9.1. Training programs.

programs have four goals: (1) orient the individual to the mission and philosophy of the institution, (2) teach administrative, language, or negotiating skills for which the individual has aptitude, (3) introduce new concepts and keep the individual abreast of developing knowledge in a specialized technical field, and (4) train the individual to work as a member of a team in solving problems.

A variety of means are used for in-service training. Government and industrial research institutes often employ regular seminars to keep their employees abreast of new developments in science. Special skills are taught in two- to six-week short courses (Rohde and Sadjimin 1980) at institutes that are organized either by the interested government division or by an educational institution (Campbell 1976) (Table 9.2). Short course may cover a variety of subjects including administrative skills, avian diseases (Veterinary Services 1974, 1976b), or mission and philosophy of the institution (Animal Plant Health Inspection Service ca. 1977). For example, about half of the four-week USDA course on foreign animal diseases deals with mission and philosophy and the other half with new skills and knowledge. Similar courses dealing with epidemiology, disease surveillance, and program planning and administration are presented by the Pan American Health Organization to veterinary personnel from Latin American countries (Pan American Foot-and-Mouth Disease Center 1980). Manuals are also used to train and indoctrinate (Animal Health Division 1971; Veterinary Services ca. 1976a). Another procedure for helping employees understand the mission of the institution is by an initial period of employment rotation through many sections of the institution or its field stations so that the employee may become acquainted both with the staff and with agency activities.

The last element of the in-service program, training the individual to work as a member of a team to solve problems and, particularly, to understand the contributions of other professionals in handling complex issues is the most important and the most difficult to implement. Three methods that can complement each other have been used to achieve this goal.

Many countries send members of their staffs to a foreign nation to assist in a declared emergency. Without question this is an important learning situation. Although methodology is invariably different and philosophies vary, goals are almost identical. The individual may gain new insights as well as experience in administration and problem solving.

Table 9.2. Training Programs of Veterinary Services in 1980

Name of Course	Duration in days	Number of Times Offered
Intermediate epidemiology training course	5	1
Brucellosis epidemiology training course for vets	4	3
Tuberculosis epidemiology training course	5	1
TB postmortem training course	4	5
Foreign animal diseases training course	22	2
Foreign animal diseases seminar for diagnosticians	3	1
Wildlife seminar for FAD diagnosticians	3	1
Military support for emergency animal disease programs	5	1
READEO epidemiologist's seminar	3	1
Foreign animal diseases seminar (universities)	2-3	2
Scabies identification and eradication training course	3	2
Tick identification and eradication training course	3-5	3
Pesticide use training course	3	3
Animal identification procedures and tracing techniques for technicians	3	2
Regulations compliance course	4	1
Biologics orientation course	3	1
Animal care-research facilities	4	1
Animal care-exhibition animals	5	1
Animal care-dealers and transportation	5	2
Animal care-horse protection	4	2
Pseudorabies training course (field) (1)	3	1
Pseudorabies training course (laboratory) (3)	5	3
Preventive veterinary medicine teachers work conference	5	1
Technical development course for animal health technicians	4	1
Veterinary administrator development program	5	1

Source: Personal correspondence, Veterinary Services, USDA, 1980.

While it is not routine, some staff members are encouraged to take a foreign assignment, usually in an international agency, as a technologist or an administrator in a foreign aid program. Likewise, a period spent in an industrial or an academic position can provide important insights. In the past, an employee who left government service to go abroad or into academia or industry was making an irreversible decision because opportunities for promotion were generally blocked if the individual returned. This is no longer true in England, the United States, and many other countries. The increased breadth of experience benefits both the individuals and their institutions.

The last method, which has been used particularly by the disease control officials in the United States and New Zealand and by armies everywhere, is a field exercise that simulates a real emergency as far as possible (Emergency Programs 1979; Perkins and Tate 1979). A well-planned field exercise tests communication networks, organizational skills, knowledge acquired through conventional instruction, and ability of individuals to work together in solving problems. In these exercises, which may be called at any time during an alert period, the participants are asked to carry out preassigned duties required to contain an exotic disease discovered in a stockyard or feedlot. Most tasks are actually carried out except destruction of the animals. In a less-expensive alternative teaching method, participants play roles in a scenario that requires use of their knowledge to satisfactorily solve a given crisis (Pan American Foot-and-Mouth Disease Center 1978, 1981). Computer programs can also be developed to provide training in problem-solving skills (Chibuzo et al. 1980).

EXAMPLES

In-service Training

Veterinary Services of the Animal Plant Health Inspection Service of the USDA conducts a Foreign Animal Diseases Training Course twice a year. Fifteen to twenty students, most of whom are employed by the USDA or its sister agencies in each of the fifty states, are admitted to each session. In addition, one or two students are nominated by foreign governments or educational institutions.

The course lasts three or four weeks, and the time is divided primarily between residence at the National Animal Disease Center in Ames, Iowa, and the Plum

Island Animal Disease Center in New York State. A day or two may be spent at the headquarters of Veterinary Services in Hyattsville, Maryland. Instructional time is devoted to illustrated lectures, videotapes, demonstrations, and laboratory exercises. Students also examine animals infected with important exotic diseases and observe the course of the disease. A typical day begins at 8:00 A.M. and ends at 5:00 P.M. Mornings are usually spent in the lecture room and afternoons in the animal rooms and laboratories.

While most of the lectures and demonstrations are given by selected members of the staff at the two laboratories, six to eight authorities from various universities present guest lectures. The Veterinary Services staff in Hyattsville organizes and supervises the course and provides lectures on administrative matters. One unstated objective is to acquaint participants with agency administrators and experts they may wish to contact at a later date.

The objective of the course, in the words of the agency, is "to orient federal, state, military, and industry veterinarians in the diagnosis of foreign animal diseases of livestock and poultry and their differential diagnosis from domestic diseases of these species. The program is designed to (1) provide information about the organization of Emergency Programs and the policies and procedures to be used in handling suspected foreign animal disease investigations, (2) provide knowledge of the clinical symptoms and gross pathology of certain foreign animal diseases and certain domestic animal diseases for which a differential diagnosis should be made, (3) provide knowledge of laboratory diagnostic procedures and the specimens required for confirmation of the disease in question, (4) provide information on research being conducted or planned, and (5) stimulate interest in technical literature pertaining to foreign animal diseases.

At the conclusion of this training, students should possess skills to:

1. Properly <u>conduct</u> and <u>report</u> a suspected foreign animal disease investigation.
2. Recognize clinical signs and lesions, know the species affected, and have knowledge of the causative agent of the foreign animal diseases discussed or demonstrated.
3. Recognize clinical signs and lesions, know the species affected, and have knowledge of the causative agent of certain domestic diseases that may be confused with a foreign animal disease.

4. Recognize clinical signs and lesions of toxicities that may be confused with a foreign animal disease.

5. Properly collect a probang specimen.

6. Conduct a systematic postmortem of equine, bovine, porcine, and avian species.

7. Collect correct diagnostic specimens, properly preserve and package the specimens, and prepare the specimens and paperwork for submission to the laboratory.

8. Recognize when and how vectors may be involved in the transmission of foreign animal diseases and how these vectors may be controlled."

A Field Training Exercise

A test exercise, Alpha 79, was held in January 1979 by the U.S. Animal Plant Health Inspection Service to see how quickly and effectively responsible individuals, on both federal and state levels, would react to a simulated outbreak of "Nada," a deadly animal disease.

The script was prepared by Emergency Programs of Veterinary Services of USDA and called for the disease, which was detected on an Iowa farm, to be introduced into the Omaha stockyards and spread from there to all major regions of the country. Specimens from the suspected herd were sent to the exotic disease laboratory at Plum Island. When confirmed by the laboratory, a docket was prepared by officials at Hyattsville. The Secretary of Agriculture was promptly briefed, and he signed the National Animal Disease Emergency Declaration, a measure required to release funds for emergency action.

Logistic teams, who rented space and equipment and took care of personnel matters and communications, were sent to establish regional headquarters in Omaha, Atlanta, Fort Worth, Riverside, and Chicago. The logistic teams were followed by personnel who directed the program activities. Information officers contacted news media. Livestock industry officials were briefed and asked to participate. The U.S. military headquarters and representatives of foreign countries were advised.

The activated staff in each region established a communication system, laid out quarantine lines, located livestock markets, found possible disposal sites, and determined availability of heavy equipment. In several areas movement of animals was traced. Contact was also made with state and federal wildlife officials

and national park officials. In one region an
"injunction" was served that prohibited destruction of
deer adjacent to an infected feedlot, and a solution to
the impasse was sought. The 7-day test covered a
simulated 30 day period.

The exercise revealed a need to improve the
staff's communication skills within the U.S. Department
of Agriculture as well as with other agencies, state
and local governments, affected industry, and the
consumer.

On June 14, 1979, the test exercise was critiqued
by the staff and many problems were brought to light.
Personnel, supplies, vehicles, contracting, and day-to-
day administration and coordination were identified as
matters that needed more attention. A suggestion was
also made that the participation of more outside observers in the critique would help in planning more
realistic exercises.

REFERENCES

Animal Health Division. 1971. Emergency animal
    disease eradication guide. Agric. Res. Serv.,
    USDA, Hyattsville, Md.
Animal Health Yearbook 1974. Rome: FAO/WHO/OIE.
Animal Plant Health Inspection Service. Ca. 1977.
    Training handbook. USDA, Hyattsville, Md.
Arambulo, P. V., III; Steele, J. H.; Beran, G. W.;
    Escudero, S. H., III; and Carey, J. F. 1976.
    Veterinary manpower in the Philippines: Supply,
    demand model and projections, and impact of animal
    diseases on human health. Manuscript. Inst.
    Public Health, Univ. of the Philippines, Manila,
    Philippines.
Bailey, W. S. 1978. Veterinary medicine and compara-
    tive medicine in international health. *Am. J.
    Trop. Med. Hyg.* 27:441-465.
Baker, T. D., and Perlman, M. 1967. Health Manpower
    in a Developing Economy: Taiwan, a Case Study in
    Planning. Baltimore: Johns Hopkins Press.
Blackmore, D. K., and Harris, R. E. 1979. Problems
    related to the formal teaching of veterinary
    epidemiology. In Veterinary Epidemiology and
    Economics. Int. Symp. Vet. Epidemiol. Econ. Proc.
    2:315-318. Canberra: Aust. Gov. Publ. Serv.
Campbell, R. S. F. 1976. Veterinary training for the
    tropics: With particular reference to the
    Australian experience. *World Anim. Rev.* 17:16-21.
Chibuzo, G. A.; Habtemariam, T.; and Carey, J. A.
    1980. A population health program for a school of

veterinary medicine. *J. Am. Vet. Med. Assoc.* 177:1227-1230.

Chrysler, E. 1977. Relationship of veterinary population to total. *J. Am. Vet. Med. Assoc.* 170:405.

Cockrill, R. W. 1964. The profession and the science: International trends in veterinary medicine. In <u>Advances in Veterinary Science</u>, vol. 9, eds. C. A. Brandly and E. L. Jungherr. New York: Academic Press, pp. 251-325.

Emergency Programs. 1979. Narration for Alpha 79 exercise "Nada." Anim. Plant Health Insp. Serv., USDA, Hyattsville, Md.

Goodfield, J. 1977. Humanity in science: A perspective and a plea. *Science* 198:580-585.

Howe, C. 1979. Toward an educational philosophy. *ASM News* 45:642-645.

Humphrey, H. H., chairman. 1961. <u>Veterinary Medical Science and Human Health</u>. Committee on Government Operations, United States Senate. Washington, D.C.: USGPO.

Joint Committee on Veterinary Education. 1975. Veterinary medicine: A national resource and a national responsibility. Am. Vet. Med. Assoc., Chicago, Ill.

Leech, F. B. 1979. What teaching is relevant to veterinary epidemiology? In <u>Veterinary Epidemiology and Economics</u>. Int. Symp. Vet. Epidemiol. Econ. Proc. 2:326-327. Canberra: Aust. Gov. Publ. Serv.

Lyle, W. E., moderator. 1969. The undergraduate, graduate and continuing education needs of diagnostic veterinary medicine. *U.S. Anim. Health Assoc. Proc.* 73:510-527.

McLaughlin, G. W.; Bard, H. E.; and Talbot, R. B. 1976. Veterinary medical manpower: Supply-demand projections to 2020. *J. Am. Vet. Med. Assoc.* 168:319-321.

Miller, E. B. 1979. Nonacademic influences on education of the veterinarian in the United States, 1887-1921. *J. Am. Vet. Med. Assoc.* 175:1106-1110.

Morey, P. E.; Mahan, B. T.; McLaughlin, G. W.; and Montgomery, J. R. 1976. Benefit-cost analysis of Colleges of Veterinary Medicine. *J. Am. Vet. Med. Assoc.* 168:855-857.

Pan American Foot-and-Mouth Disease Center. 1978. Seminar on prevention of exotic animal diseases, Dec. 11-15, Kingston, Jamaica. Rio de Janeiro, Brazil.

————. 1980. Annual Report. Rio de Janeiro, Brazil.

————. 1981. Ejercicio epidemiologico de simulacion

de un brote de fiebre aftosa, May 30–June 6, Rio Grande de Sul, Brazil. Rio de Janeiro, Brazil.

Perkins, D., and Tate, J. 1979. How will you react if . . . foot-and-mouth strikes. *The Cattleman* 65(11):36–43.

Rohde, J. E., and Sadjimin, T. 1980. Teaching epidemiology in developing countries: A field exercise. *Int. J. Epidemiol.* 9:369–373.

Sadler, W. W. 1975. Graduate training in preventive veterinary medicine in the University of California, School of Veterinary Medicine. Univ. of Calif., Davis, Calif.

Schwabe, C. W. 1969. Graduate study for regulatory veterinarians. *U.S. Anim. Health Assoc. Proc.* 73:18–30.

Swann, M. M., chairman. 1975. The committee of inquiry into the veterinary profession. Vol. 1, report; vol. 2, appendices to report. Cmnd. 6143. Her Majesty's Stationery Off., London.

Thrusfield, M. V. 1979. The scope and content of epidemiology courses in veterinary curricula. In Veterinary Epidemiology and Economics. Int. Symp. Vet. Epidemiol. Econ. Proc. 2:303–314. Canberra: Aust. Gov. Publ. Serv.

Veterinary Services. 1974. Avian medicine training course, Jan. 22–29. Anim. Plant Health Insp. Serv., USDA, Hyattsville, Md.

————. Ca. 1976a. Eradication guide for African swine fever. Anim. Plant Health Insp. Serv., USDA, Hyattsville, Md.

————. 1976b. Foreign animal disease training course, Sept. 8–17. Anim. Plant Health Insp. Serv., USDA, Hyattsville, Md.

10

Ongoing Control Programs

OBJECTIVES AND ORGANIZATION

A significant portion of the budget of animal disease control agencies is devoted to activities designed to prevent the introduction and spread of disease through commerce in animals and animal products (Fig. 10.1).

Veterinary medicine, as a discipline separate from human medicine, developed, in part, from the need for professionally trained individuals to establish a national system of border inspection and quarantine that would keep out animals carrying highly contagious diseases (Diamant 1978). The association between commerce and the movement of several important contagious diseases was demonstrated very early, and the use of quarantines and embargoes to stop the movement of disease was fully accepted. Leaders of human medicine lagged far behind veterinarians in their epidemiologic thinking and argued the futility of regulatory control long after its effectiveness for certain diseases had been scientifically proven (Matovinovic 1969; Les Benedict 1970). Regulation began with control over animal importation and was later extended to domestic commerce in animals and eventually animal products (Hendershott 1965; Ellis 1974). Control has been enforced by quarantines and condemnations, permits and licenses, and premise and product inspections. Diagnostic laboratories were established to verify field diagnoses and support condemnation of animals. These laboratories have subsequently become involved with surveys to measure the prevalence of disease (Beal 1975) and the effectiveness of control measures

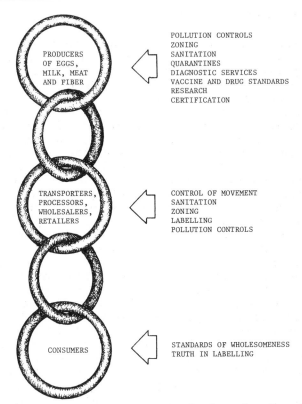

FIG. 10.1. Role of government in the food production chain.

(Organization for European Economic Co-operation 1959;
Ministry of Agriculture, Fisheries and Food 1976).
     Whether all of the regulatory functions relating
to animal disease control are located within a single-
line agency, assigned to separate agencies within an
agricultural ministry (Veterinary Services 1974) (Figs.
7.2 and 7.3), or shared with a ministry of health
varies from country to country for historic reasons.
The basic functions of the regulatory agency may be
classified as (1) supportive, which includes administration and laboratory services; and (2) regulatory,
which includes: (a) border or export-import control,
(b) supervision of livestock shipping and marketing,
(c) inspection of products for human consumption, (d)
licensing and inspection of veterinary biologicals and
drugs, and (e) programs directed to control of specific
diseases.   The last may include certification that
breeding stock or certain regions are free from specific diseases.

DIAGNOSTIC LABORATORY SUPPORT

A fully functional diagnostic service consists of (1) laboratory staff, (2) field investigation staff, and (3) personnel concerned with the maintenance, re- trieval, and analysis of records (Beal 1980).

The diagnostic laboratory plays a major role in disease surveillance (Davies 1979) and is an integral part of programs for the control of disease (Estupinan and Silva 1972; Stabenow and Jara Guillen 1972; Christiansen 1979). The laboratory staff confirms diagnoses based on clinical and epidemiological evi- dence and provides information, unobtainable in any other way, about the animals' past experience with disease. This information helps protect buyers against the false claims of sellers and thereby supports the actions taken by regulatory officials. The laboratory personnel want to know (1) if an animal is a reactor or an animal product is from a reactor, and (2) if the reactor state indicates probable resistance or lack of resistance to reinfection. These two questions imply the need to establish the identity of the agent that causes the reactivity. Consequently, most diagnostic procedures are etiology specific. In contrast, condem- nation of animals and organs is based on pathologic conditions, such as abscesses, fevers, and neoplasms, which may have different causes. Answers about reac- tors are subject to many qualifications. Depending on the disease, the reactor status of an animal may mean that the animal was either once infected and is now free of infection or remains a carrier of the disease. The serologic titer that indicates resistance to one disease may be indicative of susceptibility to another.

Evolution of Diagnostic Tests

Microbiologists and immunologists have devised a great variety of tests to answer questions about the state of infection and resistance to disease. These tests differ in sensitivity, accuracy, time required, cost and, in particular, whether they provide an appro- priate answer for a specific question.

The development of a given test starts in the lab- oratory with the application of an idea, such as the use of a Vero cell culture to measure the quantity of neutralizing antibodies in an animal serum. A host of variables must be understood before the test is useful. To measure antibodies the indicator system must provide a regular overt response, such as the development of virus-induced plaques in the Vero cell culture. Quan-

titative and temporal relationships of the test reagents (i.e., the dilution of virus and serum and the
length of time they should be allowed to interact) must
then be established.

Demonstration that the indicator system works when
the constituents are controlled is only the first step.
In order to interpret the test, the investigator needs
to know how soon the animal developed neutralizing
antibodies after infection and how long this responsiveness was retained after the animal recovered. In
some diseases antibody is retained for years or even
life (Plowright 1968); for others the response is
ephemeral, and the antibody disappears in a few weeks
(Vickers and Hanson 1979). The investigator also needs
to know whether (1) the disease agent is cleared before
antibody develops (Lancaster 1964), (2) the agent continues to persist along with the antibody (Henson et
al. 1969), or (3) the agent persists when antibody is
undetectable (Hotchin 1969). Obviously, a serologic
test for those few diseases in which the last occurs
would be of limited use in a regulatory program. The
answers to the questions just mentioned must be determined for each species of infected animals because
cows, pigs, and chickens may respond differently to a
given agent. Even within the same species, the response of different age cohorts may often be dissimilar
enough to merit further investigation before conclusions are drawn. The investigator must also be aware
that antibody in two- to six-week old animals may have
been received in the colostrum, across the placenta, or
through the yolk (Brandly et al. 1946) and does not
signify an experience with active infection.

After the validity and meaning of the test has
been established in the laboratory with experimental
reagents, field materials should be used. Samples from
a more genetically diverse population, collected and
handled under a variety of environmental conditions,
may have considerable effect on sensitivity and accuracy. At the same time, the test should be carefully
evaluated regarding time and cost factors. Such an
evaluation may show that automation would reduce the
time and decrease the labor costs, or conversion from a
bank of large test tubes to small wells in a plastic
microtiter plate would lessen the quantity of reagents
needed and lower costs significantly. Unfortunately,
any procedural changes may alter the sensitivity of the
test. When alterations must be made, parallel testing
of the original and new procedures is a wise course of
action. For example, during the Newcastle disease
eradication program, the personnel in the laboratory at

San Gabriel, California, ran the new microtiter test and the older tube-type hemagglutination inhibition test in parallel until everyone was satisfied that no loss in sensitivity or accuracy resulted from adopting the faster and cheaper microtiter method (McDaniel and Orsborn 1973).

Diagnosing the Presence of Disease

Officials who direct a task force or an on-going program usually ask their laboratory staff only one question, "Is it positive?" Whether a test result is interpreted as positive or negative depends on the program objective. Isolation of an agent does not necessarily mean that the agent is inducing disease, just as the detection of an antigen may not indicate that the agent possessing the antigen is still infective. Detection of antibody does not indicate when the infection occurred or whether the animal is a carrier, has recovered and is resistant, or is susceptible to reinfection. If the question to be posed is known, it should be answered by use of the most appropriate test so that the responsible regulatory official can be given a meaningful evaluation of the presence of disease. For example, in a situation in which an exotic agent is invading a new region, a single isolation of the agent will be an acceptable positive; however, failure to isolate the agent within a known diseased area is an inadequate basis for deciding that the area is disease free.

Demonstration that carriers are present in a herd, flock, or shipment of animals will result in their devaluation and, often, condemnation. Sometimes the test result will be contested and, consequently, should be defensible in a court of law. To stand challenge (Grumbles et al. 1975), the laboratory should:

1.   Protect the identity of the sample at all times as it moves through the laboratory, regardless of whether it is in storage or under examination. The sample should never be in an inappropriate place.

2.   Maintain in writing the experimental protocol to which the sample is subjected and be certain the protocol is followed.

3.   Determine that the protocol followed is acceptable by other laboratorians as good practice.

4.   Preserve an aliquot of the specimen for retest, if that should be necessary.

5.   Preserve the test records as they have been kept in the laboratory log book. Entries should be

dated and, preferably, signed or initialled by the observer.

Some laboratory directors, at intervals, obtain coded positive and negative samples and have them processed as unknowns. Diagnostians should not object to this practice because it helps identify faulty equipment and reagents as well as irregularities in procedure. Serologists in certain laboratories have exchanged titered serum samples and antigen lots to cross check procedures and materials. Protocols have been improved as a result. These practices, which go beyond the standard positive and negative controls employed in many tests, strengthen the position of the laboratory when any of its results are questioned in court.

False positives appear in most tests at a certain, usually low, frequency. Some are false positives only at the presumptive stage and disappear when the confirmatory test is applied. For example, the isolation in a chicken embryo of a lethal hemagglutinating agent from a suspected case of Newcastle disease can be something other than Newcastle disease virus. The antigen-identity test establishes whether it is or is not.

False positives in serologic tests are sometimes more difficult to establish. While most nonspecific reactive substances in serum are more heat labile than true antibody and are more sensitive to certain other treatments, there are exceptions. In a few instances, investigators have had to demonstrate that a heat-resistant neutralizing substance was not a specific antibody because it was not in the globulin fraction of the serum where true antibody is found (Nakamura and Easterday 1967). This is clearly impractical as a routine test procedure.

An alternative method of recognizing the nonspecificity of substances in serum that mimic antibody has been used in some large-scale serum surveys. For example, Argentina, in collaboration with the Chilean and British governments, conducted an extensive study of the sheep population of the island of Tierra del Fuego (Argentine-United States Joint Commission 1966). The objective was to determine if the island was free of foot-and-mouth disease. It was suspected that even if true antibodies were not detected, some nonspecific reactions would be found that would leave the status of the island unresolved. To determine the allowable frequency and nature of nonspecific reactors in sheep in the tests employed, sera were obtained from a genetically similar sheep population in New Zealand, a country

in the antipodes that has been under close veterinary
inspection for years, and is unquestionably free of
foot-and-mouth disease. The very low frequency of
reactors found in the New Zealand sheep was similar to
the reactor rate in the sheep from Tierra del Fuego.
Furthermore, the old dictum that nonspecific reactors
are not serotype specific was not supported because
most reactors were either A or O, and few reacted to
both antigenic types. Later studies in the United
States, where foot-and-mouth disease does not occur,
showed a similar low frequency of reactors in sera from
cattle (Andersen 1977). These animals were probably
infected with an unknown picornavirus having an antigen
that is cross reactive with that of foot-and-mouth
disease. Numerous examples of such cross reactive
antigens have been documented for both bacteria and
viruses. Nonspecific reactors generally create diagnostic and administrative problems when an eradication
program nears completion. This was particularly true
in the 1950s during the later phases of the tuberculosis eradication program in the United States (Berman et
al. 1959). A similar problem arose when the prevalence
of brucellosis was reduced (Anderson et al. 1962).

Determining the Absence of Disease Agents

Finding a negative may be just as important as
finding a positive. It means that the pathogen, one or
more of its antigens, or its antibody is not present.
However, while a negative test can mean that the pathogen is not or was not present in the animal, it can
also mean that the test was insensitive (Anderson et
al. 1962). Even when the negative test accurately
reflects the status of the tested animal, it may not
reflect the status of the herd. Before reporting a
negative, one needs to know about the sensitivity of
the test (Carmichael 1962) and the adequacy of the
sampling procedure (Shook 1979).
From a regulatory point of view, demonstrating the
negative status of a herd is important in (1) evaluating the progress of an eradication campaign, (2)
establishing the eradication of a disease agent from
the area under quarantine, (3) establishing the suita-
bility of animals to be imported or offered for export,
and (4) certifying the specific pathogen-free status of
animals used for certain purposes. The chief veterinarian of a nation that is a member of the European
Economic Community told the authors that the major endeavor of his agency is demonstrating the absence of
disease. It must be remembered that such a task is

expensive because the cost of detecting disease is
inversely proportional to its frequency (Fig. 10.2).
     Establishing the validity of a negative test de-
pends upon the sensitivity of the test and the nature
of the disease (Hitchner et al. 1975; Cottral 1978).
Isolation of some bacteria and viruses is a relatively
simple problem because the culture system is sensitive,
and if an animal is infected the agent will be found at
certain sites.   Isolation of other bacteria or viruses
is difficult because (1) a sensitive culture system is
not available; (2) the agent is not regularly present,
is hidden at an inaccessible site, or is bound in some
fashion that necessitates special procedures for its
demonstration; and (3) the isolation takes a very long
time.   A negative test for the easy-to-detect group of
agents has considerable significance, but a negative
test for the hard-to-detect group has little meaning.
     Failure to detect antibody in an animal is mean-
ingful for both those diseases in which a carrier state
is always associated with antibody and those in which a
persistent antibody titer follows full recovery. It is
of no value for those diseases that (1) produce a transient antibody response following complete recovery
(Vickers and Hanson 1979), (2) remain persistent or
intermittent carriers after the antibody response
disappears (DeTray 1957; Henson et al. 1969), and (3)
induce no antibody at all (Marsh et al. 1970).

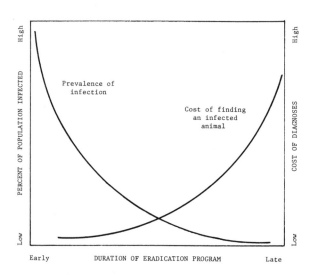

FIG. 10.2.   Inverse relationship of disease prevalence and
cost of detection.

Assuming the test is valid, the animal or herd is placed in quarantine for a period appropriate to the character of the disease. The animal is sampled both at the beginning and end of the quarantine. A negative result at both samplings usually clears the animal or herd for importation or certification (Hejl 1974).

Establishing that the animals of a region are free of a specific disease by securing a set of negative tests is a more complicated matter. Testing every individual is usually economically prohibitive and logistically impossible. The only option is to test materials obtained from a representative number of animals.

Sampling a large population in a truly random fashion that would give every individual an equal chance to be selected presumes an exact knowledge of the population and the existence of a scheme of animal identification that has not yet been developed. In addition, such a sampling would pose major logistic problems. Sampling randomly selected herds is sometimes possible. Such random selection generally takes place within a population that has first been stratified, usually on a geographical basis. After the region is divided into districts and the districts into areas, one of the areas in each district is chosen for testing. Either all or a random sample of the herds in the selected areas is then tested. Logistically and administratively, this method of sampling is easy to manage because travel is reduced and education programs can be pinpointed to participants (Shook 1979).

Whatever sampling methods are used (Leech and Sellers 1979), characteristics of the sample should be compared with characteristics of the total population to determine whether the sample is representative in terms of such epidemiologically significant characters as herd size, age structure, and animal management (open versus closed herds; confined versus range animals).

The size of the sample is determined by the size of the error one is willing to accept, a large sample having the smallest error and a small sample having the largest (Nordskog et al. 1961). However, the frequency with which reactors occur in the population must be considered. Reactor rate is a disease-determined characteristic that approaches 100 percent for some diseases but is closer to 1 percent for others. Obviously, a relatively small sample, such as 1 in 50, is more likely to reveal disease in the first instance than a large sample, such as 1 in 5, in the latter.

Tables by the APHIS staff have been developed to illustrate this problem.

Serum Banks

A set of sera or other biological material that
can be used in biological tests is a valuable resource
if it was obtained from an animal population by a sampling method that permits generalization of test results
to the population (Committee on Sampling Techniques
1954; Leech 1971). However, the cost of materials,
travel, and personnel required to amass such a set is
causing administrators to give increasing attention to
developing repositories, such as serum banks that not
only permit several studies to be conducted on a given
sample (St George 1979; Timbs 1979) but also provide
better utilization of centers, such as abattoirs where
samples can be automatically collected (Van Ness 1966;
Christiansen and Hellstrom 1979). Serum banks make it
possible for investigators to obtain a perspective
concerning the changes in prevalence and incidence of
diseases, a particularily important point in establishing whether a newly recognized disease was recently
introduced.

ANALYSIS OF DIAGNOSTIC AND FIELD REPORTS

Most regulatory services have given inadequate
attention to the establishment of a system of recall
(an institutional memory of the laboratory diagnoses
and field studies that have been conducted) that would
provide a temporal and geographic picture of the pattern and movement of disease (Hugh-Jones 1972; Davies
1979; Jackson 1979). Files of reports obtained at
great cost in terms of labor and funds lay unused.
Plotting the monthly reports of foot-and-mouth disease
cases in South America on coordinates by hand (Fig.
2.3) clearly shows patterns in the periodic surges of
that virus and enables the epidemiology staff to predict regions at risk. However, if a series of variables are to be analyzed, computer services provide the
only feasible approach to data management (Hugh-Jones
et al. 1969; Christiansen 1979; Roe 1979; Willeberg
1979). Problems encountered with the implementation of
an automated collection system (Ray 1980) can be avoided only by careful planning and training of staff prior
to its initiation and assurance that the staff will
have uninterrupted access to the system.

CONTROL OF ANIMAL MOVEMENT

Mechanisms of Control

A major part of regulatory veterinary medicine concerns the control of animal movement (Cockrill 1963; *Journal American Veterinary Association* 1976). Most governments require that animals moving from one political jurisdiction to another must be accompanied by a permit certifying that each individual animal was not only healthy at the point of origin but that it had been tested and found either free of specified diseases or had received any required course of vaccination (Anderson 1965). These records permit tracing animals that are subsequently found to be diseased to the point of origin (Fig. 10.3). In many instances, dealers who engage in the purchase and sale of animals, particularly if they transport and house them, may be allowed to ply their trade only if they are licensed. Movement of animals across an international border is more difficult than between states and provinces and regulations often require that the animals spend a period in a government-operated or supervised quarantine station where the animals are inspected and tested (Food and Agriculture Organization 1956; Hejl 1974). If a highly communicable disease appears, a quarantine is established around the diseased area to stop animal traffic and contain the disease within the smallest possible political jurisdiction. Nations may establish an embargo against a diseased neighbor who adjoins them to avoid possible introduction into their territory. Within the quarantined area the government can confiscate and destroy animals in order to eliminate the foci of infection. In all countries these procedures are detailed in regulations backed by enabling legislation, and opposition carries significant penalities.

Control of the movement of diseased animals is based on the integrity of individuals who engage in commerce and conduct the inspections that are required. Independent surveillance of the market process is obtained by such procedures as the use of back tags on market cattle so their origin can be traced (Christenberry 1979). Even pathogens can be traced through new techniques. For example, nucleic acid fingerprints of virus from an outbreak of foot-and-mouth disease were found to match those of a virus used in a vaccine, a finding that incriminated the vaccine as the cause of the outbreak (Brooksby 1981). The same method was used to convict a quarantine station operator of illegally moving birds infected with Newcastle disease (McMillan and Hanson 1982).

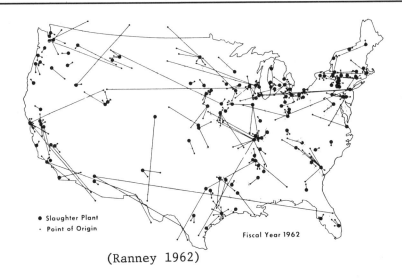

(Ranney 1962)

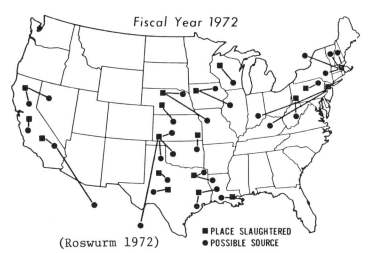

(Roswurm 1972)   ■ PLACE SLAUGHTERED
                      ● POSSIBLE SOURCE

FIG. 10.3.   Traceback of tubercular cattle from slaughter-
house to farm of origin.

Movement within a Political Jurisdiction

Regional movement of diseased livestock and poultry is largely regulated by establishing conditions of
sale.   In countries having tuberculosis and brucellosis
control programs, cattle must not only be identified by
their farm of origin but also marked to indicate their
reactor status (Ranney 1962).   This status determines

whether they can be sold as breeders, for slaughter only, or depending upon inspection, for use as human food or rendering. Permanent identification of animals by ear tags, back tags, tattoos, or responding devices is compulsory in some regions. Such regulations permit officials to trace an animal back to its herd of origin if it is discovered to be diseased after entering the market channel (Trade and Consumer Protection 1978, 1979; Watt 1979). There is increasing interest in universal animal identification systems that are inexpensive and not subject to tampering.

International Movement

All nations exercise control over animals that cross their borders (Peisley 1961; Fiennes 1964; Smith 1969). This control may include point-of-origin inspection and testing of animals to be imported and supervision of their assembly and transport (Wells et al. 1963; Swindle 1979). Regulations also usually include government-controlled or supervised quarantine in the vicinity of the port of entry for a prescribed period (Conn 1967; Hejl 1974; Pan American Health Organization 1978; Peterson 1979; Veterinary Services ca. 1979). Sometimes, release from quarantine is subject to an additional inspection. Imported animals are not all treated the same (Wells 1965) (Tables 10.1 and 10.2). Animals from countries whose regulatory systems and disease situation are similar to that of the importing country may receive only a cursory examination and move to market without quarantine.

Facilities for holding animals in quarantine near major seaports have existed for many years. However, important changes have taken place in animal movement over the past several decades (Pierce 1975). One factor has been the shift from slow-moving ocean ships to fast-moving transport planes that can land at any international airport. Other factors have been the growing pressure by livestock growers to obtain exotic blood lines for breeding programs and the pressure by importers to obtain exotic wild animals for game preserves and the expanding demand by an affluent society for unusual household pets, particularly birds.

In the 1960s, Canada refurbished a facility on an island in the St. Lawrence River that had been used to train staff to handle exotic diseases, into a center for importing cattle from European countries in which foot-and-mouth disease existed (Wells 1965). Although some cattle for the United States came through this center, pressure for a station in the United States

Table 10.1. U.S. Quarantine Regulations for Imported Animals

Category	Preentry Requirements	Entry Requirements
From countries free of exotic disease		
Livestock and poultry	None	Port inspection
Fish, reptiles, mammals, nonpsitta- cine birds	None	Port inspection
From countries with exotic disease present		
Ruminant livestock	Isolation, testing in approved stations	USDA Fleming Key quaran- tine facility
Poultry, horses, swine	None	USDA-supervised quarantine facility
Wild birds, wild mammals	Approved treatment for psittacines	USDA-supervised quarantine facility
Fish, reptiles	None	Port inspection

Table 10.2. U.S. Regulations for Imported Livestock and Poultry Products

Category	Preentry Requirements	Entry Requirements
From countries free of exotic disease		
All products	Port inspection	None
From countries with exotic disease present		
Canned meats	Port inspection	None
Products consigned to manufacturer	Port inspection	Processed products only are released
Fresh and frozen meat, eggs, milk	Total ban	

mounted. In 1979 the United States government dedica-
ted the elaborate Harry S. Truman Animal Quarantine
Center on Fleming Key off the southern tip of Florida
(Veterinary Services ca. 1979). The interest of stock-
men had changed while the center was being built, and
rather than handling European cattle as had been
anticipated, the first cattle processed through the
center came from South America. Australia is in the
process of developing a similar importation center on a
peninsula south of Melbourne.

Prior to 1972 many species of birds were imported
into the United States without being subjected to any
quarantine. However, the introduction of Newcastle
disease through this traffic (Fig. 10.4) resulted in
the requirements that all birds not classified as
poultry should be quarantined and enter either through
government facilities or government supervised, privately operated quarantine stations (Peterson 1979).
In 1979 an investigating panel looked at problems in
the privately operated stations and recommended, with
the subsequent support of several veterinary-livestock
associations, that all birds enter the country only
through federally operated quarantine facilities. An
expedient solution in the face of budgeting restraint,
such as the authorization of privately operated quarantine stations, invariably has many unanticipated manifestations. Such actions should be closely monitored
and reevaluated.

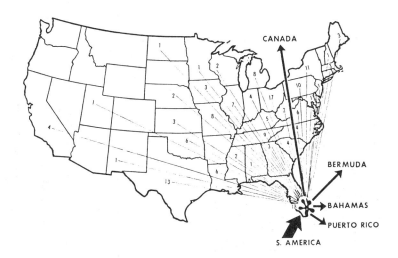

FIG. 10.4. Interstate movement of birds from the facilities
of an importer (Walker et al. 1973).

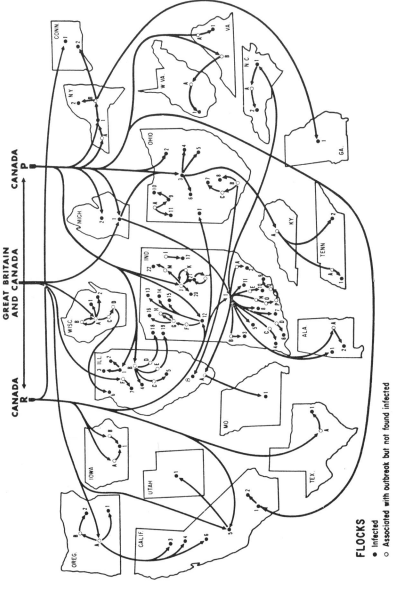

FLOCKS

● Infected
○ Associated with outbreak but not found infected

FIG. 10.5. Spread of scrapie through the movement of sheep incubating the disease (Hourrigan et al. 1979).

The strategy of regulatory veterinary medicine is to permit the movement of healthy animals and stop the movement of diseased animals. If all diseases were overt and all traders forthright, the job would be relatively easy. The requirements for animal identification, laboratory tests, complex regulations, and close government supervision of certain operations are necessitated by the latency of disease (Fig. 10.5) and the devious ways of some dealers. The introduction of new technology, such as frozen semen and ova transplants is making the assessment of hazards even more difficult.

Certification of animals for export and status as specific-pathogen free requires that the animal or herd be isolated for a predetermined period, kept under surveillance, and subjected to specified tests. The exact procedure, defined by regulations that depend on the stated objective, may require that the animals have remained clinically healthy and free of specific antibodies during the quarantine period and also that they have been systematically sampled for isolation of selected pathogens. In addition, the procedure may require that cattle from countries infected with foot-and-mouth disease be quarantined for a period in the country of export where they must be free of antibodies to foot-and-mouth disease before they can be considered for import (Veterinary Services ca. 1979). When such animals arrive at the quarantine station in the United States, they are subjected to probang sampling for live virus and allowed to mingle with susceptible animals. If the probang sample is negative and the susceptible animals remain clinically healthy and antibody free, the shipment of cattle can be admitted.

Exotic birds that are trapped in the wild and offered for U.S. importation are handled differently. No preshipment examination is required but the birds are systematically sampled during quarantine in the U.S. All live birds are swabbed cloacally, and all birds dying of any cause are submitted to the virus laboratory for attempted virus isolation. The detection of any exotic poultry pathogen in any bird in the shipment results in rejection of the entire shipment.

INSPECTION OF PRODUCTS FROM AND FOR ANIMALS

A set of laws and a large body of regulations have been established to insure that animal products used in human and animal nutrition are safe and wholesome (Payton 1966; Baker 1973). A similar set has been devised to insure the safety, purity, and efficacy of products used in animals as vaccines, reagents, or drugs. To insure compliance, the government has established inspection of premises involved in the production and processing of these products as well as random sampling and testing of the products offered for sale to determine whether they meet the minimum standards. Most regulations covering sanitary codes for specific enterprises are based on what is considered to be good practice. The permits and licenses that producers and processors must have may be revoked if violations are found. Most of these regulations deal with factors important in the control of disease.

Food of Animal Origin

Regulations distinguish between milk produced for the fluid milk trade (bottled and sold fresh) and milk used for manufacturing purposes (production of cheese, ice cream, canned and dried milk). More stringent standards are required for fluid milk. Dairies supplying fluid milk are subjected to onsite inspections that determine degree of compliance with the sanitary code (Fig. 10.6). The code covers sanitation of equipment for milking and milk cooling, cleanliness of the barn

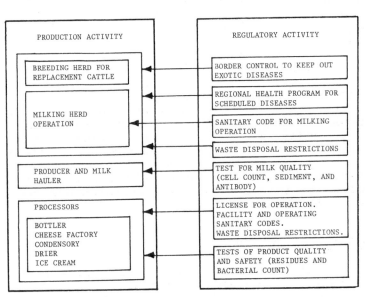

FIG. 10.6. Regulatory activities relating to milk production and manufacture.

or milking parlor, condition of the water supply, and disposal of human waste. Disease status of the herd is determined. The milk undergoes regular tests, at the farm and when it arrives at the milk plant, for the bacterial count and somatic cell count or its chemical equivalent that indicates the presence of mastitis and for the presence of adulterants such as antibiotics or other drugs. Additional specific tests, such as the ring test for presence of brucellosis, may also be conducted. The processing plant in which milk is bottled or subjected to a manufacturing process is also inspected for violations of the sanitary code. Milk that does not meet minimum requirements is downgraded or discarded and producers and processors are informed of noncompliance. Repeated noncompliance may result in government closure of the operation.

Meat packers and poultry processors are subjected to on-line carcass inspection by trained individuals who are either veterinarians or under the supervision of a veterinarian (Food and Agriculture Organization 1974). Special inspection is required of meat products that are imported (Hejl 1976) (Table 10.2). A carcass or part of a carcass can be rejected for lesions (abscesses, tumors, discolorations) and unwholesome appearance. Rejected material is usually rendered (subjected to high temperature processing that inactivates any pathogenic organism). If rejected material is suspected of containing certain pathogenic microorganisms or unwholesome chemicals, it is buried or incinerated. Specimens may be taken by the inspector for laboratory examination by pathological, microbiological, or chemical procedures, and the carcasses can be held pending laboratory findings.

Packing and processing plants are also subjected to inspection of the premises for violations of the sanitary code, particularly the water supply and adequacy of sanitary waste disposal. Adequacy of pasteurizing or canning temperatures and integrity of equipment and containers used in packaging the product are among the things examined. Training and experience of the staff are reviewed.

Feed of Animal Origin

The inedible portion of animal carcasses and animal carcasses condemned as diseased are processed in rendering plants where heating and grinding procedures produce (1) bone meal, (2) meat meal or scrap, and (3) oils and fats for manufacturing uses. The bone meal and meat meal produced by rendering plants that operate in an approved fashion are free of disease pathogens and may be safely used to supply mineral and protein in animal diets. Unfortunately, disease has often been traced to bone meal or meat scraps that has been inadequately processed to eliminate disease or recontaminated after processing. The cost of disease induced by such products can be very high. For example, steamed bone meal that had been contaminated with anthrax in shipment was fed to livestock on thousands of midwest farms and caused widespread mortality (Van Ness 1971). During inspection of the rending plant and its grounds, special attention is given to adequacy of segregation of processed and unprocessed materials to avoid recontamination and also to the operation of equipment to insure proper grinding and heating of the product. Random samples of a product may be examined to verify compliance with sanitary standards. The government also has a responsibility to see that animal feed sold interstate is free of drugs, antibiotics, or toxic chemicals (*Federal Register* 1972) that would contaminate meat, milk, or eggs if fed to livestock or poultry.

Biological and Pharmaceutical Products for Animals

Vaccines, sera, and some drugs are produced in animals and from animal substances. These products may be used in thousands of animals throughout a country and sometimes in foreign countries as well. Records show many instances in which biologicals were inadvertently contaminated with pathogens and served as vehicles to spread disease and, on occasion, were the means of introducing disease to a region or country. For example, foot-and-mouth disease virus was introduced into the United States on two occasions by importation of contaminated cultures of vaccinia virus for use in human vaccine.

Vaccines are largely produced in chicken embryos, in cell cultures, or on artificial media, and this information is indicated on the label or in the instructions accompanying the vaccine. However, the purchaser may not know that other animal products, such as bovine or swine trypsin, fetal calf or lamb serum, fetal extract from chicken embryos, bovine albumin hydrolysate, and beef protein extract, are used in the production of biologicals. During World War II, human serum used in the preparation of yellow fever vaccine introduced human hepatitis into military and civilian populations that received the vaccine (Fox et al.

1942). Trypsin and embryo extracts have introduced mycoplasmas into avian vaccines, and in-plant contamination has introduced Newcastle disease virus into avian pox vaccines (Zargar and Pomeroy 1950; Johnson et al. 1954). Mammalian cell cultures and chicken embryos containing endogenous viruses have spread lymphocytic choriomeningitis and avian leukosis (Burmester et al. 1956), and swine serum has spread pseudorabies to swine receiving simultaneous serum-virus for hog cholera (McNutt and Alice 1942).

Inspection of biological houses is directed to adequacy of their facilities, segregation of specific operations (separation of the production of one product from that of another and separation of experimentation from production) (Allan et al. 1973), and adequacy of training of the staff. The inspection also includes examination for irregularities of protocols that the staff are required to keep of production serials (Fig. 10.7). Inspectors may be required to take samples of the final product for examination by a federal laboratory for purity, safety, and efficacy (Johnson and Van Houweling 1963).

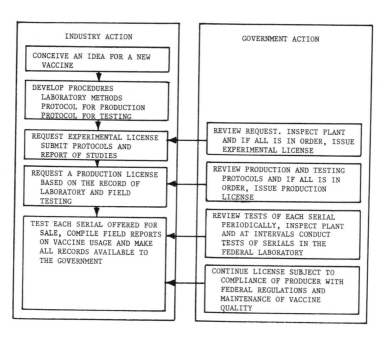

FIG. 10.7. Vaccine development, production, and evaluation.

REGULATION OF PRACTICES THAT RELATE TO CONTROL

Professional Practices

In certain fields of practice that involve human
health and welfare, the government retains the right to
insure competence standards by issuing a conditional
license to practice a profession or produce a product.
The license can be revoked if standards are not maintained. Veterinary medicine, like human medicine, is
regulated by licensing boards that issue a license
based upon proof of professional training in approved
schools and the passing of examinations conducted by
the board (Hannah 1979). Many other service groups
that have a role in disease control, such as spray
applicators and well drillers, are also licensed.

Commercial Practices

Companies must obtain a license to operate a plant
that produces vaccines as well as special licenses for
each vaccine produced. Importers need a license to
operate as an international trader, a license to operate an importation station, and a permit for each
importation.

Sanitary codes are based on federal, state, and
local regulations and are enforced through inspection
and a system of permits. Any change in waste disposal
requires a permit. Erection of a new building or major
remodeling of an old structure requires a permit. Permits may also be required to burn or bury wastes or use
aerial sprays.

This complicated system of controls has been
created to protect the public from actions by exploi-
tive businesses and aggressive neighbors who do not
care about the long-term consequences of their activities. Regulation is favored by consumer protection
groups, and even though most industrialists fear overregulation, they agree that complete deregulation may
be undesirable.

Regulations should be reviewed periodically to
evaluate their usefulness in terms of scientific knowledge and current objectives as well as the economic
impact of their continuation or termination.

When developing regulations it should always be
kept in mind that they (Anderson 1966; Kirk 1966) can
benefit or harm the producer and/or the consumer. The
outcome is determined partly by the new regulation itself, partly by the constellation of rules into which

it is placed, and partly by the rigor of enforcement
and the interpretation of the enforcing authorities.
Because of these interactions, regulations can limit
the options of both the producer and consumer far more
than the proponents of the new rule envisioned.
Furthermore, a regulation can be used to intimidate
competitors. For example, a producer might rush publication of preliminary and unsubstantiated evidence that
a chemical to be used by a competitor in a new product
has carcinogenic properties. Refutation can cost more
in delay and money than the competitor can afford, and
the new product is dropped. Consumers should be concerned when the regulatory process becomes a major
deterrent to innovation and thus deprives them of useful drugs or vaccines. The choice should not be, as
some protagonists claim, between no regulation and
stifling overregulation. Instead, costs and benefits
of each new regulation should be weighed and a balance
reached between the safety gained and the options lost.
Table 10.3 illustrates the complexity and costs involved in developing a new product for livestock and the
kinds of regulatory hurdles that must be cleared. For
example, the developers of Sevin spent seven years and
$2.5 million before the insecticide even reached the
market (Wellman 1966). Although most producers agree
that the objectives behind each requirement are good,
the time, cost, and uncertainties of completing the
process have slowed and discouraged innovation. When
new regulations are proposed or old ones modified, some
procedure for evaluation is needed that views the
entire process and considers ways of introducing
simplifications.

CERTIFICATION AND GRADING

Industry has solicited product examination that
leads to certification. The oldest example of certification for disease control is the pullorum certification program (Zamberg and Lancaster 1977) that was
instituted over 50 years ago in the United States. In
this program, flocks of cooperating chicken breeders
are randomly tested using a serologic technique to detect disease carriers (Van Roekel 1931). Using these
results, the flocks are certified at several points on
a scale from free to controlled, and the rating is used
in merchandising hatched chicks. The program has reduced disease in the flocks, protected the customer,
and rewarded the cooperating producer.
Currently, programs are under study that would

Table 10.3. Development of a New Insecticide, Antibiotic, Antiviral, or Antiparasitic Drug

Developmental Steps Undertaken by the Entrepreneur	Performance Criteria Established by the Government
Define the need for a new product	
Synthesize or search for the chemical needed	
Screen possible chemicals for desired activity	
Test promising chemicals in the prospective host species against the target organism	Determine effective dosage Determine margin of safety Determine environmental limitations Determine incompatibilities with other drugs Determine persistence in the environment Determine possible induction of resistance
Study toxicology	Do metabolic studies Determine effect of low dosages over long periods Test in individuals of high risk (pregnant females) Determine carcinogenic effects
Obtain a patent on the product or the process by which it is made	
Formulate useful products	
Register the product and obtain a government-accepted label	Register the chemical for safety and effectiveness Have the risk of residues in the food defined Consult other agencies as prescribed
Conduct a market survey on which to plan production facilities	
Proceed with product development (formulation, packaging, storage life)	
Solve the problem of transferring manufacture from the pilot plant to full-scale production	
Conduct a study of production and marketing alternatives	
Finance and construct production facilities	
Test market the product	
Initiate production and sales	Submit samples for random testing

certify specific pathogen-free-status for breeders who
supply eggs to biologics manufacturers and laboratory
animals to research institutions. Similar programs for
breeders of swine and some other species are also being
promoted. Certification programs are voluntary endeavors to control certain diseases that can be transmitted
through breeding stock.

   Although the grading of meat and eggs provides a
guide to the consumer regarding certain qualities of
the product, it has little significance in terms of
disease control.

REFERENCES

Allan, W. H.; Lancaster, J. E.; and Toth, B. 1973.
    The Production and Use of Newcastle Disease
    Vaccines. Rome: FAO.
Andersen, A. A. 1977. Cross reactions of normal
    bovine serums with foot-and-mouth disease virus.
    U.S. Anim. Health Assoc. Proc. 81:264-269.
Anderson, R. J. 1965. United States policy on live-
    stock imports. Paper read at 2nd Annu. Charolais
    Congr., Oct. 16, Kansas City, Mo.
————. 1966. Official registration of pesticides.
    In Scientific Aspects of Pest Control. NAS-NRC
    Publ. 1402. Washington, D.C., pp. 385-391.
Anderson, R. K.; Pietz, D. E.; Nelson, C. J.;
    Kimberling, C. V.; and Werring, D. F. 1962.
    Epidemiologic studies of bovine brucellosis in
    problem herds in Minnesota. U.S. Livest. Sanit.
    Assoc. Proc. 66:109-118.
Argentine-United States Joint Commission on Foot-and-
    Mouth Disease. 1966. Studies on Foot-and-Mouth
    Disease. NAS-NRC Publ. 1343. Washington, D.C.
Baker, E. D. 1973. Report of the committee on meat
    and poultry hygiene. U.S. Anim. Health Assoc.
    Proc. 77:138-140.
Beal, V. C., Jr. 1975. The cost-benefit aspects of
    various types of animal disease monitoring
    activities. In Animal Disease Monitoring, eds.
    D. G. Ingram, W. R. Mitchell, and S. W. Martin.
    Springfield, Ill.: Charles C. Thomas, pp. 72-79.
————. 1980. Recordkeeping systems and computer ap-
    plications in disease prevention and control with
    emphasis on having a valid purpose for their exis-
    tence. Paper read at Work Conf. Teachers Prev.
    Med., Epidemiol., Public Health, Feb. 4-6, Fort
    Worth, Tex.
Berman, D. T.; Tervola, C. A.; and Erdmann, A. A.

1959.   Preliminary report of investigations of
tuberculin sensitivity in Wisconsin cattle.   *U.S.*
Livest. Sanit. Assoc. Proc. 63:197-204.
Brandly, C. A.; Moses, H. E.; and Jungherr, E. L.
1946.   Transmission of antiviral activity via the
egg and the role of congenital passive immunity to
Newcastle disease in chickens. *Am. J. Vet. Res.*
7:333-342.
Brooksby, J. B.   1981.   Tracing outbreaks of foot-and-
mouth disease. *Nature* 293:431-432.
Burmester, B. R.; Cunningham, C. H.; Cottral, G. E.;
Belding, R. C.; and Gentry, R. F.   1956.   The
transmission of visceral lymphomatosis with live
virus Newcastle disease vaccines. *Am. J. Vet. Res.*
17:283-289.
Carmichael, L. E.   1962.   Factors that influence the
neutralization test.   *U.S. Livest. Sanit. Assoc.*
Proc. 66:59-70.
Christenberry, C. C.   1979.   Traceback.   Paper read at
Conf. Concepts Tech. Control Erad. Anim. Dis.,
Sept. 10-14, Auburn, Ala.
Christiansen, K. H.   1979.   Laboratory management and
disease surveillance information system.   In
Veterinary Epidemiology and Economics.   Int. Symp.
Vet. Epidemiol. Econ. Proc. 2:59-64.   Canberra:
Aust. Gov. Publ. Serv.
Christiansen, K. H., and Hellstrom, J. S.   1979.   The
collection of data from New Zealand abattoirs and
slaughterhouses.   In Veterinary Epidemiology and
Economics.   Int. Symp. Vet. Epidemiol. Econ. Proc.
2:168-176. Canberra: Aust. Gov. Publ. Serv.
Cockrill, W. R.   1963.   The changing status of animal
quarantine. *Br. Vet. J.* 119:338-349.
Committee on Sampling Techniques. 1954. On the use of
sampling in the field of public health.   *Am. J.*
Public Health 44:719-740.
Conn, E.   1967.   Organization and regulations for quar-
antine establishments set up in northern Ireland
for the sanitary control of importations and
exportations of animals and products of animal
origin. *Bull. Off. Int. Epizoot.* 68:331-337.
Cottral, G. E., ed.   1978.   Manual of Standardized
Methods for Veterinary Microbiology.   Ithaca, N.Y.:
Cornell Univ. Press.
Davies, G.   1979.   Animal disease surveillance.   In
Veterinary Epidemiology and Economics.   Int. Symp.
Vet. Epidemiol. Econ. Proc. 2:3-10.   Canberra:
Aust. Gov. Publ. Serv.
DeTray, D. E.   1957.   Persistence of viremia and
immunity in African swine fever. *Am. J. Vet. Res.*
18:811-816.

Diamant, G. 1978. Regulatory veterinary medicine: And they blew a horn in Judea. *J. Am. Vet. Med. Assoc.* 172:45-54.

Ellis, P. R. 1974. The development of animal health services. *Agric. Adm.* 1:199-219.

Estupinan, J. A., and Silva, O. M. 1972. The animal diagnostic service in Colombia. *Boletin de la Oficina Sanitaria Panamericana* 6(3):69-76.

Federal Register. 1972. Antibiotic and sulfonamide drugs in animal feeds. 37(21):2444-2445.

Fiennes, R. N. T. W. 1964. Animal disease and quarantine regulations. *Bull. Epizoot. Dis. Africa* 12:93-96.

Food and Agriculture Organization. 1956. Report of the meeting on the appraisal of quarantine regulations for the importation and exportation of livestock, Feb. 13-17, FAO, Paris.

Food and Agriculture Organization. 1974. <u>Manual on Standards of Veterinary Services, Meat Hygiene and Meat Inspection, Post-mortem Judgement of Slaughter Animals and Establishment of Specific Disease-free Zones.</u> Rome: FAO.

Fox, J. P.; Manso, C.; Penna, H. A.; and Para, M. 1942. Observations on the occurrence of icterus in Brazil following vaccination against yellow fever. *Am. J. Hyg.* 36:68-116.

Grumbles, L. C.; Bankowski, R. A.; Beard, C. W.; and Hanson, R. P. 1975. Report of special committee to evaluate veterinary services diagnostic virology laboratory: Ames, Iowa. Anim. Plant Health Insp. Serv., USDA, Hyattsville, Md. (Internal document.)

Hannah, H. W. 1979. Professional licensing under siege. *J. Am. Vet. Med. Assoc.* 175:1162.

Hejl, J. M. 1974. Fleming Key animal import center. *Fed. Regist.* 39(42), FR Doc. 74-4875.

————. 1976. Importation of meat and meat products from countries infected with certain animal diseases: Clarification and relief of restrictions; importation of test samples. Anim. Plant Health Insp. Serv., USDA, Washington, D.C., Apr. 6.

Hendershott, R. A. 1965. The history of regulatory veterinary medicine in the United States. *U.S. Livest. Sanit. Assoc. Proc.* 69:1-6.

Henson, J. B.; Gorham, J. R.; Kobayashi, K.; and McGuire, T. C. 1969. Immunity in equine infectious anemia. *J. Am. Vet. Med. Assoc.* 155:336-343.

Hitchner, S. B.; Domermuth, C. H.; Purchase, H. G.; and Williams, J. E., eds. 1975. <u>Isolation and Identification of Avian Pathogens.</u> Ithaca, N.Y.: Am. Assoc. Avian Pathol.

Hotchin, J. 1969. Lymphocytic choriomeningitis virus. In International Virology, vol. 1, ed. J. L. Melnick. Basel: S. Karger, pp. 109-112.

Hourrigan, J.; Klingsporn, A.; Clark, W. W.; and de Camp, M. 1979. Epidemiology of scrapie in the United States. In Slow Transmissible Diseases of the Nervous System, vol. 1, eds. S. B. Prusiner and W. J. Hadlow. New York: Academic Press, pp. 331-356.

Hugh-Jones, M. E. 1972. Causes of death diagnosed during 1971 at veterinary investigation centres in Great Britain. Paper read at World Assoc. Buiatrics Congr., July 31, London.

Hugh-Jones, M. E.; Ivory, D. W.; Loosmore, R. M.; and Gibbins, J. 1969. Veterinary investigation diagnosis analyses: A system of information recording and retrieval for Veterinary Diagnostic Laboratory in the Ministry of Agriculture, Fisheries, and Food. *Vet. Rec.* 84:304-307.

Jackson, C. A. W. 1979. The value of serological surveillance of disease in intensive poultry production. In Veterinary Epidemiology and Economics. Int. Symp. Vet. Epidemiol. Econ. Proc. 2:81-86. Canberra: Aust. Gov. Publ. Serv.

Johnson, E. P.; Hanson, R. P.; Rosenwald, A. S.; and Van Roekel, H. 1954. The responsibility of state and federal agencies in the improvement of poultry vaccines. *J. Am. Vet. Med. Assoc.* 125:441-446.

Johnson, G. O., and Van Houweling, C. D. 1963. Veterinary biologics: A summary of product, methods of examination, and testing results. *U.S. Livest. Sanit. Assoc. Proc.* 67:58-69.

Journal of the American Veterinary Medical Association. 1976. Poultry health committee urges tighter import regulations. 169:1292.

Kirk, J. K. 1966. Role of the Food and Drug Administration in regulation of pesticides. In Scientific Aspects of Pest Control. NAS-NRC Publ. 1402. Washington, D.C, pp. 392-398.

Lancaster, J. E. 1964. Newcastle disease-control by vaccination. *Vet. Bull.* 34:57-76.

Leech, F. B. 1971. A critique of the methods and results of the British national surveys of disease in farm animals. I. Discussion of the surveys. *Br. Vet. J.* 127:511-522.

Leech, F. B., and Sellers, K. C. 1979. Statistical Epidemiology in Veterinary Science. New York: Macmillan Publ. Co., Inc.

Les Benedict, M. 1970. Contagion and the Constitution: Quarantine agitation from 1859 to 1866. *J. Hist. Med.* 25:177-193.

McDaniel, H. A., and Orsborn, J. S., Jr. 1973. Diagnosis of velogenic viscerotropic Newcastle disease. *J. Am. Vet. Med. Assoc.* 163:1075-1079.

McMillian, B. C., and Hanson, R. P. 1982. Differentiation of exotic strains of Newcastle disease virus by oligonucleotide fingerprinting. *Avian Dis.* 26:332-339.

McNutt, S. H., and Alice, F. J. 1942. Doenca de Aujeszky (pseudoraiva) em suinos. *Bol. Soc. Brasil Med. Vet.* 11(3):61-66.

Marsh, R. F.; Pan, I. C.; and Hanson, R. P. 1970. Failure to demonstrate specific antibody in transmissible mink encephalopathy. *Infect. Immun.* 2:727-730.

Matovinovic, J. 1969. A short history of quarantine. *Univ. Mich. Med. Cent. J.* 35:224-228.

Ministry of Agriculture, Fisheries, and Food. 1976. Animal disease surveillance in Great Britain: The report of a MAFF working party, 1975-76. Weybridge, UK.

Nakamura, R. M., and Easterday, B. C. 1967. Serological studies of influenza in animals. *Bull. WHO* 37:559-567.

Nordskog, A. W.; David, H. T.; and Eisenberg, H. B. 1961. Optimum sample size in animal disease control. *Biometrics* 17:617-625.

Organization for European Economic Co-operation. 1959. Livestock diseases and the organization of veterinary services in Europe. Documentation in Food and Agriculture, 1959 Ser. 5.

Pan American Health Organization. 1978. Animal quarantine stations in the Americas. 11th Inter-Am. Meet. Foot-and-Mouth Dis. Zoonoses Control, Apr. 11-14, Washington, D.C.

Payton, J. 1966. The role of meat inspection in public health. *U.S. Livest. Sanit. Assoc. Proc.* 70:376-395.

Peisley, H. R. 1961. The development of the animal quarantine service of the commonwealth of Australia. *Aust. Vet. J.* 37:243-252.

Peterson, I. L. 1979. Background materials for Newcastle disease review group: Bird quarantine stations. Anim. Plant Health Insp. Serv., USDA, Hyattsville, Md.

Pierce, A. E. 1975. An historical review of animal movement, exotic disease and quarantine in New Zealand and Australia. *NZ Vet. J.* 23:125-136.

Plowright, W. 1968. Rinderpest virus. *Virol. Monogr.* 3:25-110.

Ranney, A. F. 1962. The status of state-federal

bovine tuberculosis eradication. *U.S. Livest. Sanit. Assoc. Proc.* 66:193-203.

Ray, W. C. 1980. Recordkeeping and computer application. Paper read at Work Conf. Teachers Prev. Med., Epidemiol., Public Health, Feb. 4-6, Fort Worth, Tex.

Roe, R. T. 1979. Features of the Australian national animal disease information system. In Veterinary Epidemiology and Economics. Int. Symp. Vet. Epidemiol. Econ. Proc. 2:26-34. Canberra: Aust. Gov. Publ. Serv.

Roswurm, J. D. 1972. The status of the state-federal tuberculosis eradication program. *U.S. Anim. Health Proc.* 76:412-422.

St George, T. D. 1979. The technology and application of sentinel herds and serum banks. In Veterinary Epidemiology and Economics. Int. Symp. Vet. Epidemiol. Econ. Proc. 2:69-75. Canberra: Aust. Gov. Publ. Serv.

Shook, J. C. 1979. Field and laboratory diagnosis in disease control and eradication. Paper read at Conf. Concepts Tech. Control and Erad. Anim. Dis., Sept. 10-14, Auburn, Ala.

Smith, C. A. 1969. Protecting the United States against foreign animal diseases. *J. Am. Vet. Med. Assoc.* 155:2212-2216.

Stabenow, M. B., and Jara Guillen, B. 1972. The national network of diagnostic laboratories in the republic of Mexico. *U.S. Anim. Health Assoc. Proc.* 76:605-614.

Swindle, B. D. 1979. Keeping disease out of the United States. Paper read at Conf. Concepts Tech. Control and Erad. Anim. Dis., Sept. 10-14, Auburn, Ala.

Timbs, D. V. 1979. The New Zealand national bovine serum bank. In Veterinary Epidemiology and Economics. Int. Symp. Vet. Epidemiol. Econ. Proc. 2:76-80. Canberra: Aust. Gov. Publ. Serv.

Van Ness, G. B. 1966. The role of meat inspection in a disease reporting system. *U.S. Livest. Sanit. Assoc. Proc.* 70:396-402.

————. 1971. Ecology of anthrax. *Science* 172:1303-1307.

Van Roekel, H. 1931. Eleventh annual report on eradication of pullorum disease in Massachusetts. Mass. Agric. Exp. Stn. Control Serv. Bull. 58, Amherst.

Veterinary Services. 1974. Veterinary services activities organization: Responsibilities and cooperative programs. Anim. Plant Health Insp. Serv., USDA, Hyattsville, Md.

————. Ca. 1979. Tests to be conducted on cattle imported through Fleming Key Animal Import Center. Anim. Plant Health Insp. Serv., USDA, Hyattsville, Md.

Vickers, M. L., and Hanson, R. P. 1979. Experimental Newcastle disease virus infection in three species of wild birds. *Avian Dis.* 23:70–79.

Walker, J. W.; Heron, B. R.; and Mixson, M. A. 1973. Exotic Newcastle disease eradication program in the United States. *Avian Dis.* 17:486–503.

Watt, G. E. L. 1979. Studies on the development of an abattoir traceback system for sheep. In Veterinary Epidemiology and Economics. Int. Symp. Vet. Epidemiol. Econ. Proc. 2:177–180. Canberra: Aust. Gov. Publ. Serv.

Wellman, R. H. 1966. Industry's role in the development of pesticides. In Scientific Aspects of Pest Control. NAS-NRC Publ. 1402. Washington, D.C., pp. 355–366.

Wells, K. F. 1965. Method of importation of animals from countries in which exotic diseases may be prevalent. *U.S. Livest. Sanit. Assoc. Proc.* 69:274–283.

Wells, K. F.; Gasse, H.; and Vittoz, Dr. 1963. The technical role of veterinary quarantine regulations in the protection of the health of animals as both national and international projects. In Animal Health Yearbook 1963. Rome: FAO/WHO/OIE, pp. 283–288.

Willeberg, P. 1979. Epidemiological applications of Danish swine slaughter inspection data. In Veterinary Epidemiology and Economics. Int. Symp. Vet. Epidemiol. Econ. Proc. 2:161–167. Canberra: Aust. Gov. Publ. Serv.

Wisconsin Department of Agriculture, Trade, and Consumer Protection. 1978. Market cattle identification manual. Madison, Wis.

————. 1979. Market swine identification manual. Madison, Wis.

Zamberg, Y., and Lancaster, J. E. 1977. Veterinary control and sanitary routine in hatchery operations. *World Anim. Rev.* 21:36–41.

Zargar, S. L., and Pomeroy, B. S. 1950. Isolation of Newcastle disease virus from commercial fowl pox and laryngotracheitis vaccines. *J. Am. Vet. Med. Assoc.* 116:304–305.

11

Environmental Impact

NATURE OF PROBLEM

Every action used in disease control, livestock production, and manufacturing has some harmful as well as beneficial consequences if one examines the entire scene in a thorough manner. If the harmful consequences are immediate and marked, such as overindulgence at a party, they are easily recognized. But if one consequence is delayed or can be measured only by close comparison with controls, its recognition may take years even though it is eventually considered to be very significant. The teratogenic action of thalidomide on the fetus (Sunday Times 1973) and the pneumonic effects of quarry dust on the lungs (Davies 1969) are examples of delayed effects that were belatedly recognized to be important.

The public now expects and demands that the impacts of proposed actions be determined in advance, and that the search for them should not be limited to the immediate and obvious adverse effects. Deciding whether the harmful consequences of an action are an acceptable price for the benefits then can be based on information that is reasonably complete (Schwing and Albers 1980).

NATURAL ENVIRONMENT

Adverse Effects of Animal Disease

Before measuring the adverse environmental effects of human intervention in controlling disease, the

effect of uncontrolled disease on the natural environment should be understood so that the trade-offs can be
put into perspective.

Human and animal diseases may have adverse effects
upon wildlife (Thomas and Neitz 1933; de Villiers 1943;
Fletch 1970; Hedger et al. 1972) by threatening the
survival of endangered species and reducing or re-
stricting the population of more abundant species to
limited areas (Scott 1970). For example, duck enteritis virus causes the highest mortality in species of
waterfowl having small natural populations and the low-
est mortality in abundant mallards and domestic pekins
(Spieker 1978). Similarly, although Newcastle disease
causes high mortality in most pheasants, chickens, and
some rare species of parrots, it causes no mortality
in most other birds (Hanson 1974; Pearson and McCann
1974). Heavy mortality can also be caused by diseases
limited to wildlife, such as hemorrhagic disease of
deer (Trainer and Karstad 1970) and chlamydiosis in
snowshoe hares (Spalatin and Iversen 1970). The
adverse effects of disease go beyond mortality, however. For example, when tularemia reduces an abundant
rodent population in a community (Jellison et al.
1958), natural predators of rodents are forced to prey
upon alternative hosts, and plants formerly eaten by
the rodents increase greatly. The effect is beneficial
if these are cultivated plants, but if they are a weed
species, the result can be environmental degradation.

Adverse Effects of Disease Control Measures

Reduction of reservoir-vector populations. Measures
that are used to reduce or destroy reservoir and vector
populations may reduce or destroy nontarget populations
as well (Yuill and Kuns 1973). Chemical insecticides,
such as organic phosphates, are particularly harmful
because much of the compound, which is sprayed on land
or water, fails to reach the target insects (Chapin and
Wasserstrom 1981) and is ingested from soil and surface
waters by other invertebrates, which are eaten in turn
by higher animals (Hill et al. 1975). With each step
up the food chain (Woodwell 1967), the toxic substance
becomes more concentrated until predators near the top
of the food pyramid, such as the peregrine falcon, receive a sterilizing or even fatal dose. Other actions,
such as draining, flooding, or clearing land for the
purpose of destroying certain pest species, also eliminate many nontarget species (Borg and Hugoson 1979).

Many examples of unanticipated problems from these
two types of interventions exist. In southeast Asia,
DDT sprayed into thatched-roofed houses to control

malarial vectors killed predacious insects that kept
thatch-consuming insects under control; consequently,
the roofs deteriorated (Cheng 1963).   In Beni, a
Bolivian province in the upper Amazon basin, DDT used
to control malaria moved up the food chain to cats.
Unchecked by feline predation, a field rodent, *Calomys
callosus*, moved into dwellings during the rainy season
and spread hemorrhagic fever to the human population
(Kuns 1965).   In the United States, DDT, which was used
to control pests of fruit trees and certain field
crops, entered a complex food chain (Buck 1969) by
leaching into surface waters where it contaminated fish
and eventually impaired the reproduction of both mink
and falcons (the fish's predators) at the top of the
food pyramid (Stephenson 1966).   As a result, the
falcon has virtually disappeared from the continental
United States (Hickey 1969), and most of one season's
mink production was lost before the contaminated fish
in their diet was incriminated and eliminated. Persistent poisons that reach nontargeted species, like the
mink and falcon, can cause significant and sometimes
catastrophic decreases in animal populations as well as
disrupt the entire ecological fabric.
     Unfortunately, many of the target species develop
resistance to chemicals (Crow 1957; World Health
Organization 1963).   Wide and indiscriminate use of an
antibiotic as a therapeutic drug or a dietary stimulant
(1) provides an environment that selects for resistant
organisms and renders that antibiotic useless as a specific therapeutic agent, and (2) may suppress enteric
bacteria that are necessary for nutrition and health
(Swann 1969; *Federal Register* 1972; Food and Drug
Administration Task Force 1972).   The possibility of
resistance occurring in serious pathogens is greatly
increased, because resistance can be transferred between bacteria by transduction as well as be acquired
by direct exposure to drugs (Sojka et al. 1977).
     Decades ago, low and wet fields were ditched and
tiled primarily to permit cultivation and also to reduce the hordes of biting insects that bred in temporary pools.   The disappearance of malaria from the
central portion of the United States is probably
attributable to the conversion of these marginal wetlands into croplands and pastures (Williams 1963).
Unfortunately, these changes, which were beneficial to
agriculture and public health are believed to have led
to the extinction of some native species of plants and
animals.   As another example, industrialization, which
has been of economic benefit to the human population,
has had detrimental effects on wildlife and livestock
(Burns and Allcroft 1964).

Control of vectorborne diseases has been the major consideration in renovating irrigation projects. Repairing ditches and leveling land to prevent pooling of irrigation water are effective ways of reducing unwanted vectors that otherwise breed in these pools. Solutions to some other problems created by irrigation have not been found. For example, irrigation projects that improved agricultural production in arid countries of the tropics also brought schistosomasis, a crippling human disease (Hughes and Hunter 1972; May 1972). Impoundments for irrigation inundate river valleys, destroying plants and animals that lived there, but at the same time, create new habitats for waterfowl and other species that previously may have been rare.

Controlling vectors by removing cover was described in agriculture publications as far back as the eighteenth century. Government policies in several African countries require brush removal by physical or chemical means to control tsetse flies (Ormerod 1976). In the United States, brush is often removed to improve pastures. Some methods of removing cover, particularly the aerial spraying of herbicides, have been severely criticized. In fact, allegations have been made (Lang 1974) that aerial spraying caused harmful effects in the civilian and military populations in southeast Asia during the war (1965-1972).

Another program, tried at various times, attempts to reduce or eliminate an animal population believed to be a reservoir of disease or of no benefit (Lewis 1975; Zuckerman 1981). Predator control programs, often entitled as rabies control programs, have been directed against foxes, wolves, and coyotes (McCabe 1966). Population reduction programs for pigeons, starlings, sparrows, and blackbirds have cited psittacosis and fungal infections that these birds can carry. Specific programs, sometimes successful, have been directed toward the white-tailed deer in the Stanislas National Forest in California during an epizootic of foot-and-mouth disease (Fletch 1970) and toward bison infected with anthrax in western Canada (Novakowski et al. 1963). Many other species, such as insectivorus and vampire bats infected with rabies (Kverno and Mitchell 1976) and songbirds believed to carry St. Louis encephalitis, have also received attention. In instances in which numbers are reduced, the decrease may be the result of cyclic decrease in the population and not the consequence of measures taken (Anderson et al. 1981).

Population reduction campaigns seldom endanger the survival of the target species and are usually ephemeral and often ineffectual (Emlen et al. 1948; Wynne-

Edwards 1964; Bogel 1976). Poisoning and trapping can
be unselective, killing nontargeted species as well.
Hunting is generally too expensive. A few chemical
methods have been developed that are quite specific;
the best is a chemical that selectively destroys lam-
preys of the Great Lakes in the small streams where
they go to spawn. Antifertility drugs are being studied for use in predators that are considered pests
(Balser 1964; Lewis 1975). The population of a vampire
bat that feeds on cattle was reduced by 90 percent
through the use of an anticoagulant drug. No other bat
species were disturbed in this program that treated
cattle with a dosage harmless to them but fatal to the
bats (Thompson et al. 1972). Earlier attempts to control bats by poisoning, dynamiting caves, and infecting
bats with pathogens were unselective and ineffective
(Greenhall 1968). Although the attempt in Australia to
eradicate the European rabbit from cattle and sheep
ranges by introducing a virus lethal to the rabbit did
not fully succeed, the rabbit population has been
appreciably reduced (Fenner and Ratcliffe 1965). Such
population reductions can disrupt the ecological balance and cause unanticipated consequences. For instance, removal of large predators from the Kaibab
plateau in the southwestern United States allowed the
white-tailed deer population to increase until suitable
browse was destroyed. Many of the deer starved, and
for several decades the region's deer population remained far below its original level (Leopold 1943).
        Successful control of a disease that has caused
high livestock mortality, such as rinderpest, allows
that population to increase rapidly. In some countries
in Africa and the Middle East where possession of animal numbers is more important than income from selling
surplus animals, the unrestricted, increasing cattle
population has overbrowsed and overgrazed the pastures
causing habitat degeneration and erosion (Ormerod
1976). Similarly, the lack of major forests in the
mountains of the Mediterranean region is largely
attributed to the unchecked browsing of goats and
cattle in ancient times.

Disposal of Carcasses and Wastes

        Animals that die of disease or are destroyed
because they are carriers and the wastes of these
diseased animals (bedding, manure, contaminated feed,
and water) must be buried, burned, or disposed of in
some other fashion to eliminate the hazard created by
their presence. Wastes can create new hazards by con-

taminating the water table when buried, polluting the air when burned, and introducing toxic substances into food chains when salvaged (Atwell 1975).

Burial of large quantities of wastes, depending on soil and drainage, can pollute the water table and render well water unfit for human or animal use. Pollution caused by concentrated wastes can be avoided by spreading manure containing short-lived organisms over fields to fertilize crops, but manure from animals infected with long-lived organisms or highly contagious diseases can seldom be safely disposed of in this way. Composting in covered pits is sometimes satisfactory. Heating and disinfecting treatments are very expensive, and since the latter method can introduce soil-water pollutants if the manure is buried, the disinfected waste cannot be used as fertilizer. When the water table and the filtration rate through the soil is low, burial may be the least expensive solution for safe disposal of both the manure from diseased animals and the carcasses of dead animals. If the water table is high or the soil is deeply frozen, incineration of animals and wastes should be considered. Unfortunately, burning creates smoke, particularly if oil or automobile tires are used to provide the heat required to dry the wastes to the point of combustion, and many communities have regulations prohibiting incineration because of the production of solid particulates (soot and fly ash), odors, and gases.

The remaining alternatives, such as rendering dead animals, canning meat of healthy contacts, and incinerating animal wastes in plants with adequate burners and smokestacks, create less pollution and provide a measure of salvage but require facilities that may not be readily available (Animal Protein Conservation Work Group ca. 1974). In addition, some trucking is required to use these facilities. Unless this is done in watertight and covered vehicles, disease can spread. As additional restraints are imposed, the allover costs of disposal are inevitably increased.

While incineration in facilities with smokestacks does not eliminate pollution, the quantity of smoke is reduced and better dispersed. However, organisms can still be spread during the burning of animal carcasses, even in incinerators. For example, chlamydia were isolated in Oregon some distance downwind from the stack effluent of an incinerator in which turkeys with psittacosis were being burned (Spendlove 1957). Unless a special heater in the stack maintains a continuously high temperature lethal to all organisms, there is a period after the incinerator is charged with dead animals when pathogens are uplifted in the warm air and escape into the community.

INSTITUTIONS AMD HUMAN WELFARE

Adverse Effects of Animal Disease

Human health. Many agents of animal disease, from helminths to viruses, are capable of infecting people and inducing disabling or even fatal diseases (Meyer 1955; Abdussalam 1970; Ellis 1972). These diseases, the zoonoses, are sometimes acquired by animal handlers through vector bites or contact with aerosols and animal feces. Other infections of animal origin are acquired when the animal is killed and its tissues are handled or consumed. Because zoonoses acquired from food products are a primary concern of public health officials, a high priority has been assigned to their elimination (Held et al. 1958). Regardless of origin, the effect of human disease on economic development is measurable by appropriate methods (Weisbrod et al. 1973).

Diseases that do not affect people directly can, if they seriously curtail animal production and lead to food scarcities, cause human malnutrition (Kaplan 1966; Post 1977; National Research Council 1977). Protein deficiency diseases, attributable in many instances to a scarcity of animal products, are a major human health problem in many developing countries. In addition, increasing evidence indicates that severe protein deficiency in the neonatal period results in irreversible mental retardation.

Scarcities and institutional maladjustments. The short-falls in projected food production that result from disease not only cause internal problems for the nation by disrupting the processing and food distributing industries but also often make it difficult for the nation that traditionally exports livestock products to meet its balance of payments.

Agricultural systems. The impact of disease on the agriculture of a nation is best illustrated (Fig. 11.1) by the restriction the tsetse fly imposes on land use in many African countries (du Toit 1959; Lambrecht 1972; West 1972; Ford 1971, 1977). Even though African nations are in dire need of agricultural land, millions of acres have been left untamed because domestic cattle cannot withstand disease carried by the tsetse fly.

CHANGES IN THE GRASSLAND ECOSYSTEM OF EAST AFRICA 1890 TO 1980		
PERTURBATION	RESULTANT CHANGE	IMPACT ON HABITAT
RINDERPEST EPIZOOTIC OF 1890	UNGULATE POPULATION REDUCED 50% TO 90%	GRASSLANDS ABANDONED BY CATTLE REVERT TO ACACIA SAVANNAS. TSETSE FLY AREAS REDUCED FOR 10 TO 25 YEARS
TRIBAL WARS OF LATE 1800 AND HUMAN DISEASE OF EARLY 1900	HUMAN POPULATION REDUCED. PATTERN OF PLANNED BURN-ING OF GRASSLAND DIS-RUPTED	USE OF GRASSLANDS FOR CATTLE HERDING REDUCED. ACACIA INVADE
PREEMPTION OF GRASSLAND FOR FARMING BY WHITES AFTER 1900. HEDGEROWS INTRODUCED	NATIVE HERDSMEN DRIVEN INTO FOREST EDGES AND WETLANDS	TSETSE FLIES OF WOODLANDS ATTACK CATTLE AND HERDSMEN, REINVADE SAVANNA, AND UTILIZE HEDGES
HUNTING AND TRAPPING OF WILD UNGULATES BEGINNING IN 1930	TRANSIENT REDUCTION IN WILD UNGULATES	REDUCTION OF HOST POP-ULATIONS OF THE TSETSE FLY
EFFECTIVE RINDERPEST VACCINATION AFTER 1940	RAPID INCREASE IN CATTLE POPULATION. ALSO INCREASE IN HUMAN POPULATION	OVERSTOCKING OF CATTLE. DETERIORATION OF RANGE
INTERMITTENT DROUGHT	INCREASED RATE OF PASTURE DETERIORATION. DEATH OF CATTLE	ACACIA INVADE GRASSLANDS
PASTURE IMPROVEMENT BEGINNING IN 1960	MECHANICAL OR CHEMICAL CLEARING OF ACACIA AND BRUSH FROM SAVANNAS	REDUCTION OF TSETSE FLY. REDUCTION OF TRYPANOSO-MYASIS
AERIAL AND HAND SPRAY-ING OF INSECTICIDES SINCE 1965	REDUCTION OF TSETSE FLY POPULATIONS	ALSO REDUCTION OF NON-TARGET INVERTEBRATE SPECIES

FIG. 11.1. Consequences of environmental and social change on cattle disease in Africa (Mack 1970; Lambrecht 1972; West 1972; Ormerod 1976).

More subtle effects of animal diseases include in-creased capital costs and loss of feed efficiency, managerial options, and access to markets.

Adverse Effects of Disease-Control Measures

Disruption of life patterns. Although disease-control measures inevitably have temporary adverse effects on certain segments of the population, they can also have long lasting effects on the welfare of a few individu-als. Quarantines disrupt the movement of animals or goods and interrupt human living patterns by restric-ting access to recreational opportunities and preferred routes of travel (Cothern 1972; Bell 1973). As an illustration, the Newcastle disease eradication effort in southern California conflicted with the activities of homing pigeon fanciers, the stocking of game by pheasant-hunting clubs, and the travel of families with pets. Forced compliance met with considerable resistance and some illicit actions (Animal Plant Health Inspection Service 1978).

Human health hazards. Most chemicals that are used in disease control, such as insecticides, predator poisons, herbicides, and drugs are also toxic, in varying degrees, to the human population. If misused, some of these chemicals are very dangerous (Buck 1969) and, in certain instances, accidental exposure has caused illness, permanent disability, or death (Davies 1972). For this reason certain chemicals have been banned, others are restricted (special clearance being required before their use is approved), and still others, which are deemed safe, are generally available.

Controversy surrounds the use of many herbicides and insecticides. Two scientific panels that studied the impact of the use of herbicides on the people and environment in Vietnam concluded that it was significant but differed on the gravity of the situation (Lang 1974). In other instances, lawsuits have been filed in an attempt to either halt their use or claim damages based on impairment of human health caused by aerial spraying for control of insects causing crop or forest damage.

Elimination of dependent occupations. When a disease is successfully eradicated or controlled, industries and occupations that depended upon the presence of the disease disappear. Companies that produced hog cholera virulent virus and serum were prohibited from marketing their product after the eradication program was initiated and subsequently ceased operation unless they also produced other biologicals. Similarly, eradication of the screwworm from Texas had some adverse effects that were not fully anticipated. The ranch hands or cowboys had spent a large percentage of their working time finding and treating cattle with wounds that were already infected or likely to become infected with screwworms. Eradication eliminated the need for this work and hundreds of men were discharged. In 1975, when the screwworm temporarily reestablished itself in Texas, field hands were not available to treat the affected animals and the results were devastating. Unanticipated social and economic consequences have also been caused when people must be resettled as the result of land inundation by impounded water, creation of irrigation districts, and severance of pasture rights, all of which are sometimes done in the name of disease control (Darling and Farvar 1972).

Creation of political division. Controversies that develop into divisive political issues can lessen the effectivness of disease-control programs or delay their completion. For example, efforts to create political division in Mexico during the foot-and-mouth disease eradication program were quite effective. Some politicians, with the assistance of newspaper personnel, exploited the inefficiencies of the program and fears concerning not only the use of unusual and misunderstood procedures, but also foreign intervention by the powerful northern neighbor who cooperated in the program. Attempts to placate this opposition seriously jeopardized the campaign on several occasions (Machado 1968).

The effectiveness of political action programs mounted by special interest groups have eliminated certain options in disease control, such as the use of insecticides like DDT or the reduction of certain reservoir populations. Outcries have been raised not only against a government program to kill coots infected with fowl cholera that is transmissible to ducks but also against programs to eliminate vampire bats infected with rabies, a virus that kills cattle and man. In these two instances, the activists were protectionists, but in other cases, the activists can be consumer groups concerned with residues in foods or groups that champion individual freedom and fight what they believe are government expenditures that benefit only a few.

Not all protests yield the desired results, however. For example, authorities and certain industry personnel disagreed over the decision to eradicate the viserotropic Newcastle disease in southern California (Bell 1972). Although a few politicians were sympathetic to the vocal dissenters, the eradication program had strong support from the industry and the protest was prevented from becoming a political issue (Animal Plant Health Inspection Service 1978). Furthermore, state and local officials worked together closely. Harmony among officials coupled with industry support effectively deterred the political assault. Whenever differences about control procedures become an issue, leadership has been provided by a group that is effective because of its size, resources, an articulate speaker, or some dramatizable event. On occasion, a group opposed to an existing policy has changed that policy through litigation based on scientific evidence (Dunlap 1981).

Backlash of success. Successful control and eradication of animal disease can create problems that existing institutions are unable to handle (Fig. 11.2). For instance, the effective control of rinderpest in East Africa removed the primary restraint on livestock population (McKelvey 1973), and caused an increase in cattle population that resulted in overgrazing and erosion. It is also reputed to have decreased the value of cattle, which in turn inflated the bride price and led to increased conflict between young men trying to gain resources and old men trying to retain resources. Other examples even include attempts to improve human nutrition by distribution of high protein foodstuffs that had unanticipated adverse effects by stimulating the growth of parasites and the severity of disease in heavily parasitized children (Bunce 1972).

Successful disease control can increase opportunities for exploitation and competition for limited resources, and the problems that result can have an impact on human institutions as well as the natural environment.

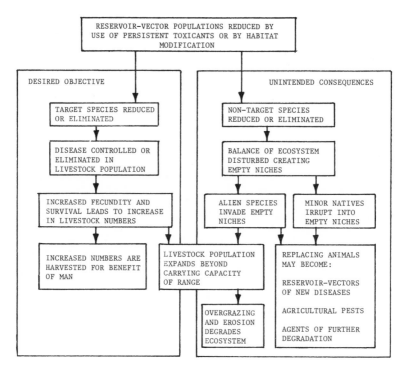

FIG. 11.2.   Effect of disease control measures on the natural environment.

SOCIETAL CONSIDERATIONS

Impact of Alternative Methods and Schedules

More than one strategy may be scientifically feasible for the control of a disease, but even if there is only one, alternative methods and a number of schedules can be employed to carry it out. The criteria for selecting the method to be used should not be limited to determination of the most scientifically elegant or economic method but should also include evaluation of the control technique's impact on natural and human environments. The latter can be done by searching the literature, using consultants with appropriate areas of expertise, and in some instances, developing and testing models. Choices are then made with all criteria in mind.

Impact upon Natural Environment

Obvious questions about the safety of any method should be subjected to test. If it is suspected that a live virus vaccine can spread from the animal to be vaccinated to associated animals, the virus should be tested in those animal species; if it is hazardous to any of them, its use should be restricted or banned. Toxicants, such as insecticides, that are rapidly biodegradable and have a narrow specificity are clearly to be preferred to those that degrade slowly and have a broad specificity, even if the first toxicant is more expensive than the latter. In general, a method that has the narrowest target (kills only the vector mosquito) is preferred to one that hits a broad target (all insects including honeybees) (Laird 1980; Batra 1982). Similarly, a procedure that removes reservoirs by rendering them noninfective or at least nonreproductive (sterile male technique used to eradicate screwworm fly [Bushland 1978]) is better than one that necessitates killing and burying reservoir animals. As previously mentioned, killing a reservoir animal can disrupt other populations, and burial of carcasses may pollute the water table.

Impact upon Institutions

A thorough understanding of the sequence of events that are set off by each action of a control program is fundamental to minimizing its impact and avoiding unnecessary disruptions. For example, alternatives should be made available before banning materials in current use, such as insecticides (Batra 1982), or halting procedures, such as open livestock auctions that are necessary for the distribution of food. Substitutes for draft animals should be at hand before work oxen or horses are slaughtered (Machado 1968). If diseased animals are to be rendered, sanitary trucks and rendering facilities must be ready. If the importation of meat scrap is to be banned, an alternate source of protein for animal feed must be found.

Since preparation for some alternatives may take several years, the prevalence of an infectious disease may be reduced by supervised vaccination until it is feasible to eliminate the remaining carriers (Schomisch 1967). Without sufficient preparation, elimination of the livestock carrier would disrupt agricultural production and cause major shortages in meat.

Dissension can be minimized by insuring that compliance is uniform for all groups and no one is given special privileges. Producers need to be assured that they will receive a price deferential for complience or their competitors must also bear increased capital and labor costs and meet the same improved product standards.

Inevitability of Change

Opposition to control measures based on the fear of adverse effects to the natural environment or human institutions can be met with the argument that it is impossible to preserve anything from change. The objective should be to control change so that the rate is tolerable and the benefits exceed the losses (De Soet 1974).

REFERENCES

Abdussalam, M. 1970. Zoonoses as occupational diseases: Some general features. Work. Pap. 7, WHO, Geneva.
Anderson, R. M.; Jackson, H. C.; May, R. M.; and Smith, A. M. 1981. Population dynamics of fox rabies in Europe. *Nature* 289:765-771.
Animal Plant Health Inspection Service. 1978. Eradication of exotic Newcastle disease in southern California, 1971-74. 91-34. USDA, Hyattsville, Md.
Animal Protein Conservation Work Group. Ca. 1974. Animal protein conservation report. Anim. Plant Health Insp. Serv., USDA, Hyattsville, Md.

Atwell, J. 1975. Animal protein conservation work group report. *U.S. Anim. Health Assoc. Proc.* 79:336-341.

Balser, D. S. 1964. Management of predator populations with antifertility agents. *J. Wildl. Manage.* 28:352-358.

Batra, S. W. T. 1982. Biological control in agroecosystems. *Science* 215:134-139.

Bell, D. 1972. Southern California poultry industry reactions to the Newcastle disease eradiction program. Univ. Calif. Agric. Ext., Davis, Calif.

————. 1973. The socio-economic impact of the VVND problem on the poultry industry of southern California. Univ. Calif. Agric. Ext., Davis, Calif.

Bogel, K. 1976. Assessment of fox control operation on wildlife rabies. In Wildlife Diseases, ed. L. A. Page. New York: Plenum Press, pp. 487-490.

Borg, K., and Hugoson, G. 1979. Wildlife as an indicator of environmental disturbances. In Veterinary Epidemiology and Economics. Int. Symp. Vet. Epidemiol. Econ. Proc. 2:250-253. Canberra: Aust. Gov. Publ. Serv.

Buck, W. B. 1969. Pesticides and economic poisons in the food chain. *U.S. Anim. Health Assoc. Proc.* 73:221-226.

Bunce, G. E. 1972. Aggravation of vitamin A deficiency following distribution of non-fortified skim milk. In The Careless Technology, eds. M. T. Farvar and J. P. Milton. New York: Doubleday, pp. 53-60.

Burns, K. N., and Allcroft, R. 1964. Fluorosis in cattle, part 1. Occurrence and effects in industrial areas of England and Wales, 1954-57. Anim. Dis. Surv., Rep. 2, Weybridge, UK.

Bushland, R. C. 1978. Eradication and suppression of the screwworm fly by the sterile male technique, ed. Comm. Jt. US/USSR Acad. Study Fundam. Sci. Policy. NAS, Washington, D.C.

Chapin, G., and Wasserstrom, R. 1981. Agricultural production and malaria resurgence in Central America and India. *Nature* 293:181-185.

Cheng, F. Y. 1963. Deterioration of thatch roofs by moth larvae after house spraying in the course of a malaria eradication programme in North Borneo. *Bull. WHO* 28:136-137.

Cothern, J. 1972. Economic impact of alternative Newcastle disease depopulation strategies in southern California. Univ. Calif. Agric. Ext., Davis, Calif.

Crow, J. F. 1957. Genetics of insect resistance to chemicals. *Annu. Rev. Entomol.* 2:227-246.

Darling, F. F., and Farvar, M. A. 1972. Ecological consequences of sedentarization of nomads. In The Careless Technology, eds. M. T. Farvar and J. P. Milton. New York: Doubleday, pp. 671-682.

Davies, C. N. 1969. Health Conditions in the Ceramic Industry. London: Pergamon Press.

Davies, J. E. 1972. Pesticides and the environment. Bol. Of. Sanit. Panam. 6(3):24-32.

De Soet, F. 1974. Agriculture and the environment. Agric. Environ. 1:1-15.

de Villiers, S. W. 1943. An outbreak of anthrax amongst Koedoes. J. South African Vet. Med. Assoc. 14:17-18.

Dunlap, T. R. 1981. DDT: Scientists, Citizens, and Public Policy. Princeton, N.J.: Princeton Univ. Press.

du Toit, R. M. 1959. The eradication of the tsetse fly Glossina pallidipes from Zululand, Union of South Africa. In Advances in Veterinary Science, vol. 5, eds. C. A. Brandly and E. L. Jungherr. New York: Academic Press, pp. 227-240.

Ellis, P. R. 1972. Principles for socio-economic studies of the zoonoses. WHO Consultations on Socioeconomic Aspects of Zoonoses, Nov. 21-25, Reading, UK.

Emlen, J. T., Jr.; Stokes, A. W.; and Winsor, C. P. 1948. The rate of recovery of decimated populations of brown rats in nature. Ecology 29:133-145.

Federal Register. 1972. Antibiotic and sulfonamide drugs in animal feeds. 37(21):2444-2445.

Fenner, F. J., and Ratcliffe, F. N. 1965. Myxomatosis. Cambridge: Cambridge Univ. Press.

Fletch, A. L. 1970. Foot-and-mouth disease. In Infectious Diseases of Wild Mammals, eds. J. W. Davis, L. H. Karstad, and D. O. Trainer. Ames, Ia.: Iowa State Univ. Press, pp. 68-75.

Food and Drug Administration Task Force. 1972. The use of antibiotics in animal feeds. Bur. Vet. Med., FDA, Rockville, Md.

Ford, J. 1971. The Role of the Trypanosomiasis in African Ecology: A Study of the Tsetse Fly Problem. Oxford, UK: Clarendon Press.

———. 1977. Integration of rural development and tsetse control. Trans. R. Soc. Trop. Med. Hyg. 71:12.

Greenhall, A. M. 1968. Problems and ecological implications in the control of vampire bats. Int. Union Conserv. Nature Nat. Resour., IUCN Publ., New Ser. 13:94-102.

Hanson, R. P. 1974. The reemergence of Newcastle disease. In *Advances in Veterinary Science and Comparative Medicine*, vol. 18, eds. C. A. Brandly and E. L. Jungherr. New York: Academic Press, pp. 213-229.

Hedger, R. S.; Condy, J. B.; and Golding, S. M. 1972. Infection of some species of African wildlife with foot-and-mouth disease virus. *J. Comp. Path.* 82: 455-461.

Held, J. R.; Bauer, H.; and West, R. L. 1958. Effect of eradicating brucellosis in cattle on incidence of human cases. *USPHS Public Health Rep.* 73:1096-1100.

Hickey, J. J., ed. 1969. *Peregrine Falcon Populations: Their Biology and Decline*. Madison, Wis.: Univ. Wis. Press.

Hill, E. F.; Health, R. G.; Spann, J. W.; and Williams, J. D. 1975. Lethal dietary toxicities of environmental pollutants to birds. Spec. Sci. Rep.-Wildl. 191. U.S. Fish Wildl. Serv., Washington, D.C.

Hughes, C. C., and Hunter, J. M. 1972. The role of technological development in promoting disease in Africa. In *The Careless Technology*, eds. M. T. Farvar and J. P. Milton. New York: Doubleday, pp. 69-101.

Jellison, W. L.; Bell, J.F.; Vertrees, J. D.; Holms, M. A.; Larson, C. L.; and Owen, C. R. 1958. Preliminary observation on disease in the 1957-58 outbreak of microtus in western United States. *North Am. Wildl. Conf. Trans.* 23:137-145.

Kaplan, M. M. 1966. Social effects of animal diseases in developing countries. Int. Agric. Ser. 3. Inst. Agric., Univ. Minn., St. Paul, Minn.

Kuns, M. L. 1965. Epidemiology of Machupo virus infection. II. Ecologic and control studies of hemorrhagic fever. *Am. J. Trop. Med. Hyg.* 14:813-816.

Kverno, N. B., and Mitchell, G. C. 1976. Vampire bats and their effect on cattle production in Latin America. *World Anim. Rev.* 17:1-7.

Laird, M. 1980. Biocontrol in veterinary entomology. In *Advances in Veterinary Science and Comparative Medicine*, vol. 24, eds. C. A. Brandly and C. E. Cornelius. New York: Academic Press, pp. 145-177.

Lambrecht, F. L. 1972. The tsetse fly: A blessing or a curse? In *The Careless Technology*, eds. M. T. Farvar and J. P. Milton. New York: Doubleday, pp. 726-741.

Lang, A. 1974. Chairman of committee on effects of herbicides in Vietnam. In The Effects of Herbicides in South Vietnam: Part A. Summary and Conclusions. Washington, D.C.: NAS.

Leopold, A. 1943. Deer irruptions. *Wis. Conserv. Bull.* 8(8):3-11.

Lewis, J. C. 1975. Control of rabies among terrestrial wildlife by population reduction. In The Natural History of Rabies, vol. 2, ed. G. M. Baer. New York: Academic Press, pp. 243-259.

McCabe, R. A. 1966. Vertebrates as pests: A point of view. In Scientific Aspects of Pest Control. NAS-NRC Publ. 1402. Washington, D.C., pp. 115-134.

Machado, M. A., Jr. 1968. An Industry in Crisis: Mexican-United States Cooperation in the Control of Foot-and-Mouth Disease. Univ. Calif. Publ. Hist., vol. 80. Berkeley and Los Angeles: Univ. Calif. Press.

Mack, R. 1970. The great African cattle plague epidemic of the 1890's. *Trop. Anim. Health Prod.* 2:210-219.

McKelvey, J. J., Jr. 1973. Man against Tsetse: Struggle for Africa. Ithaca, N.Y.: Cornell Univ. Press.

May, J. M. 1972. Influence of environmental transformation in changing the map of disease. In The Careless Technology, eds. M. T. Farvar and J. P. Milton. New York: Doubleday, pp. 19-34.

Meyer, K. F. 1955. The Zoonoses in their Relation to Rural Health. Berkeley and Los Angeles: Univ. Calif. Press.

National Research Council. 1977. World Food and Nutrition Study. Washington, D.C.: NAS.

Novakowski, N. S.; Cousineau, J. G.; Kolenosky, G. B.; Wilton, G. S.; and Choquette, L. P. E. 1963. Parasites and diseases of bison in Canada. II. Anthrax epizooty in the Northwest Territories. *North Am. Wildl. Nat. Resour. Conf. Trans.* 28:233-339.

Ormerod, W. E. 1976. Ecological effect of control of African trypanosomiasis. *Science* 191:815-821.

Pearson, G. L., and McCann, M. K. 1974. The role of indigenous, wild, semidomestic and exotic birds in the epizootiology of exotic Newcastle disease in southern California. Position paper, U.S. Fish Wildl. Serv. and Anim. Plant Health Insp. Serv., USDA, Hyattsville, Md.

Post, J. D. 1977. The Last Great Subsistence Crisis in the Western World. Baltimore: Johns Hopkins Univ. Press.

Schomisch, T. P.   1967.   Wisconsin brucellosis cam-
     paign.   M.S. thesis, Univ. Wis., Madison.
Schwing, R. C., and Albers, W. A., Jr., eds.   1980.
     Societal Risk Assessment: How Safe is Safe
     Enough?   New York: Plenum Publ.
Scott, G. R.   1970.   Rinderpest.   In Infectious
     Diseases of Wild Mammals, eds. J. W. Davis, L. H.
     Karstad, and D. O. Trainer.   Ames, Ia.:   Iowa
     State Univ. Press, pp. 20-35.
Sojka, W. J.; Wray, C.; and Hudson, E. B.   1977.   A
     survey of drug resistance in Salmonellae isolated
     from animals in England and Wales during 1973 and
     1974.   Br. Vet. J. 133:292-311.
Spalatin, J., and Iverson, J. O.   1970.   Epizootic
     chlamydiosis of muskrats and snowshoe hares.   In
     Infectious Diseases of Wild Mammals, eds. J. W.
     Davis, L. H. Karstad, and D. O. Trainer.   Ames,
     Ia.:   Iowa State Univ. Press, pp. 304-308.
Spendlove, J. C.   1957.   Production of bacterial
     aerosols in a rendering plant process.   Public
     Health Rep. 72:176-180.
Spieker, J. O.   1978.   Virulence assay and other stud-
     ies of six North American strains of duck plague
     virus tested in wild and domestic waterfowl.
     Ph.D. thesis, Univ. Wis., Madison.
Stephenson, R. G.   1966.   Chemicals and pesticides as
     they affect mink.   Am. Fur Breeder, June, pp.
     14-17.
Sunday Times.   1973.   The Thalidomide Children and the
     Law.   London: Andre Deutsch.
Swann, M. M., chairman.   1969.   Joint committee on the
     use of antibiotics in animal husbandry and veteri-
     nary medicine.   Cmnd. Rep. 4190.   Her Majesty's
     Stationery Off, London.
Thomas, A. D., and Neitz, W. O.   1933.   The importance
     of disease in wild animals.   South African J. Sci.
     30:419-425.
Thompson, R. D.; Mitchell, G. C.; and Burns, R. J.
     1972.   Vampire bat control by systemic treatment
     of livestock with an anticoagulant.   Science
     177:806-808.
Trainer, D. O., and Karstad, L. H.   1970.   Epizootic
     hemorrhagic disease.   In Infectious Diseases of
     Wild Mammals, eds. J. W. Davis, L. H. Karstad, and
     D. O. Trainer.   Ames, Ia.:   Iowa State Univ.
     Press, pp. 50-54.
Weisbrod, B. A.; Andreano, R. L.; Baldwin, R. E.;
     Epstein, E. H.; Kelley, A. C.; and Helmeniak, T.
     W.   1973.   Disease and Economic Development: The
     Impact of Parasitic Diseases in St. Lucia.
     Madison, Wis.:   Univ. Wis. Press.

West, O. 1972. The ecological impact of the introduc-
    tion of domestic cattle into wildlife and tsetse
    areas of Rhodesia. In The Careless Technology,
    eds. M. T. Farvar and J. P. Milton. New York:
    Doubleday, pp. 712-725.
Williams, L. L. 1963. Malaria eradication in the
    United States. *Am. J. Public Health* 53(1):17-21.
Woodwell, G. M. 1967. Toxic substances and ecological
    cycles. *Sci. Am.* 216(3):24-31.
World Health Organization. 1963. WHO expert committee
    on insecticides: Insecticide resistance and
    vector control. WHO Tech. Rep. Ser. 265, Geneva.
Wynne-Edwards, V. C. 1964. Population control in
    animals. *Sci. Am.* 211(2):68-74.
Yuill, T. M., and Kuns, M. L. 1973. Environmental
    concerns and disease control programs. Animal
    disease eradication: Evaluating programs. Proc.
    NAS Workshop, Apr. 12-13, Univ. Wis. Ext.,
    Madison, Wis.
Zuckerman, Lord. 1981. The great badger debate.
    Nature 289:628-630.

12

Economic Benefits
and Social Priority

USE OF MODELING

Assessing Benefits

The projected cost of a disease-control program is
based on time estimates and the anticipated inputs required to achieve the stated goals. Construction of a
model that can be used to simulate the course of the
program is the best way to assess the probability that
many interacting events will result in a desired goal
within a given period of time. In simple terms, a
model is a budget of the inputs and outputs involved in
a process.

Modeling begins with the development of a structural model of the pathogen's epidemic behavior. This
epidemic model (Fig. 12.1) is a statement of the relationships of epidemic elements and shows what effect
changes in the value of any of the elements will have
on the course of the epidemic.

According to Lehman et al. (1976), the first
epidemiological model used to study relationships of
various parameters was created by Sir Ronald Ross in
the early 1900s. He sought an estimate of the critical
mosquito population density required for malaria maintenance. A series of workers followed this lead in
exploring functional relationships between various
epidemiological and entomological parameters and
created models that attempted to describe more of the
process. By the mid 1950s, the World Health Organization tried to use the best of these models to plan
malaria control programs. The use of insecticide
application as the only intervention did not succeed;
later, mass administration of drugs only gave ambiguous

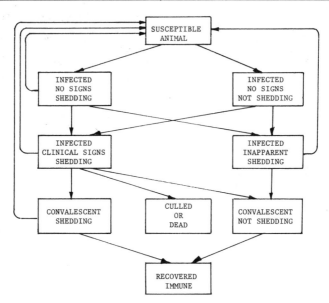

FIG. 12.1. Simple epidemic model.

results. In the 1960s, the World Health Organization established a project in northern Nigeria to develop and test an improved malarial model. This model included the human population's age and immune status, provision for heterogeneity of the vector mosquito population, and a provision for nonrandom allocation of drug therapy. This new model gave a good prediction of the effect of such an intervention as area insecticide treatment.

A major benefit of model building is the general sharpening of perception that arises as precise questions are raised, formulated, and organized in logical fashion during the exercise. Development of such a model requires close communication between the model builder, statistician, epidemiologist, and field worker. Available laboratory and field data (Groot 1972) should be used but consideration must be given to the design limitations of the laboratory data and sampling errors in field data (Hugh-Jones 1979).

When building a model, the purpose of the model must be kept in mind. It may be simply a statement of the relationship between two elements or an attempt to describe (1) the relationships of all the elements that are essential for the development or abatement of an epidemic, or (2) the development of a vector population involved in an epidemic (Moon 1976) or its control

(Jobin 1979). In any case, the purpose must be stated clearly, and the parameters being used must be specified in understandable biological terms to facilitate measurement in the field.

Epidemiological models (Dietz 1972) deal not only with rates by which processes proceed but also with thresholds above which processes can be sustained and breakpoints below which they cannot. An elegant model is the simplest expression possible, and an awkward model is encumbered by unnecessary parameters. However, the first objective must be to develop a model that works; it can be refined later. No matter how carefully the model is structured, the builder should remember that it can never be better than an approximation of reality.

Program planners depend upon an epidemiological model that gives a reasonable simulation of the disease's behavior in a population when using available laboratory and field data to test alternative control measures (Ferguson 1969; Hugh-Jones 1976). Once a model is built, dynamic interaction over a period of time can be predicted. The probability of events are treated in either a deterministic or stochastic (Monte Carlo) fashion. The scenario can be developed by hand, but a computer is usually used to follow the interaction because of the complexity of the elements. The best control measures are selected and subjected to economic analysis (Ellis 1972; Johnston 1979). With an estimate of the time required to reach certain program goals, the size of various inputs can be calculated and an estimate of program costs determined (Astudillo et al. 1976). Physical measurements of disease losses can be given economic values that must be (1) adjusted for compensating factors and (2) augmented by the value of indirect losses to calculate loss abatement benefits (Weisbrod et al. 1973; James and Ellis 1979; McCauley 1979). Using different strategies or different rates of investment, several alternative programs can be compared at low cost in an economic model that is based on the disease and program costs gained from the epidemic and control models (Waaler 1968; Power and Harris 1973; Anderson et al. 1976; Bootes and Gilchrist 1979; Dietrich et al. 1979; Harris et al. 1979; Kryder 1980).

Cost-benefit analysis dates back to 1768 when an exact accounting of costs and expected returns was required before monies were made available to construct the Forth and Clyde Canal in Scotland (Grindle 1979). It was also applied to water resource projects in the United States in the 1930s and was used in many countries in the 1960s. The World Bank has often used this technique in assisting developing countries.

Problems of Risk and Uncertainty

        Standard cost-benefit assessment techniques do not
adapt well to the evaluation of uncertainties of
whether a program can be completed successfully. The
simplest approach is presentation of the most probable
outcome followed by a sensitivity analysis in which the
calculations are reworked to determine what would
happen under different assumptions and corresponding
alternative outcomes. Unfortunately, the extended
discussions of risk and uncertainty in project
appraisal literature has diverted attention from the
fundamental problem, which in many situations is really
an ignorance of the basic facts and relationships
within the epidemic and economic models. "Ignorance"
does not have the scientific aura of "risk and uncertainty," but according to Grindle (1979), it describes
accurately the lack of knowledge that often exists on
many animal disease-control projects, particularly, in:

        1. Livestock numbers--lack of up-to-date census
data.
        2. Disease prevalence--primarily when estimating
the potential effect of an exotic disease.
        3. Economic impact--failure to allow for compen-
satory factors.
        4. Future prices--present prices may be a poor
guide to future prices in a fluctuating market.
        5. Related projects--inadequate appreciation of
the interrelatedness of disease control and such areas
as livestock nutrition and marketing.

        The position that risk must be eliminated before a
program can be implemented is not only impractical and
probably impossible, but it may also remove the safest
and most feasible options from consideration (Wildavsky
1979). Because of the limited and possible inaccurate
information that is available to the planners of most
programs (Funder 1979), a monitoring system of the
program's progress as well as a means of providing
operational flexibility should be required to avoid the
disasters that would otherwise be the inevitable result
of the initial miscalculations. In support of this
idea, Nelson (1977) argued that emphasis should be
focused on the organizational framework for making
decisions as new information becomes available rather
than any particular cost-benefit analysis presumed to
fit the future course of action.

THE CASE FOR CONTROL

Governments operating within limited budget resources continuously are beset with numerous alternative demands on those resources. Much of the budget is needed to maintain the government itself (defense, judiciary, legislative, and revenue obligations), but a portion is allocated to national development (transportation, agriculture, commerce, and education). Obviously, some method of analysis must be utilized to determine objectively which developmental needs merit funding. The basic concept used in an economic analysis of programs requiring capital expenditures is a comparison of program alternatives in terms of their proposed costs and expected benefits to determine which alternative gives the best return for the money spent (Carpenter 1979).

After costs and benefits have been quantified by modeling, a comparison must be made of projects having differently shaped future cost-and-benefit streams (Anderson et al. 1978; Aulaqi and Sundquist 1979). Discounting is the method usually used for this comparison. For the individual who is not trained in economics, the process of discounting and the merits of several different discounting methods need a brief description.

If we lend money to someone, we can expect to be paid interest for the use of that money. Economists explain interest as (1) payment received for deferring the use of money for present pleasure. In other words, interest is related to current income foregone (loaned). The person borrowing the money must therefore pay the lender for its use. If $1,000 is lent for two years (or put into a savings account) at 9 percent interest, the amount due (or in the account) at the end of the first year would be $1,090; at the end of the second year it would be $1,188.10 (value due = $P(1 + i)^t$ where P = principal, i = interest, and t = time; $1,188.10 = $1,000(1 + 0.09)^2$).

Now suppose we look at this from a different perspective. If someone promises to pay $1,000 in five years (assuming a 9 percent interest rate), how much is that promise worth today? To determine this the amount due must be divided by $1.09 per year. Today that promise is worth $650 (see Table 12.1). The process of finding the present worth of a future value is called discounting. The interest rate assumed for discounting is the discount rate.

Using the same figures of $1,000, 9 percent discount rate, and five years, suppose the recipient is

Table 12.1. Present Worth of Future Value

Year	Amount Promised at End of Year	Interest Rate	Worth at Beginning of Year
5	$1,000	1.09	$917
4	917	1.09	842
3	842	1.09	772
2	772	1.09	708
1	708	1.09	650
0	650		

Present value = (amount due)$/(1 + i)^t$; $650 = $1,000/1.09^5$.

to receive a stream of income instead of being paid a single amount in some future year. What is the present value of that stream of income?

According to Table 12.2, a promised income of $1,000 per year for five years has a present value of $3,889. In other words, if $3,889 were invested at 9% interest, $1,000 could be removed from that account each year for five years leaving no balance in the account.

We are now able to look at the three methods of project analysis: (1) discounted benefits, (2) benefit-cost, and (3) net present value. In Table 12.3, the discounted benefits of the three projects A, B, and C are the same as the benefit-cost ratios. However, the net present values differ, with project A giving the best return and project C the poorest. The difference is found in the cost items of the two projects. If the benefit items had also differed over time, as they usually do, the analysis, although more complicated, would be calculated in the same way with each method of analysis giving a different value.

Presentation of the case for control must take into consideration not only the total costs and total benefits but also the effects of discounting of those costs and benefits because the individuals who compare the projects will pay attention to all these factors.

Table 12.2. Present Value of Income Stream

Year	Income to be Received	Discount Factor	Present Worth
1	$1,000	.917	$ 917
2	1,000	.842	842
3	1,000	.772	772
4	1,000	.708	708
5	1,000	.650	650
			$3,889

Discount factor = $1/(1 + i)^t$; i.e., $1/1.09^t$.

Table 12.3. Example of Discounting by Three Methods of Analysis

Project	Year	Cost	Discounted Present Cost (9%)	Benefits	Discounted Present Benefits (9%)	Benefit–Cost*	Net Present Value**
A	1	$ 1,000	$ 917	$ 4,000	$ 3,668	$3,000	$2,751
	2	2,000	1,684	4,000	3,368	2,000	1,684
	3	3,000	2,316	4,000	3,088	1,000	772
	4	4,000	2,832	4,000	2,832	0	0
	5	5,000	3,250	4,000	2,600	−1,000	−650
	6	6,000	3,576	4,000	2,384	−2,000	−1,192
		$21,000	$14,575	$24,000	$17,940	$3,000	$3,365
B	1	$ 3,500	$ 3,209	$ 4,000	$3,668	$ 500	$ 459
	2	3,500	2,947	4,000	3,368	500	421
	3	3,500	2,702	4,000	3,088	500	386
	4	3,500	2,478	4,000	2,832	500	354
	5	3,500	2,275	4,000	2,600	500	325
	6	3,500	2,086	4,000	2,384	500	298
		$21,000	$15,697	$24,000	$17,940	$3,000	$2,243
C	1	$ 6,000	$ 5,502	$ 4,000	$ 3,668	$−2,000	$−1834
	2	5,000	4,210	4,000	3,368	−1,000	−842
	3	4,000	3,088	4,000	3,088	0	0
	4	3,000	2,124	4,000	2,832	1,000	708
	5	2,000	1,300	4,000	2,600	2,000	1,300
	6	1,000	596	4,000	2,384	3,000	1,788
		$21,000	$16,820	$24,000	$17,940	$3,000	$1,120

*Benefit–cost = benefit minus cost.
**Net present value = benefit–cost discounted 9%.

ESTABLISHING SOCIAL PRIORITY

     Regional programs for control of animal diseases,
whoever conceives them, are developed and implemented
by the government and funded largely or entirely by
society. Consequently, decisions regarding the amount
and source of funding depend on social priorities and
become part of the political process. At top decision
levels, the choice is between funding a disease control
program or some totally unrelated program (Gittinger
1972; McGregor 1973; Stoops 1973) because high administrators confronted with alternative disease programs
are not likely to fund either of them. Consequently,
proponents of the program must dispose of competitive
disease-control programs before seeking final approval.
The experienced official carefully prepares the case
for the selected disease program by (1) citing its
benefits to society as a whole, (2) justifying cost,
and (3) documenting the need to initiate the program
without delay (World Health Organization 1970). During
this preparation, efforts are also made to gain the
support of a wide spectrum of interested groups who can
play a crucial role in influencing decision-making
politicians.
     If justification for animal disease-control pro-
grams is narrowly defined, the program is unlikely to
be funded. However, control of animal disease becomes
a matter of primary importance when it is shown to have
an effect on the availability of food (Horsfall 1975).
From the earliest times it has been clear that survival
of a nation is as dependent upon its food supply as
upon availability of arms. In the past, blockades that
cut off food supplies have forced nations to surrender,
and policies that destroyed the base of agricultural
productivity (soil erosion, salination, and disease)
have ruined still more nations. To insure the health
of its citizens and maintain an essential working
force, a nation needs an ample food supply that is free
of disease organisms, products of disease, and harmful
additives. Today's political realities dictate that a
nation must either protect its productive land and
provide a favorable climate for agricultural production
or engage in economic and military struggle with its
neighbors for food supplies (Ruttan 1973).
     In developing the case for disease-control, two
questions must be answered: (1) who suffers from the
presence of animal disease, and (2) who benefits from
its control? All members of the chain--the producers
of animal products; the people who transport, process,
and retail animal products; and the consumers--may suf-

fer losses as the result of animal disease (Gordon 1967; Scott 1970). The risk of different members of the chain may vary with the disease, but rarely is any one member immune. This fact is important and must be made clear. When production is decreased or interrupted, the costs of production, transport, and processing are increased. The consequences are increased prices for the product, possible periods of unavailability of the product, and increased chances of the consumer receiving an inferior and occasionally potentially dangerous product. In spite of the far-reaching effects of animal disease, some members of the chain are able to avoid the costs of disease, in one way or another, and consequently have no interest in disease-control. Farmers who are able to pass the offsite costs of disease to others will resist any disease-control program that increases their operational costs but not their onsite benefits. They are unwilling to pay for measures that will benefit their competitors or consumers but bring them no direct gain.

If true perspective is to be achieved, the social costs and benefits of a program must always be compared with the social costs and benefits of no program. However, the analysis should not be limited to economic issues because human and animal welfare are important issues to the public.

Inevitably, programs to control and eradicate disease restrict animal movement, can inflict some pain and introduce certain hazards when the animals are captured or handled for the taking of diagnostic samples, vaccination, or treatment with vector destroying chemicals. In programs that remove infected animals and their contacts by slaughter, pain of death is certainly inflicted. The transitory pain of many animals and death of a few is unfortunate, but the pain and death that are an inevitable consequence of an unimpeded spread of disease must not be overlooked. The choice is not between the existence or absence of pain and death but between differing frequencies or levels of pain and death. Although planners emphasize the economic benefits of disease-control to livestock producers and the advantages of increased hunting success to sportsmen, they fail to speak to other people who are interested in the welfare of animals about the beneficial effects disease elimination has on domestic and wild animal populations. Among these benefits are pain reduction and extended life span. For example, one immediate effect of the screwworm eradication was a decrease in mortality in both cattle (to which the program was directed) and deer (with which the program was not concerned). The population of the latter group increased dramatically. Few observers emphasized that prior to the program the fawns, whose umbilical cords were attacked by the egg-laying fly, were slowly eaten to death by the developing maggots--a frequent, miserable, and unlovely death. Although disease in all forms is painful when it blinds, lames, starves, or quickly kills, some infectious diseases are notoriously painful. Obviously, a cow dying from pseudorabies whose bellowing can be heard a mile away suffers intensely. The decision maker is not faced with applying onerous disease-control measures on a pain-free animal population but with exacting some discomfort and an occasional death to free a large population from more intense pain and premature death.

Animal diseases can have a devastating impact. Losses of cattle from rinderpest were so great during the great African panzootic of the late 1800s, that entire nations were reduced to starving remnants, and none of the Rift Valley civilizations survived as self-governing peoples (Mack 1970; McKelvey 1973). More often, uncontrolled disease adversely affects the international trade of the nation (Brooksby et al. 1972) or results in deprivation of the nation's poorer classes who cannot afford to pay the increased prices when scarcities develop (Jahnke 1974; Horsfall 1975). Moreover, all the citizens are affected by the social unrest that results when food supplies are inadequate for the poor or the nation has a crisis in its balance of payments. Ruttan (1973) has detailed the far-reaching affect this social unrest can have not only on a nation's policies but also on its relations with the world community.

Control of an animal disease seldom provides the farmer with more than a transient gain because reduced costs are passed on to processors and wholesalers and, eventually, the consumer. It obviously makes little sense to charge the cost of disease control to the farmers unless its benefits are real and sustained (Purchase and Schultz 1979). In almost all instances, the ultimate beneficiaries are the consumers, who pay less for a better product that is always available at the market, and the government which gains from social stability and increased revenue on a larger volume of products.

The social implications of disease-control programs that have just been discussed are no less decisive in the final judgment than the economic implications, but they are not as easy to quantify. Less obvious benefits include the contribution disease control makes to national security by reducing social unrest, insuring an adequate supply of an essential resource free of alien control, and strengthening the economic viability of the country. Consideration should also be given to the program's political accept- ability, which should be based partly on its appeal to community leaders and the general public and partly on its ability to fit into the perception of societal goals held by various segments of the population and their leaders (Burger 1980).

ECONOMIC ANALYSES OF CONTROL PROGRAMS

The National Brucellosis Technical Commission Report to the U.S. Department of Agriculture

In 1978 the National Brucellosis Technical Com- mission (NBTC), appointed by the U.S. Secretary of Agriculture, published a study of the USDA's control program for brucellosis (Anderson et al. 1978; Dietrich et al. 1979). The commission compared three earlier studies (England and Wales, Australia, and the United States) of the benefits of brucellosis control (Hugh- Jones et al. 1975; Roe and Morris 1976; Beal and Kryder 1977a, 1977b) with a model that they developed (Table 12.4). The models used for the NBTC study and the Australian study are shown in Figs. 12.2 and 12.3. The comparison showed positive benefit-cost ratio for each of the control programs examined and the net benefits of the four proposed, alternative programs were pre- sented in a graph (Fig. 12.4). While all four programs eventually gave positive benefits, only one program gave a net benefit from its initiation. Other studies on the economics of brucellosis control have been made (Carpenter and Heron 1975; Carpenter 1976; Esuruoso 1979; Shepherd et al. 1979), but the NBTC study of the economic impact and control of a disease was, with one exception (McCauley et al. 1979), the first published report based on a dynamic rather than static economic model. The effect of a changing meat and milk supply and the interactions with competing commodities of these changes on prices paid to farmers were considered by the NBTC in calculating benefits of control. Such compensating interactions in determining benefits must be considered or the methodology will be unacceptable to economists. The National Brucellosis Technical Commission also examined both the biological and social restraints on the brucellosis control program, and this analysis merits review. The USDA has commissioned Texas A & M University to do further studies of dynamic

Table 12.4. Benefit-Cost Studies of Brucellosis Control Programs

	1978 U.S. NBTC	1973 Australia Roe, Morris	1975 UK. Hugh-Jones, Ellis, Felton	1977 U.S. Beal, Kryder, McCallan
1. Program				
2. Population	8 regions, survey of herds in each region	Selected regions, 10% sample of herds in region	1 region, 100-herd sample	5 regions, survey of herds in each region
3. Disease model	Deterministic simulation (Fig. 12.2)	Stochastic simulation (Fig. 12.3)	Stochastic simulation	Deterministic simulation
4. Discount rate	10%	10%		10%
5. Benefit-cost Number of programs compared	5	2	2	7
Highest ratio	complex (Fig. 12.4)	5.0	2.2	10.6
Lowest ratio		2.9	1.1	1.6

Source: Anderson et al. 1978.

248

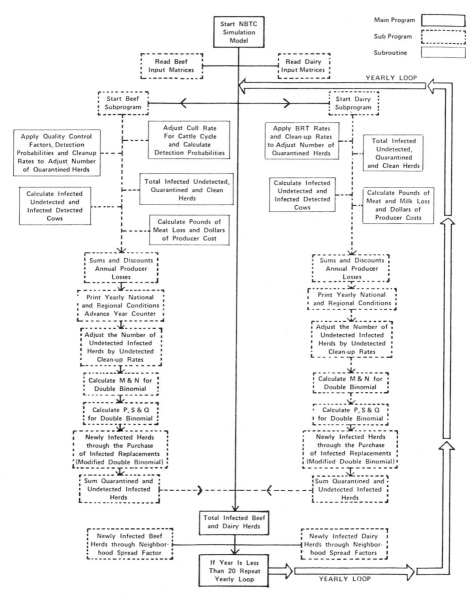

FIG. 12.2. National Brucellosis Technical Commission simulation model (Anderson et al. 1978). See note at end of chapter.

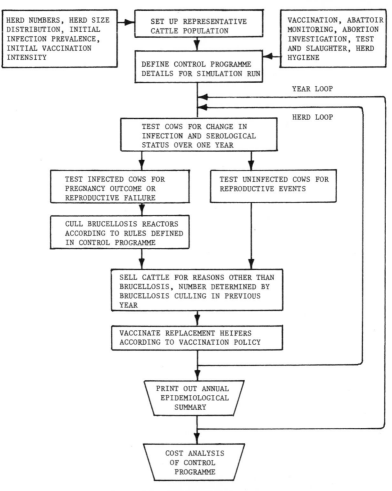

FIG. 12.3. Simplified flow diagram of brucellosis simulation model covering dairy and beef industries in an Australian state (Roe and Morris 1976).

economic models in evaluating the cost-benefits of disease control in the United States.

Cost-benefit Analysis of a Program in Tanzania

At the request of the Tanzanian government, an English team led by Brooksby (1972) prepared a proposal for the creation of a disease free zone that would permit Tanzania to develop export trade in carcass meat. The primary factor limiting beef export from that coun-

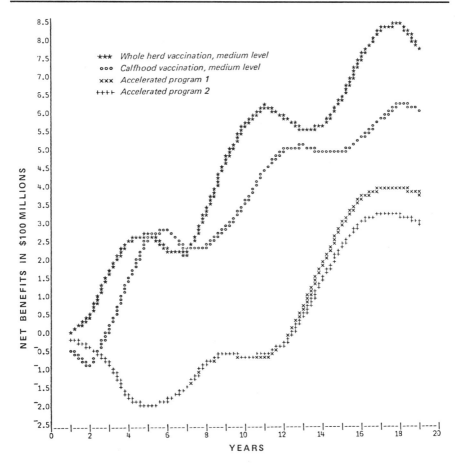

FIG. 12.4.   National Brucellosis Technical Commission
simulation model: Comparison of net benefits for selected
programs by year (Anderson et al. 1978).

try was the presence of foot-and-mouth disease.   After
studying the infrastructure, nature of the losses, and
measures for control, the consultants prepared a cost-
benefit analysis of a program that would create a
disease-free zone.

A description of the control program and an
account of the costs were given in chapter 1.   Benefits
were projected in six categories (Table 12.5), and the
assumptions underlying each category can be found in
the proposal prepared by Brooksby and his associates.
The cost-benefit analysis (Table 12.6) was based on a
twenty-year period and used the method of internal rate
of return to give a value of 19 percent.

Table 12.5. Anticipated Benefits of a Program to Establish a Disease-Free Zone in Tanzania

Nature of Benefits	Year					
	1	2	3	4	5	6-20
			(Tanzanian dollars)			
Exports to Zambia	0	0	0	0	$5,730,000	$5,730,000
Reduction in trade losses	0	0	0	0	0	967,500
Replacement present controls	0	$ 60,000	$ 72,000	$223,300	291,800	562,500
Reduction in holding costs	0	40,000	48,000	155,500	194,500	375,000
Decrease in calf deaths	0	160,000	160,000	370,000	370,000	800,000
Improved productivity	0	0	0	0	0	750,000
Total benefits	0	$260,000	$280,000	$748,800	$6,586,300	$9,185,000

Source: Brooksby et al. 1972.

Table 12.6. Cost Benefit Analysis of Program to Establish a Disease-free Zone in Tanzania (19 Percent Internal Rate of Return over 20-Year Period)

Year	Costs	Benefits	Balance
		(Tanzanian dollars)	
1	1,903,762	0	-1,903,762
2	4,924,858	260,000	-4,664,858
3	3,131,376	280,000	-2,851,376
4	4,253,325	748,800	-3,504,525
5	6,874,804	6,586,300	- 288,504
6	6,304,574	9,185,000	2,280,426
7	4,652,535	9,185,000	4,532,465
8	4,916,535	9,185,000	4,268,465
9	5,048,535	9,185,000	4,136,465
10	4,520,535	9,185,000	4,664,465
11	4,652,535	9,185,000	4,532,465
12	4,916,535	9,185,000	4,268,465
13	5,048,535	9,185,000	4,136,465
14	4,520,535	9,185,000	4,664,465
15	4,652,535	9,185,000	4,532,465
16	4,916,535	9,185,000	4,268,465
17	5,048,535	9,185,000	4,136,465
18	4,520,535	9,185,000	4,664,465
19	5,652,535	9,185,000	4,532,465
20	4,916,535	9,185,000	4,268,465

Source: Brooksby et al. 1972.

Other Cost-Benefit Analyses

The actual costs and benefits as well as analyses of the cattle scabies eradication program in the United States has been presented by Kryder (1980). When the actual costs were discounted at 10 percent the present value of the costs over the 10-year period was $22.92 million (Table 12.7) with benefits of $63.53 million and a benefit-cost ratio of 2.77 (B-C ratio = $63.53/ $22.92 = 2.77). The net present value over 10 years is then $40.61 million (NPV = $63.53 - $22.92 = $40.61). If the process is taken further, different discount rates can be tried until one is found that equalizes the total discounted cost and benefits. For the scabies program a 35.5 percent discount rate resulted in a net present value of 0 and a benefit-cost ratio of 1.00. This discount rate is called the internal rate of return. The benefit-cost ratio is used in describing the impact of a program and the rate of return is used in comparing competitive programs.

The cost-benefits of programs to control or eradicate foot-and-mouth disease have been studied to justify (1) loans to developing nations (Stoops 1973; World

Table 12.7. Annual Costs and Benefits of Cattle Scabies
Eradication Program Discounted at 10 Percent

	Millions of Dollars				
Year	Actual Costs	Actual Benefits	Discounted Costs	Discounted Benefits	Discount Factor
1	3.1	0.0	2.82	0.00	1.100
2	4.6	0.1	3.82	0.08	1.210
3	4.3	0.3	3.23	0.23	1.331
4	4.2	0.6	2.86	0.41	1.464
5	4.1	1.5	2.54	0.93	1.611
6	4.1	3.8	2.30	2.13	1.772
7	4.1	10.5	2.09	5.36	1.949
8	3.0	19.7	1.41	9.26	2.144
9	3.0	40.3	1.26	16.93	2.358
10	1.5	72.3	0.59	28.20	2.594
Total	36.0	149.1	22.92	63.53	

Source: Kryder 1980.

Bank 1977) and (2) the allocation of monies by developed nations to prevent introduction of the disease (McCallon 1973; Carpenter and Thieme 1979; Hubbert 1979). One of the major studies for the latter purpose was conducted by a group from the University of Minnesota (McCauley et al. 1979). Several groups in South America have considered the rationale for allocation of monies for control of foot-and-mouth disease in developing nations (Rubinstein and Beltran 1975; Gomez et al. 1976; Rubinstein 1976, 1977; Rubinstein et al. 1978; Hugh-Jones 1979).

Disease-control officials in most major countries have developed models in an attempt to determine the cost-benefits of control programs. However, various critics do not accept the validity of some program models because of the assumptions upon which they are based and the analysis methods that are used. Beal (1980) examined 17 program analyses prepared by the Animal Plant Health Inspection Service of USDA (Table 12.8) and rated 6 as good or excellent. In his study

Table 12.8. Benefit-Cost Ratio of USDA Animal Disease-Control
Programs Rated Good or Excellent

Disease	Year	Type of Model	Benefit-Cost Ratio
Mastitis	1968	Simple	4-1
Bovine tuberculosis	1969	Modified double binomial	4-1
Cattle fever ticks	1969	Modified double binomial	99-1
Brucellosis	1975	Modified double binomial	5-1
Brucellosis	1976	Modified double binomial	8-1
Cattle scabies	1976	Modified double binomial	27-1

Source: Beal 1980.

he distinguished between true epidemic models that can be used to predict the course of disease in a changing world and pseudoepidemic models that fit a given situation in the past. The double binomial mathematic model has shown practical value in these studies.

NOTE ON FIGURE 12.2:
THE SIMULATION MODEL AND BASIC DATA INPUTS

The Beef and Dairy Simulation Model

The basic model (NBTC model) used to measure the impact of various brucellosis policy alternatives upon the spread, control, and/or eradication of brucellosis upon the beef and dairy sectors of the cattle industry in the United States was a computer simulation model.

The NBTC model determined simultaneously the effect of various policy alternatives upon the beef and dairy sector and was structured such that the disease was transmitted among and between beef and dairy herds in approximately the same manner as presently occurs within the cattle industry. In addition, the model was designed such that infected and detected herds could be placed in a "quarantine" status while undetected infected herds remained on a nonquarantined status. The subdivision of infected herds into quarantined and nonquarantined herds has a major impact upon physical losses, spread of the disease, and cleanup rates.

Some of the major mathematical components of the NBTC model are (1) the probability of detection, (2) the double binomial, and (3) the neighborhood spread formula.

The Probability of Detection

To calculate the number of newly quarantined herds in the beef population, the probability of undetected infected herds being detected has to be estimated. These detection probabilities were calculated by an approximation of a hypergeometric distribution. Detection probabilities varied by region, herd size, year of infection, cull rate cycle, market cattle inspection rate, and level of vaccination:

$$DP = 1 - (\frac{A - I - S/2 + 0.5}{A - S/2 + 0.5})^S$$

Source: Note from Anderson et al. (1978).

where DP = detection probability
  A = number of cows culled
  I = number of infected cows culled
  S = number of cows culled under surveillance system

The Double Binomial

A double binomial was used to simulate the spread of the disease through the purchase of infected replacements. Due to the nature of the cattle industry, parameters p, s, q, m, and n defined below were necessary for calculating the double binomial, which is defined as

$$1 - (q + ps^m)^n$$

where

$$p = \frac{\text{number of cows in infected herds in region}}{\text{total number of cows in region}}$$

$$q = \frac{\text{number of cows in brucellosis-free herds in region}}{\text{total number of cows in region}}$$

$$s = 1 - \frac{\text{total number of infected cows in region}}{\text{total number of cows in infected herds in region}}$$

n = number of sources from which replacements were purchased

$$m = \frac{\text{number of replacements purchased annually}}{\text{number of sources}}$$

Parameters p, s, and q were dependent on the number of undetected infected cows and herds in the region. Therefore, p, s, and q changed from year to year as the undetected infected population expanded or contracted.

Parameters m and n were calculated in the initial year of the model by region and herd size group and were held constant for the rest of the years of the simulation.

The double binomial was modified in order to allow for interregional movement of breeding stock. Each region had a certain probability of purchasing from within their own region and each of the seven other

regions. These probabilities always summed to 1 for
any given purchasing region and were held constant
throughout the simulation.

$$PP_{hij} = LL \; \Sigma = [(\text{regional purchase probability})_{hiLL} \times 1 - (q + PS)_{hij}^{mn}]$$

where

> PP = probability of a region purchasing one or
>   more infected replacements
> h = 1, 2 species (1 = beef, 2 = dairy)
> i = 1, 8 purchasing regions
> LL = 1, 8 regions from which replacements are
>   purchased
> j = 1, 7 herd size groups

To arrive at the number of newly infected herds,
the probability of a herd purchasing one or more infected replacements by herd size and region was multiplied
by the number of clean herds in that herd size group
and region.

$$NI_{hij} = PP_{hij} \text{ times NCLEAN}_{hij}$$

where

> NI = number of newly infected herds
> PP = probability of purchasing one or more
>   infected replacements
> NCLEAN = number of clean herds in the region
> h = 1, 2 species
> i = 1, 8 regions
> j = 1, 7 herd sizes

Neighborhood Spread

The second method in which a clean herd could be
infected was through contact with a neighboring infected herd. The first step in determining the number of
newly infected herds through neighborhood spread was to
calculate the weighted total infected herds. A quarantined herd was assumed to have one-half the spread of a
first year undetected infected herd (equation 1).
The newly adjusted undetected infected herds were

then weighted by their year of infection and totaled over herd size, year of infection and species for the region (equation 2).

$$INF_{hijL} = \sum_{L}^{L=1,3} \sum_{k}^{k=1,3} QUAR_{hijkL} \tag{1}$$

$$T_i = \sum_{h}^{h=1,2} \sum_{j}^{j=1,7} \sum_{k}^{k=1,3} (INF_{hijk} \text{ times } WINF_{hik}) \tag{2}$$

where

INF = undetected infected herds
QUAR = quarantined infected herds
T = total weighted infected herds
WINF = weighted infected rate where $WINF_{hik} = INFR_{hik}/INFR_{hi}$
INFR = within herd infection rate
i = 1, 8 regions
j = 1, 7 herd sizes
k = 1, 3 yr of infection
L = 1, 3 yr of quarantine
h = 1, 2 species

Newly infected herds due to neighborhood spread were then calculated by multiplying the weighted total infected herds (T) by the probability of a herd becoming infected (NS), which varied by region and species. These newly infected herds were distributed to the herd size groups on the basis of their weighted population proportions (WPP):

$$INF_{hijl} = T_i \times NS_{hi} \times WPP_{hij}$$

where

NS = neighborhood spread factor
INF = undetected infected herds
T = weighted total infected herds
$$WPP = \frac{\text{number of herds by herd size group and species in region}}{\text{total number of herds in region}}$$
h = 1, 2 species
i = 1, 8 regions
j = 1, 7 herd sizes
k = 1, 3 years of infection

REFERENCES

Anderson, N.; Morris, R. S.; and McTaggert, I. K. 1976. An economic analysis of two schemes for the anthelmintic control of helminthiosis in weaned lambs. *J. Aust. Vet. Assoc.* 52:174-180.

Anderson, R. K.; Berman, D. T.; Berry, W. T.; Hopkin, J. A.; and Wise. R. 1978. Report National Brucellosis Technical Commission. Anim. Plant Health Insp. Serv., USDA, Washington, D.C.

Astudillo, V. M.; Gauto, M. T.; Wanderley, M.; and Caballero, B. 1976. The cost of foot-and-mouth disease vaccination in Paraguay. Bol. Cent. Panam. Fiebre Aftosa 23-24:17-24.

Aulaqi, N. A., and Sundquist, W. B. 1979. A benefit-cost analysis of foot-and-mouth disease spread and control in the United States. In A Study of the Potential Economic Impact of Foot-and-Mouth Disease in the United States, eds. E. H. McCauley, N. A. Aulaqi, J. C. New, Jr., W. B. Sundquist, and W. M. Miller. Tech. Rep. 5. Washington, D.C.: USGPO, pp. 71-102.

Beal, V. C., Jr. 1980. Cost-benefit analysis in national animal disease control and eradication programs: A historical review with emphasis on the requirements for good analysis. Paper read at Work Conf. Teachers Prev. Med. Epidemiol. Public Health, Feb. 4-6, Fort Worth, Tex.

Beal, V. C., Jr., and Kryder, H. A., Jr. 1977a. Brucellosis program analysis. Anim. Plant Health Insp. Serv., USDA, Hyattsville, Md.

————. 1977b. Double binomial methodology for brucellosis program analysis. Anim. Plant Health Insp. Serv., USDA, Hyattsville, Md.

Bootes, B. W., and Gilchrist, P. T. 1979. Economics of alternative plans for Newcastle disease eradication. In Veterinary Epidemiology and Economics. Int. Symp. Vet. Epidemiol. Econ. Proc. 2:471-475. Canberra: Aust. Gov. Publ. Serv.

Brooksby, J. B.; Stubbins, A. J. G.; and Petrzik, J. 1972. Report to the government of Tanzania control of foot-and-mouth disease and the establishment of a disease-free zone. TA 3146. FAO, Rome.

Burger, E. J., Jr. 1980. Science at the White House: A Political Liability. Baltimore: Johns Hopkins Univ. Press.

Carpenter, T. E. 1976. The application of benefit-cost analysis to compare alternative approaches to the brucellosis problem in California. In New Techniques in Veterinary Epidemiology and

Economics.   Proc.   Int.   Symp.,   July   12-15.
    Reading, UK: Univ. Reading, pp. 122-125.
Carpenter, T. E.   1979.   The use of decision analysis
    in an eradication program: A case study of the
    eradication   of   *Mycoplasma meleagridis*   at   the
    commercial turkey breeder level.   In Veterinary
    Epidemiology and Economics.   Int.   Symp.   Vet.
    Epidemiol. Econ. Proc. 2:531-535.   Canberra:
    Aust. Gov. Publ. Serv.
Carpenter, T. E., and Heron, B. R. 1975. Benefit-cost
    study of brucellosis program.   A report on the
    bovine   brucellosis   eradication   program   in
    California.   Dep. Food Agric. Health Ind. Relat.,
    Sacramento, Calif., pp. 187-264.
Carpenter, T. E., and Thieme, A. 1979. A simulation
    approach to measuring the economic effects of
    foot-and-mouth disease in beef and dairy cattle.
    In Veterinary Epidemiology and Economics.   Int.
    Symp. Vet. Epidemiol. Econ. Proc. 2:511-516.
    Canberra: Aust. Gov. Publ. Serv.
Dietrich, R. A.; Amosson, S. H.; and Hopkin, J. A.
    1979.   Epidemiologic and economic analysis of the
    USA bovine brucellosis program and selected pro-
    gram alternatives via an open ended simulation
    model.   In Veterinary Epidemiology and Economics.
    Int. Symp. Vet. Epidemiol. Econ. Proc. 2:623-632.
    Canberra: Aust. Gov. Publ. Serv.
Dietz, K.   1972.   A supplementary bibliography on
    mathematical models   of   communicable diseases.
    Div. Res. Epidemio. Commun. Sci., WHO, Geneva.
Ellis, P. R.   1972.   Principles for socio-economic
    studies of the zoonoses.   WHO Consultations on
    Socioeconomic Aspects of Zoonoses, Nov. 21-25,
    Reading, UK.
Esuruoso, G. O.   1979.   Current status of brucellosis
    in Nigeria and a preliminary evaluation of the
    probable   costs   and   benefits   of   a   proposed
    brucellosis control program for the country.   In
    Veterinary Epidemiology and Economics.   Int. Symp.
    Vet. Epidemiol. Econ. Proc. 2:644-649.   Canberra:
    Aust. Gov. Publ. Serv.
Ferguson, W. 1969. Periodicity of epidemics and cost-
    benefit of vaccination programmes.   *Vet. Rec.*
    85:420-421.
Funder, J. 1979. All really great lies are half true.
    Science 206:1139.
Gittinger, J. P.   1972.   Economic Analysis of Agricul-
    tural Projects.   Baltimore: Johns Hopkins Univ.
    Press.
Gomez, G.; Espinoza, M.; Jimenez, J. M.; Bernal, C.;
    Suarez, E.; and Castaneda, J. 1976. Foot-and-

mouth disease economical effects on pig farm. Paper read at Int. Swine Symp., Ames, Ia.

Gordon, R. F. 1967. The economic effect of disease on the poultry industry. *Vet. Rec.* 80:101-107.

Grindle, R. J. 1979. Appropriate methodology in economic analysis of disease control projects. In Veterinary Epidemiology and Economics. Int. Symp. Vet. Epidemiol. Econ. Proc. 2:506-510. Canberra: Aust. Gov. Publ. Serv.

Groot, H. 1972. The health and economic impact of Venezuelan equine encephalitis (VEE). Sci. Publ. 243:7-27. Pan Am. Health Organ., Washington, D.C.

Harris, R. E.; Revfeim, K. J. A.; and Heath, D. D. 1979. A decision-oriented simulation for comparing hydatid control strategies. In Veterinary Epidemiology and Economics. Int. Symp. Vet. Epidemiol. Econ. Proc. 2:613-616. Canberra: Aust. Gov. Publ. Serv.

Horsfall, J. G., chairman. 1975. Agricultural Production Efficiency. Washington, D.C.: NAS.

Hubbert, W. T. 1979. Socioeconomic aspects of disease control. Paper read at Conf. Concepts Tech. Control Erad. Anim. Dis., Sept. 10-14, Auburn, Ala.

Hugh-Jones, M. E. 1976. Cost-benefit studies in relation to vaccination and immunization programmes. Pan Am. Health Organ. Sci. Advis. Comm. on Dengue, Yellow Fever and *Aedes aegypti*, Mar. 22-26, Panama City.

————. 1979. Some effects of foot-and-mouth disease in Brasilian cattle. Paper read at 2nd. Int. Symp. Vet. Epidemiol. Econ., May 7-11, Canberra, Aust.

Hugh-Jones, M. E.; Ellis, P. R.; and Felton, M. R. 1975. An assessment of the eradication of bovine brucellosis in England and Wales. Study 19. Dept. Agric. Hortic., Univ. Reading, Reading, UK.

Jahnke, H. E. 1974. The Economics of Controlling Tsetse Flies and Cattle Trypanosomiasis in Africa Examined for the Case of Uganda. Munchen IFO-Institut fur Wirtschaftsforschung.

James, A. D., and Ellis. P. R. 1979. The evaluation of production and economic effects of disease. In Veterinary Epidemiology and Economics. Int. Symp. Vet. Epidemiol. Econ. Proc. 2:363-372. Canberra: Aust. Gov. Publ. Serv.

Jobin, W. R. 1979. Cost of snail control. *Am. J. Trop. Med. Hyg.* 28:142-154.

Johnston, J. H. 1979. Decision making and veterinary epidemiology. In Veterinary Epidemiology and Economics. Int. Symp. Vet. Epidemiol. Econ. Proc. 2:523-530. Canberra: Aust. Gov. Publ. Serv.

Kryder, H. A., Jr. 1980. Animal health and economics. Paper read at general session Office International des Epizooties, May 26-31, Paris.

Lehman, J. S.; Bradley, D. J.; Hirsch, W. M.; and Fine, P. E. M. 1976. Mathematical models of schistosomiasis. Proceedings of a workshop held at The Rockefeller Foundation's Villa Serbelloni Study and Conference Center, May 9-14, Bellagio, Italy.

McCallon, W. R. 1973. Determining the economic feasibility of a disease control program. Animal disease eradication: Evaluating programs. Proc. NAS Workshop, Apr. 12-13, Univ. Wis. Ext., Madison, Wis., pp. 17-19.

McCauley, E. H. 1979. Estimation of the physical loss in animals infected with foot-and-mouth disease. In A Study of the Potential Economic Impact of Foot-and-Mouth Disease in the United States, eds. E. H. McCauley, N. A. Aulaqi, J. C. New, Jr., W. B. Sundquist, and W. M. Miller. Tech. Rep. 2. Washington, D.C.: USGPO, pp. 23-32.

McCauley, E. H.; Aulaqi, N. A.; New, J. C., Jr.; Sundquist, W. B.; and Miller, W. M., eds. 1979. A Study of the Potential Economic Impact of Foot-and-Mouth Disease in the United States. Washington, D.C.: USGPO.

McGregor, R. C. 1973. Government criteria for evaluating competing programs. Animal disease eradication: Evaluating programs. Proc. NAS Workshop, Apr. 12-13, Univ. Wis. Ext., Madison, Wis, pp. 22-23.

Mack, R. 1970. The great African cattle plague epidemic of the 1890's. *Trop. Anim. Health Prod.* 2:210-219.

McKelvey, J. J., Jr. 1973. Man against tsetse: Struggle for Africa. Ithaca, N.Y.: Cornell Univ. Press.

Moon, T. E. 1976. A statistical model of the dynamics of a mosquito vector (*Culex tarsalis*) population. *Biometrics* 32:355-368.

Nelson, R. R. 1977. The Moon and the Ghetto. Fels Lectures on Public Policy Analysis. New York: W. W. Norton.

Power, A. P., and Harris, S. A. 1973. A cost-benefit evaluation of alternative control policies for foot-and-mouth disease in Great Britain. *J. Agric. Econ.* 24:573-600.

Purchase, H. G., and Schultz, E. F., Jr. 1979. The economics of Marek's disease control in the United States. *World's Poult. Sci. J.* 34(4):198-204.

Roe, R. T., and Morris, R. S. 1976. The integration of epidemiological and economic analysis in the planning of the Australian brucellosis eradication programme. In New Techniques in Veterinary Epidemiology and Economics. Proc. Int. Symp., July 12-15. Reading, UK: Univ. Reading, pp. 75-88.

Rubinstein, E. M., de. 1976. Economic losses from foot-and-mouth disease in pigs. Paper read at Int. Swine Symp., Ames, Ia.

──────. 1977. The economics of foot-and-mouth disease control and its associated externalities. Ph.D. diss., Univ. Minn., Minneapolis, Minn.

Rubinstein, E. M., de, and Beltran, L. E. 1975. Economic losses from foot-and-mouth disease: A case study on a pig farm in Colombia. *Trop. Anim. Health Proc.* 7:149-151.

Rubinstein, E. M., de; Ariga, D.; Aycardi, E.; and Lopera, J. 1978. Analisis economico de alternatives para erradicacion de fiebra aftosa en la region de Uraba, Colombia. Instituto Colombian Agropecuario, Bogota, Colombia.

Ruttan, V. W. 1973. Induced technical and institutional change and the future of agriculture. Dev. Counc. Inc., New York.

Scott, J. T., Jr. 1970. The hog cholera eradication program. *Ill. Res.* 12(3):8-9.

Shepherd, A. A., Simpson, B. H., and Davidson, R. M. 1979. An economic evaluation of the New Zealand bovine brucellosis eradication scheme. In Veterinary Epidemiology and Economics. Int. Symp. Vet. Epidemiol. Econ. Proc. 2:443-447. Canberra: Aust. Gov. Publ. Serv.

Stoops, D. 1973. Funding disease control programs in developing nations. Animal disease eradication: Evaluating programs. Proc. NAS Workshop, Apr. 12-13, Univ. Wis. Ext., Madison, Wis.

Waaler, H. T. 1968. Cost-benefit analyses of BCG vaccination in various epidemiological situations. WHO TB Tech. Inf. 68.61, Geneva.

Weisbrod, B. A.; Andreano, R. L.; Baldwin, R. E.; Epstein, E. H.; Kelley, A. C.; and Helmeniak, T. W. 1973. Disease and Economic Development: The Impact of Parasitic Diseases in St. Lucia. Madison, Wis.: Univ. Wis. Press.

Wildavsky, A. 1979. No risk is the highest risk of all. *Am. Sci.* 67(1):32-37.

World Bank. 1977. Basic issues emerging from the Bank's experience with animal health project loans. Washington, D.C.

World Health Organization. 1970. Administrative management's considerations as to the assessment of the socio-economic consequences of zoonoses. Work. Pap. 2. WHO, Geneva.

13

Rural Communication

Public's Need to Know

All nations carry out some activities in secrecy, but today, government agencies in most free countries must keep the public informed about any actions they plan to take (Animal Plant Health Inspection Service 1972b; Benarde 1975). In some countries even the process of planning and decision making must be open. Although such openness may increase developmental costs, it should reduce public opposition (Chain 1979) and litigation possibilities, thereby decreasing implementation time and expense. Nevertheless, administrators view openness with misgivings because, historically, many facts have been distorted by special interest groups who wish to stop programs (Machado 1968) that the majority has already decided are in the publics' best interest. Even though present-day administrators realize that it is easier to conceal information than control its dissemination, they are also aware that any escape from communicating with the public is only temporary. Eventually they will have to speak and consequently, must know how to present the material and what channels to use.

Substance of the Message

The success of a director of a disease-control task force depends upon personal communication skills or assistants talented in that area. The director deals not only with field problems, staff operations,

264

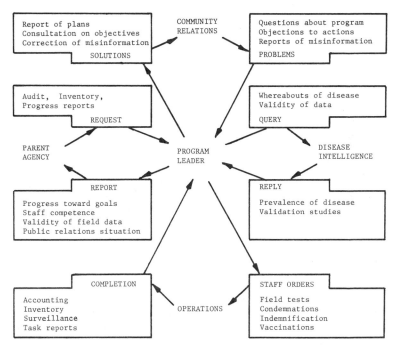

FIG. 13.1. Communication feedback loops maintained during a program.

and disease intelligence (Fig. 13.1) , but also with relations of the task force to the parent agency and impact of the program on the general public. In all instances, the information must flow two ways to form communication loops rather than one way as a directive. The emphasis of this chapter is on one of these loops: the relation between the task force and the community.

The message from the director of a disease-control task force to the public depends upon what the task force must do, who will be affected, and how proposed plans can be altered. The message should clearly state the nature of the problem the program is intended to solve, who will benefit from its solution, and what it will cost. It should also be clearly stated that the costs of a program include not only governmental out-lays for implementation but also the economic costs created by the program's impact on human and natural environments. The last two costs are often the most controversial, and consequently, it is tempting to conceal information to forestall distortions that are sure to arise. In addition to cost and benefit infor-

mation, the public should be given the projected timetable so that other plans can be coordinated.

Presentation of the message should be dynamic
rather than static, so opportunities must be provided
for feedback as well as development of impact statements and critiques (Schomisch 1967; Armstrong 1976).

Resolving Individual and Public Good

An animal disease-control program, if it is
successful, should benefit many people: livestock
producers, who are spared the uncertainties of disease;
processors, whose supply of animals is insured; and
consumers, who receive a better quality product at less
cost. However, people will not all benefit equally;
some may receive no benefit at all and some may even
be harmed. The last two consequences are generally
accepted by the public if it is clear that most of the
people involved will benefit.

Many administrators do not fully understand that
individuals and, sometimes, entire segments of the
population perceive benefits in different ways.
Beliefs regarding what is right, important or needed
for a good life are not uniform (Harris 1967). For
instance, the promise of a long-term gain in exchange
for a short-term loss is readily accepted by some
people but totally rejected by others. In a region
where the majority rejects this promise, it will be
very difficult to gain acceptance of a disease eradication program that is likely to impose a period of
sacrifice. This thinking is similar to that of individuals who say that they want to preserve their health
and improve it if possible. However, their behavior
contradicts their statements (Diehl 1969). Some will
refuse to leave a job even when they know the job is
harming their health and will shorten their life;
others continue habits that they admit are detrimental
to their health. Short-term economic advantages and
ephemeral pleasure are more important to many people
than long-term considerations. However, other individuals will remain in a community and at a job that
offers them little immediate economic return in their
pursuit of a long-term goal.

Everyone accepts information more readily from
individuals they know and sources they have found to be
dependable (Pasturino 1975). Therefore, it should not
be surprising that information offered by strangers,
whose appearance and speech may be somewhat different,
is usually viewed with suspicion and rarely accepted.

Furthermore, strangers who are government employees may encounter even more resistance to their message because they represent outside authority. Even so, those administrators who do not understand the habits and customs of the people or how to motivate them to change continue to be surprised when the public rejects what the administrators perceive to be good for them (Horowitz 1979).

However, a new idea will be accepted by even the most conservative segments of the population when they become convinced of its merit (Rogers and Shoemaker 1971; Morley et al. 1979; Shepherd 1979). On occasion, the process of effective communication must involve argument as well as delivery, and both the science and, art of persuasion must be applied (Hovland et al. 1953).

The acceptance of proposed programs is also conditioned by culture. In discussing eradication programs in his annual report for 1877, G. T. Brown, chief veterinarian of the United Kingdom, described the extreme measures that were adopted in Germany for control of rinderpest during the mid 1800s.

> All domestic animals excepting horses, mules, and asses were kept shut up. If found running about they were seized and slaughtered. Dogs and cats were killed and buried. The bringing in and sending away of cattle, hay, straw, and other infestable things was forbidden. If the disease extended to many farms in the locality, it was entirely surrounded by military sentinels; none but indispensable intercourse with the inhabitants was allowed. Divine service, school, and other assemblies were suspended, beershops and taverns closed. All roads through the locality were barred for the time. If the place was near a railway station, no train stopped there unless the station was entirely isolated from the infected place.

Brown pointed out that the English were different.

> If the proposition were fairly put that our herds could only be saved from extermination by adoption of these (German) measures the conclusion would necessarily be "so much the worse for the herds" but happily we have succeeded . . . by measures which do not seriously interfere with the liberty of the subject, on condition that more time be expended in the effort.

IDENTIFICATION OF AFFECTED PUBLICS

A special public is any group that is distinguish-
able from the general population because of an interest
that is common to its members. Because of its common
interest, the group usually has some system of internal
communication such as meetings, newsletters, or journals. If this particular public is important to the
disease-control program, its members can be reached
through these special communication channels by using a
message directed to the group's interests in its own
idiom (Bickford and Rosenwald 1976). For the message
to be heard, it must be presented to any group on its
own ground. Consequently, it is imperative to identify
all of the affected publics early in program planning
in order to develop communication with them (Abelson
1976).

The individual in charge of program communications
(Guss 1974) is responsible for identifing the special
interest groups and learning how to deliver messages to
them (Fig. 13.2). In a disease-control program, the
livestock or poultry producers are first in importance
because the task force will be dealing directly with
them. Livestock groups may be divided into subgroups,
such as breed associations and cooperatives. The supportive enterprises--truckers, packers, warehousers,
and retailers, as well as their labor unions and
creditors--are second in importance. Third are all the
other groups interested in animals: fanciers, hobby-
ists, wildlife preservationists, hunters, and all individuals who are concerned about any animal that might
be an alternative host for the disease. Fourth are
other groups, such as consumers, scientists, and tax-
payers, that have an interest in the program's success
or failure.

All of the affected groups are alike in their
independence, their own established channels of communications, their own considerable lexicon of special
terms, and their particular beliefs that cannot be
flouted (*Journal American Veterinary Medical
Association* 1976). Speakers who do not know the difference between a pullet and a broiler not only adver-
tise their incompetence on all poultry subjects to a
group of poultry producers but also reflect adversely
upon the organization that they represent. Similarly,
editors of medical journals would not reprint an article or editorial from a chiropractic journal even if
they agreed with it. The message, the style, the tone,
and the language must fit the audience and not flout
its strongly held beliefs.

Questions must be asked about each affected

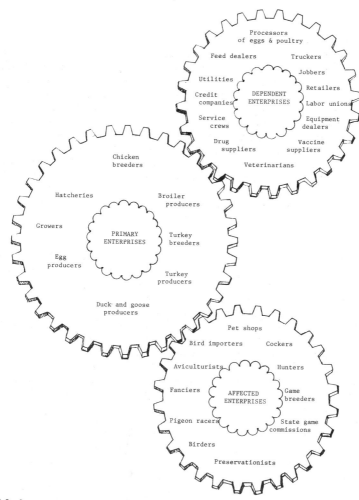

FIG. 13.2. Special interests groups concerned with the 1971-1972 Newcastle disease epizootic in southern California.

public. How is its vested interest endangered by the program (Animal Plant Health Inspection Service 1972a)? Would slaughter of animals cut off the income of its members or threaten them with loss of property or even bankruptcy? Would the program disrupt activities such as hunting or showing? If a group refuses to cooperate, how would the disease-control program be affected? For instance, birds that were raced by a pigeon fancier, in spite of a ban against movement of poultry and captive birds, could spread disease to outlying areas

as would birds smuggled into the region by an unethical
dealer.   If an animal-interest group resisted the program, the increased need for surveillance would slow
down the program and increase the costs.   Similarly,
the alienation of certain groups could have an important indirect impact.   For example, strikes by labor
unions and political meddling could make progress very
difficult.
     Clearly, it is exceedingly important to convince
the affected publics that the disease control program
is in their long-term interest.   To do that several
kinds of messages are needed.   The publics need to know
what the proposed program is, what effect it will have
on them, and what they will be asked to do (Benarde
1975).   The message should be presented clearly and
completely in a language that recognizes the unique
problems of each group and should provide assurances
that the group's concerns will be heard (Pasturino
1975).

COMMUNICATION CHANNELS

     As part-time residents of a rural area, we con-
tinue to be impressed with the speed and general
efficiency of oral communication.   Surprisingly, the
inaccuracy inherent in sequential transmission does not
seem to be much greater than the errors that occur in
mass media.   In addition, our rural mailbox is a recep-
tacle for community shoppers, newsletters, and circu-
lars from farmer co-ops, local schools, and a dairy
breeder association--all free, all presenting news, and
all relating it to their group.   Furthermore, our radio
brings us agricultural extension programs.   To this
assortment of information we add a daily newspaper, a
news journal, and a series of specialty journals.   As a
result, requests and demands come to us and our neighbors through a myriad of channels.
     Every study of communication has shown that people
listen to some channels more than others (Read 1972;
Tellez-S. 1975).   Whatever they listen to or read, some
voices are believed more than others, and even a given
voice may be believed on one subject and not another
(Victoria-L. and Arevalo-A. 1970).   Clearly, a publi-
cist must know the advantages and limitations of alternative channels and the ability of publics to discrimi-
nate between them.

Agricultural Extension

     Throughout the world, nations have used their
departments of agricultural and rural development to

create information dissemination systems that usually recognize the need for technician-farmer feedback (Duncan 1974). The system generally includes (1) a network of demonstration farms and experiment stations that people can visit to see new practices, (2) meetings and short courses conducted in cooperation with schools and colleges or fact-finding questionnaires and interviews (Elder et al. 1979), and (3) the production of printed materials (Rooney and McKeen 1972; Price and Rosenwald 1976), radio, television, and movie programs (Animal Plant Health Inspection Service 1978a). The emphasis differs from one part of the world to another. In developing countries where printed materials are of marginal value, films that demonstrate how to carry out certain procedures are effective and well accepted (Arevalo-A. and Alba-R. 1974).

Agricultural Extension has had a tremendous impact on rural development (Ruthenberg 1975). Even though the effect has been diminished by the commercial interests that employ intensive, professionally planned advertising campaigns to deliver messages, Agricultural Extension retains one important strength: a network of community-based agents who know the leaders in the community and can arrange local meetings with many kinds of groups. Local meetings are the most effective way to get a hearing of factual information on a controversial issue (Armstrong 1976). These meetings can be structured to provide not only for communication between the agency and any public but also for the public's participation in certain decisions regarding the course of the program (Chain 1979).

Special-Interest Organizations

The newsletters and journals of farmer co-ops, hunters, preservationists, and professionals carry authoritative messages to the members of these various groups. Since the members are influenced more by the information presented in these publications and at their meetings than they are by any other source, every effort should be made to disseminate information through the publications and meetings of special interest groups (Perkins and Tate 1979). General news releases are seldom effective for special-interest groups. For instance, during the California program for eradication of Newcastle disease, the most significant news event was a visit by a group of editors representing the poultry journals to the program headquarters (Animal Plant Health Inspection Service 1978a). The editors toured the offices, interviewed the program staff, and some also went into the field with the crews. The openness of the program administrator paid off in the editors' very favorable evaluation of the aims and methods of the program and the resulting extensive coverage in the journals.

Mass Media

Mass media (press, radio, and television) can create awareness of a disease problem in the mind of the general public and report actions such as the creation of a disease-control task force. However, interest of the mass media is fickle--sometimes intense, often apathetic--and may center on certain persons or become enamored with special angles. In-depth stories that treat central issues in either a critical or laudatory manner rarely appear. Attempts by task force leaders to use the media to disseminate anything other than the fact of their existence is fraught with danger (Fig. 13.3). Even if the reporter

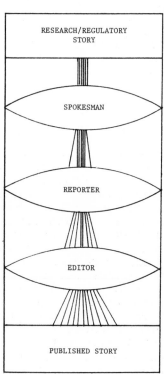

FIG. 13.3. Characteristics that interfere with objective journalism.

presents the correct information, the editor may alter it or the printer may garble it. Nevertheless, the communications staff must prepare task force leaders to meet the press and make radio and TV appearances since noncooperation invites direct attack on the program effort and, therefore, must be avoided.

An adversary relationship has often arisen between regulatory officials and the cooperating scientific community on one hand and the mass media on the other. The conflict appears to stem from a historic inability to speak the same language and mutual suspicion over objectives (Goodfield 1981). The press, assuming that regulatory officials and scientists make mistakes (which they do) and wish to protect themselves and their colleagues from embarrassing disclosures, interpret delays in the release of information as well as restricted access to areas or people as coverups that should be exposed (Cummings and Fetherston 1976). The regulatory officials and scientists, on the other hand, believe that (1) most of the informational delays they cause protect the public from unfounded information, and (2) the access restrictions they impose are necessary to stop the escape of dangerous organisms, chemicals, or radiation. They suspect that the press is less interested in informing the public than it is in selling papers, since advertising profits are based on circulation. Furthermore, regulatory officials suspect not only that the biases editors and reporters have toward certain causes and institutions determine what they will publish (Gosting 1968; Division of Vector Biology and Control 1976) but that reporters, when given freedom, do not have enough background on scientific matters to conduct an intelligent interview and write a factual story.

A few examples illustrate the nature of the problem. Some years back a reporter interviewed several members of an epidemiologic team studying an encephalitic disease in the midwest. The reporter worked hard, did background reading, and wrote a readable account that the epidemiologists checked for accuracy. The paper published the story without cutting it, but the editor distorted the message by releasing it the week before deer hunting season with the title "Disease of Deer Threatens State Hunters." The article did not even mention hunters, and the only sentence concerning deer stated that antibodies had been detected in some animals. Because of the title, hundreds of worried wives and mothers bombarded their physicians and the conservation department with calls about the risk to their husbands and sons. The resulting furor jeopardized cooperation between the researchers and the state conservation department.

More recently, an eastern paper did a series of articles, subtitled "Research For or Against Mankind," about a federal laboratory's research on foreign animal diseases (Cummings and Fetherston 1976). The writers did not visit the laboratory, discuss their charges with the director, or present any of the laboratory's accomplishments. The writers, apparently unfamiliar with biological research, criticized the staff for using procedures that are standard in laboratories throughout the country and interpreted the scientific community's common hiring and visiting practices as sinister connections.

In Mexico, the long, expensive, and eventually successful eradication program for foot-and-mouth disease was accomplished in spite of a campaign of distortion and villification carried on by several large newspapers that were politically inspired attempts to undermine the international effort (Machado 1968). It is suspected that this attack delayed the conclusion of the program even though there is no documentation to prove such a charge.

Failure to report newsworthy information or publication of distorted accounts sometimes occurs because newspapers depend upon part-time stringers or volunteer sources in distant localities who are loyal to the community and not the paper. For example, in 1962 it appeared that reports sent to the *New York Times* were delayed and lacked detail regarding an epidemic of St. Louis encephalitis in Florida, a tourist retreat for New Yorkers (Table 13.1). Reports of controversies in the later stages of the Florida epidemic, including accounts of the dismissal of a public health officer who talked to the local press, supported this inference of calculated delay and withholding of information

Table 13.1. *New York Times* Coverage of Two Epidemics of St. Louis Encephalitis

Coverage	Florida 1962	Texas 1963
Confirmed cases reported, %	90	291*
Confirmed deaths reported, %	32	120*
Timing of the first report in the *New York Times* in relation to epidemic peak	6 days after	7 days before
Lines of coverage	1,520	677
Coverage in first week, %	1.4	40.3

Source: Gosting 1968.

*Many other conditions were erroneously reported to be St. Louis encephalitis.

(Table 13.2). Such tactics were not used during a similar epidemic in 1963 in Texas, where the business interests were unconcerned about the New York tourist trade.

If the public is to receive general information through mass media, greater efforts should be made by both press and the task force (Margerison 1955; Garver 1958). The regulator or scientist should keep the story simple and be as direct and open as possible (Animal Plant Health Inspection Service 1976; Marx 1976) and editors should assign coverage to a reporter who has some specialized knowledge about animal diseases and their control. The writer should be willing to double-check the story by going over it with the persons interviewed or, if that is not feasible, having someone who is knowledgeable in the field read it for accuracy (Ogg 1978).

Television's capacity to transmit the emotional content of news events and thereby intensify their impact must not be overlooked by task force directors. The deliberate killing of animals for disease-control is a dreary chore that must be done. When the event is watched by a sad-faced family that knew those animals by name, it is emotionally draining, indeed. Machado (1968) told of Mexican women dressed in mourning who stood silently, their faces resigned, as army bullets dropped work oxen exposed to foot-and-mouth disease into the pit. Ashley (1977) described how Mrs. Thompson of West Virginia watched tearfully as the ewes and lambs that had been exposed to scrapie were given curare, died, and were buried. Her husband could not bear to come and watch.

Television crews can show these events on the evening news. The grizzly task of killing, slitting bellies, powdering with lime, and the spurt of intestinal coils as the bulldozers push soil onto the dead animals can now be caught on film in color. Further-

Table 13.2. Content Analysis of Newspaper Coverage of Epidemics of St. Louis Encephalitis (% of Total Lines of Coverage)

Content Category	New York Times on Houston Epidemic	Houston Chronicle on Houston Epidemic	New York Times on Florida Epidemic
Epidemic news	45.8	24.8	13.5
Control measures	14.8	41.8	20.1
Nature of disease	35.3	18.3	39.7
Assurances	4.1	3.2	0.4
Controversies and Impact	0.0	11.9	26.3
Total	100.0	100.0	100.0

Source: Gosting 1968.

more, the camera can probe the faces of the farm family, carrying their emotion to the living room screen.

Many messages are given with such scenes: the slaughter of innocent beasts, a family's grief, the power of government, the unfairness of calamity, and the terrible waste. Although the impact is mixed, overall it leaves most viewers feeling that all killing is bad and should be stopped (except at the butcher). When the swell of public opinion, whether it is emotional or reasoned, reaches the politicians, it often weakens their support for a necessary but controversial program.

Task force directors are faced with a dilemma when confronted with demands for television coverage of unpleasant tasks. If they prohibit filming they run the risk of increasing antagonistic commentary. Instead, they can make available an interpreter-host who can provide a perspective to the story (Animal Plant Health Inspection Service 1976). If the outcry over slaughter is to be muted, the long-term solution may be to develop alternative methods of disposal, such as meat salvage and carcass rendering. This suggests that the priorities administrators give research objectives may have to be determined by social and ethical considerations as well as managerial, scientific, and logistic needs. In order to develop better programs, the effectiveness of alternative means of communication and the identification of past communication failures should be carefully studied (Northumberland 1968).

PREPARING THE MESSAGE

Identification of material to be communicated and determination of the method of communication to be used requires the effort of a team (Lugo-Nasser 1973; Division de Comunicacion Social 1974; Animal Plant Health Inspection Service 1978b) whose members should include: (1) a representative of the program who is knowledgeable in technical and scientific matters, (2) a specialist in communication methods, and (3) an individual who is familiar with the public for whom the message is being prepared. This group should be organized when the program planning begins so that the messages as well as their form can be tested in the field.

Eric Ashby (1980) said that the public is now at the midstage of Arnstein's six levels of participation in government decision making:

1.   Manipulation--the government provides the public with selected information that makes the proposal look good.

2.   Therapy--the government uses persuasion in an attempt to convince opponents of the programs that their arguments are only ignorant prejudices.

3.   Informing--the government tells the whole story as it is, giving both pros and cons.

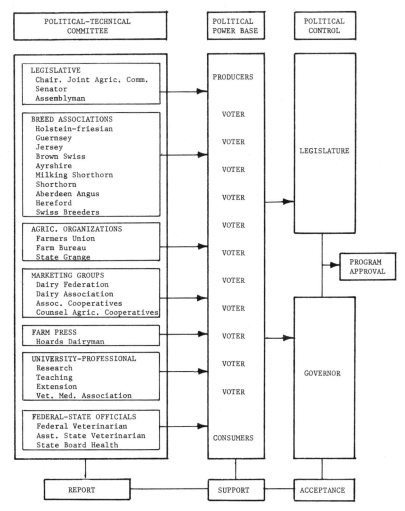

FIG. 13.4.   Twenty-eight man Wisconsin brucellosis committee (Schomisch 1967).

4. Consulting--the government asks the public to provide suggestions concerning selected matters.

5. Delegating power to participants--the government gives the public the right to make selected decisions concerning the program.

6. Citizen control--the government gives the public the right to make all decisions.

According to Ashby, the public now demands the whole story and expects to be consulted on some matters. Task force directors and communication teams must keep this in mind when preparing information programs.

Although most governments or administrators are not willing to move to the consultation level and share power with the public, some have tried it and a few have been successful. For example, the Wisconsin Director of Agriculture delegated the responsibility for developing a brucellosis eradication program to a citizen panel (Fig. 13.4) that transformed a politically unacceptable plan into a politically acceptable one (Schomish 1967). The panel helped with community education and communication and produced a regulatory program that was very similar to one drawn up earlier by the director's staff.

Today, administrators must be sensitive to the fact that the public wants to be informed and also wishes to be consulted on certain matters.

REFERENCES

Abelson, P. H. 1976. Communicating with the publics. *Science* 194:565.
Animal Plant Health Inspection Serivce. 1972a. Communication with "neglected" farmers on regulatory programs. Inf. Div., USDA, Hyattsville, Md., Jan. 26-27.
————. 1972b. Public information. USDA, Hyattsville, Md., June 23.
————. 1976. Information guidelines: Dealing with the news media. USDA, Washington, D.C., June 25.
————. 1978a. Eradication of exotic Newcastle disease in southern California, 1971-74. APHIS 91-34. USDA, Hyattsville, Md.
————. 1978b. EPIC: An information center for animal disease emergencies. Emergency Programs, USDA, Hyattsville, Md.
Arevalo-A., M., and Alba-R., V. 1974. Analisis de comprension de una pelicula pecuaria. Boletin

de Investigacion 4. Instituto Colombiano Agropecuario, Bogota, Colombia.

Armstrong, J. B. 1976. Brucellosis: Revised thoughts on issue after attending Texas A & M brucellosis symposium in July 1976. Mimeographed.

Ashby, E. 1980. Participating in planning: The public needs better information. *Nature* 283:712-713.

Ashley, S. 1977. Blood money: Sheep slaughter at government rates. *Harper's* 254(1520):28-31.

Benarde, M. A. 1975. The public's need to know. *ASM News* 41(8):625-627.

Bickford, A. A., and Rosenwald, A. S. 1976. Peripheral avian populations and poultry disease control. *West. Poult. Dis. Conf. Proc.* 25:20-22.

Brown, G. T. 1877. Annual report of Veterinary Department for 1877 cited by Francis, J. 1948. The contributions that quarantine, sanitary measures, and eradication can make to preventive medicine. *Vet. Rec.* 60:361-367.

Chain, P. 1979. Public participation and communication in Latin American disease control programs. In <u>Veterinary Epidemiology and Economics</u>. Int. Symp. Vet. Epidemiol. Econ. Proc. 2:335-340. Canberra: Aust. Gov. Publ. Serv.

Cummings, J., and Fetherston, D. 1976. The laboratory on Plum Island: Research for mankind or against it? *Newsday*, Nov. 14, Long Island, New York.

Diehl, H. S. 1969. <u>Tobacco and Your Health: The Smoking Controversy</u>. New York: McGraw-Hill.

Division de Comunicacion Social. 1974. Plan de divulgacion de la compana contra la fiebre aftosa. Instituto Colombiano Agropecuario, Bogota, Colombia.

Division of Vector Biology and Control. 1976. WHO-supported collaborative research projects in India: The facts. *WHO Chronicle* 30:131-139.

Duncan, R. J. 1974. Small farmer communication. Symposium Int. Res. Cent., Nov. 18-21, Bogota, Colombia.

Elder, J. K.; Morris, R. S.; and Knott, S. G. 1979. The choice of survey methods for eliciting livestock producers' attitudes of cattle tick control. In <u>Veterinary Epidemiology and Economics</u>. Int. Symp. Vet. Epidemiol. Econ. Proc. 2:341-350. Canberra: Aust. Gov. Publ. Serv.

Garver, W. B., moderator. 1958. Public relations in agriculture and agricultural research. NAS-NRC Publ. 644. *Agric. Res. Inst. Proc.* 7:61-79. Washington, D.C.

Goodfield, J. 1981. Reflections on Science and the Media. Washington, D.C.: Am. Assoc. Adv. Sci.

Gosting, D. 1968. Preliminary report on a content analysis of the press coverage of three encephalitis epidemics. Environ. Sci. Inst., Univ. Wis., Madison.

Guss, S. B. 1974. Communications problems. *U.S. Anim. Health Assoc. Proc.* 78:47-50.

Harris, M. 1967. The myth of the sacred cow. *Nat. Hist.* 76(3):6-12.

Horowitz, M. M. 1979. The sociology of pastoralism and African livestock projects. Agency for International Development Program Evaluation Discussion Paper 6. Bur. Program Policy Coord., AID, Washington, D.C.

Hovland, C. I.; Janis, I. L.; and Kelly, H. H. 1953. Communication and Persuasion. New Haven: Yale Univ. Press.

Journal of the American Veterinary Medical Association. 1976. Swine flu misnamed. 169:689.

Lugo-Nasser, O., coordinator. 1973. Seminario sobre tecnicas de divulgacion y educacion de la comunidad para los programas de control y prevencion de la fiebre aftosa, vol. 1. Instituto Colombiano Agropecuario, Bogota, Colombia, July 20.

Machado, M. A., Jr. 1968. An Industry in Crisis: Mexican-United States Cooperation in the Control of Foot-and-Mouth Disease. Univ. Calif. Publ. Hist, vol. 80. Berkeley and Los Angeles: Univ. Calif. Press.

Margerison, T. A. 1955. Dissemination of scientific information. *Nature* 176:1008-1009.

Marx, J. L. 1976. Science and the press: Communicating with the public. *Science* 193:136.

Morley, F. H. W.; Mitchell, R.; Napthine, D.; Gillick, J.; and Hass, C. 1979. Attitude of farmers to adoption of the Mules operation. In Veterinary Epidemiology and Economics. Int. Symp. Vet. Epidemiol. Econ. Proc. 2:354-357. Canberra: Aust. Gov. Publ. Serv.

Northumberland, Duke of. 1968. Report of the Committee of Inquiry on Foot-and-Mouth Disease, 1968, part 2, Cmnd. 4225. London: Her Majesty's Stationery Off.

Ogg, J. E. 1978. Professional relations with the communications media. *ASM News* 44(11):580-582.

Pasturino, C. 1975. Some comments on the experience of Uruguay foot-and-mouth disease campaings: The work of field veterinarians. *Bol. Centro Panamer. Fiebre Aftosa* 17-18:23-26.

Perkins, D., and Tate, J. 1979. How will you react if . . . foot-and-mouth strikes. *The Cattleman* 65(11):36-43.

Price, F. C., and Rosenwald, A. S. 1976. Preventing avian pox. Leaflet 2871. Univ. Calif. Coop. Ext., Davis, Calif.

Read, H. 1972. Communication: Methods for All Media. Urbana, Ill: Univ. Ill. Press.

Rogers, E. M., and Shoemaker, F. F. 1971. Communication of Innovations: A Cross-Cultural Approach, 2nd ed. New York: The Free Press; London: Collier Macmillan Publ.

Rooney, W. F., and McKeen, W. D. 1972. Extension effort in a Newcastle quarantine area. *West. Poult. Dis. Conf. Proc.* 21:61-63.

Ruthenberg, H. 1975. Agricultural extension as an economic investment. *Agric. Adm.* 2:1-27.

Schomisch, T. P. 1967. Wisconsin brucellosis campaign. M.S. thesis, Univ. Wis., Madison.

Shepherd, R. 1979. Technology transfer study reveals factors that influence adoption of innovations. *Trop. Med. Hyg. News* 28(3):15-16.

Tellez-R., J. 1975. La comunicacion en el oriente antioqueno: Disponibilidad de medios. Boletin de investigacion 34. Instituto Colombiano Agropecuario, Bogota, Colombia.

Victoria-L., F., and Arevalo-A., M. 1970. Canales de comunicacion que utilizan los campesinos del proyecto de desarrollo del norte del cauca. Boletin de Investigacion 16. Instituto Colombiano Agropecuario, Bogota, Colombia.

14

Disease Control
Task Force

NATURE OF TASK FORCE

Whether a task force is created in response to an emergency (Mulhern 1955) or as the most practical administrative structure for handling an existing program (Wise 1979a), plans must be laid well in advance. In order to respond to an emergency (Panamericano de Fiebre Aftosa, Centro 1962; Adlam 1979), a prior decision must have been made that certain predetermined circumstances will trigger the formation of a task force with a certain organizational plan (Figs. 14.1 and 14.2) and mode of operation (Fig. 14.3).

A task force established to carry out a disease-eradication program is similar to a military unit ordered to occupy a region (Sharman 1973; Davidson 1979b; Omohundro 1979). The person in command has a headquarters unit that is located to make the best use

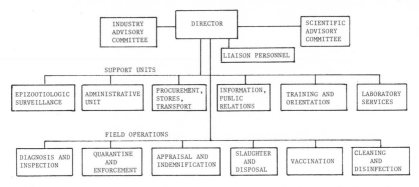

FIG. 14.1. Organization of an emergency task force (adapted from Animal Plant Health Inspection Service 1978).

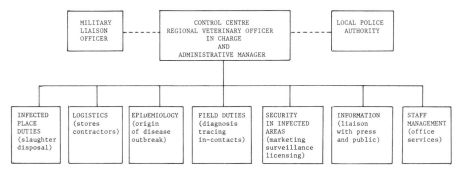

FIG. 14.2. Organizational chart: Foot-and-mouth disease-control team (adapted from Northumberland 1968).

of communication channels and supply routes in order to keep supporting services and field forces informed and operational. The supporting services provide supplies and transportation and maintain facilities. Each field unit has an assigned function and, in general, follows established procedures learned by drill. Orders and reports for all field actions descend and rise through the chain of command from headquarters to field and back again. However, this does not preclude a degree of autonomy in field units that permits diversity to meet field situations.

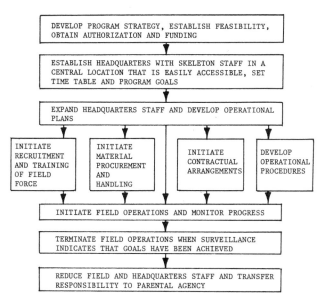

FIG. 14.3. Flow chart for an animal disease-control program.

STRUCTURING THE TASK FORCE

The details of the organizational structure vary according to the task assigned and the nature of the region in which it is to be accomplished. In all instances, however, a task force has three components: (1) a headquarters unit, (2) supporting services, and (3) field units (Animal Plant Health Inspection Service 1978).

The headquarters unit has administrative responsibilities. The director needs an administrative assistant second in command; a secretary; and several officers, some of whom may have a staff of one or more depending upon the size of the task force. In general, these officers are responsible for the identified support services and field units. The support units include: (1) an administrative unit for personnel and finance; (2) a logistics unit that provides transport, handles procurement, and manages supplies; (3) a public relations and information unit; (4) an assessment unit that conducts epizootiologic surveillance; and, depending on the campaign, (5) a laboratory services unit (McDaniel 1976) and (6) a training and orientation unit. These last two functions may be provided by contract if they are not an integral part of the task force. Operational field units differ from one campaign to another and may function only during part of the campaign. For example, a vaccination unit is not needed in some campaigns, and the slaughter and disposal unit as well as the cleaning and disinfecting unit begin to function only after the appraisal and indemnification team has been in the field. All task forces need a diagnosis and inspection team as well as a quarantine and enforcement team. The number of the various units depends upon the timetable, size of the region, and nature of the terrain. In large campaigns the director may have one assistant who supervises support units and another who directs field units.

In recent campaigns, task force commanders have learned the value of liaison personnel and advisory groups (Animal Plant Health Inspection Service 1978; Davidson 1979a). Full-time liaison personnel are attached to the task force to coordinate the activities of a group (military personnel who have been integrated into the task force) or facilitate communication on policy with a sister agency (health department) or a special industry group (affected livestock producers). Advisory groups meet when called to discuss task force problems. Scientific as well as industry advisory bodies have been particularly helpful in this regard

(Animal Plant Health Inspection Service 1978). Such groups are able to rate the feasibility of alternative actions in terms of their expertise, sometimes suggest innovative approaches, and also serve as effective communicators and defenders of campaign policy (Advisory Committee 1976).

The way a task force functions depends on administrative rules (World Health Organization 1973) and the director's style. Administrative style consists largely of the manner in which decision making, communications, and personnel questions are handled. Although the director has the responsibility for decisions, input can be obtained from supervisors, staff, and outside consultants (Sharman 1973). The director may centralize decision making or delegate it. Both recorded and off-the-record communications are utilized, but the balance between the two is determined by the director who also decides the extent to which actions are documented. Communication techniques and systems for information flow may vary (Fig. 13.1), but wise directors make every effort to insure communication that is truly two-way and includes all reports of program failures and adverse public reactions as well as program successes.

Personnel recruitment and training are ongoing tasks that are made more difficult by the urgent deadlines the organization must meet, the temporary nature of the program, and demands for expanding and contracting program units. These problems can be compounded by job dissatisfaction, which accelerates turnover, and inadequate communications with headquarters, which occurs frequently and alienates the field staff. Such a situation graphically described by Sharman (1973) in a "communique" from a disgruntled employee in the Mexican campaign. These problems can be softened by a director who understands personnel management and can help employees perceive their functions.

Training courses for administrators generally include three major areas: (1) personnel management, (2) task analysis, and (3) materials management. Personnel management includes all aspects of interpersonal relationships. One aspect, sensitivity training, provides insight regarding the effect of personal background on worker efficiency. Another fundamental management concept is the "span of control," a term describing the number of individuals--rarely exceeding six to ten--that one person can directly supervise (Delbecq 1968). However, if command is pyramided through the use of deputies, section heads, and supervisors, the number of persons one individual can super-

vise is almost unlimited.   In such a situation, there
is no escape from the delegation of responsibility.
Unfortunately, leaders can be tempted to take over the
neglected responsibilities of an incompetent subordinate and delay the search for a competent replacement.   The higher operational obligations are always
jeopardized by such expediencies.   Relationships
between people take several shapes: (1) linear and
branching linkages--superior-subordinate chains, (2)
coordination--chair-coordination relationships, and (3)
consultation--interrelationships of peers (Fig. 14.4,
Scott 1967).   Formal relationships shown on organizational charts seldom reflect operational realities that
are determined by personalities and continually changing work problems.   While growth and institutional
responsiveness depends upon the freedom of the staff to
use informal relationships, these relationships create
a certain amount of tension that a good director can
keep within bounds.

Task analysis procedures examine the methods used
in defining and organizing administrative operations
and include: (1) network analysis, (2) decision trees,
and (3) queueing theory.   In network analysis (Manger
1972), a procedure recommended by many administrative
authorities, specific events that occur during a project are identified and diagrammatically symbolized as
circles.   The activities or undertakings that consume
resources and take finite units of time to bring about
these identified events are symbolized by arrows.   The
longest path to a goal is symbolized by a double-lined

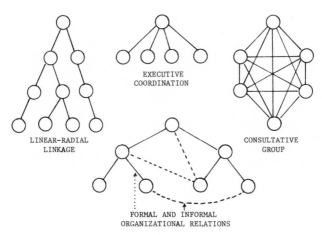

FIG. 14.4.   Organizational relationships (adapted from Scott
1967).

arrow, shorter paths by a single-lined arrow. Numbers above the arrow signify units of time. Such diagrams are used to determine the best way to achieve a given goal.

A decision tree is a device that enables a planner to consider various courses of action in terms of probability and cost. A probability from 1 (absolute certainty) to 0 (absolute impossibility) is assigned to each action. The planner obtains a value figure by multiplying the assumed cost of the action by its probability. Using this approach, the planner can determine whether the best organizational decision is to prepare for the most likely event or for one that may be somewhat less likely. If the most likely event does not involve an emergency, consideration should still be given to the possible consequences of an unexpected emergency for which the organization is not prepared.

Queueing theory deals with minimizing the costs of delays that occur at any limiting orifice. It is assumed that a program is the sum of a set of definable tasks, each of which has an inherent duration, and many of which must be done in a prescribed order. Furthermore, some of the tasks must be done within a set time of the preceding task or the entire sequence must be redone. When there is a prescribed sequence, a delay in the completion of a task at any point creates a delay in all subsequent tasks. Such delays become bottlenecks that can jeopardize the entire program. The old rhyme stated it very well:

For the want of a nail the shoe was lost
For the want of a shoe the horse was lost
For the want of a horse the rider was lost
For the want of the rider the battle was lost.

The last administrative area concerns materials management and deals largely with (1) logistics, (2) inventory control, and (3) material replacement. In military operations, logistic restraints limit the delivery of supplies to the battlefield. The supplies must be those that are needed, and the deliveries must be uninterrupted. Fulfillment depends on the equipment that moves the supplies as well as the operation of storage depots and maintenance shops. Inventory control deals with idle resources and the costs that result from overinventory (storage costs, obsolescence, and waste); underinventory (inability to meet demand or delays in meeting demands); and failure to optimize orders, such as loss of discounts. Material replacement deals with the problems of continuing operation when component parts of equipment and facilities wear out or fail. The strategy of replacement when failure occurs minimizes the number of items that will be replaced but maximizes associated costs; the strategy of replacement before failure reverses the type of costs. The preferred policy depends upon the nature of the program.

The identification of various administrative responsibilities--decision making, communication, inventory control, resource replacement, personnel training, record keeping, sequencing, or queueing--assist in the recognition of problems that arise from mishandling any one of them and delineates the value that is inherent in their mastery (Heyel 1973). Without some understanding and experience in administrative skills, few individuals can bring a well-conceived program to completion.

STAFF RECRUITMENT AND TRAINING

The task force leader's problem of recruitment and training is greatly reduced if the parental agency has a program for training field officers in administrative methodology, logistical problems, and epizootiology (by study in periodic institutes or short-term assignments to foreign programs or sister agencies) and conducts periodic field exercises (Zweigart 1973). Such anticipatory programs provide a core staff of administrative officers that can function immediately. This staff can be augmented by the loan of trained people from the agricultural departments of states or provinces and assignment of officers and sergeants from the veterinary services of the Armed Forces. Universities and veterinary schools can contribute technical and scientific experts, and in some emergencies, foreign governments send personnel to observe and assist in the program.

In addition to the trained people recruited from the sources described, certain specialists will be needed as well as a large body of laborers who are usually recruited locally. With a working force of diverse origin, it is most important, both for legal reasons and good relations with the general public, that task force actions are taken in a uniform manner (Animal Health Division 1971; Panamericano de Fiebre Aftosa, Centro 1975). This can be done only if there are standardized procedures of operations. Manuals covering foreseeable actions should be prepared in advance, and crews should be drilled in procedures before going into the field. Changes in procedures and procedures for new actions should be issued as directives. It is important that any change be implemented simultaneously after all the affected staff has been informed.

Training of personnel should never be considered to be finished. Test exercises, one-day refreshers, and special seminars can be employed to verify compliance with standards and instruct and stimulate the staff.

MARSHALLING EQUIPMENT AND SUPPLIES

Any large established enterprise uses many pieces of equipment and needs a continuous flow of supplies. Some of the equipment must be ordered weeks or even months prior to its use, and spare parts for its repair must be stockpiled weeks in advance, especially if they are available only seasonably. An experienced procurement officer uses a continuous inventory and central or regional warehouses to simplify the process.

Procurement for a task force that is established to meet an emergency is difficult because time is critical and government procedures are seldom geared for emergency situations. Stockpiling equipment and supplies in advance of an emergency is rarely practical because of the cost and the difficulty (or impossibility) of obtaining the necessary funds. Even more important, most items rapidly get out-of-date or deteriorate. Locating the storage depot to provide ready transport of goods to an unknown place of use is also a problem.

The need for a vaccine to cope with an emergency illustrates these concerns. It takes five or six years to erect a plant to produce a vaccine for a disease such as foot-and-mouth disease. Clearly, this is not an option in an emergency. If a suitable operating vaccine plant is available, conversion from one product to another can take anywhere from a few months to two years depending upon the equipment needed. A plant erected to be maintained on a standby basis can be put into use immediately, but it will still be about six months before the product can be delivered for field use. Stockpiled vaccines are available immediately, but their relatively short life (one to two years) requires continuous and, consequently, costly replacement.

What alternatives are there? Vaccines may be pur-

chased from other nations if they have available stores
and the vaccine meets the minimum standards set by the
buyer (Callis et al. 1975). There is no way of knowing
in advance whether vaccine will be available from such
sources when needed unless a contract provides for a
stockpile. For some vaccines, a better alternative is
the preparation of an antigen concentrate that can be
stored for periods as long as 10 years, and converted
in about one month to a vaccine that is bottled and
ready for use.

The alternatives for procurement of equipment and
other supplies are almost as diverse. Until purchases
can be made through commercial channels, equipment and
many supply items can be diverted from other government
uses if proper authority can be obtained. Again,
states or provinces and even foreign countries can
help. Substitution and innovation are often necessary.
For instance, in the California Newcastle disease-
eradication program, an isolation cage was needed for
housing the chickens used in properly identifying virus
isolates. Because the conventional isolation cage used
in laboratories is stainless steel and fabricated to
order, a delivery time of three to four months or more
is required. In this case, cardboard shippers, used by
dealers to transport animals, were converted by the
addition of disposable filters and used as isolators.
These disposable units were available within one week.

In advance of an emergency, procurement lists,
which should be updated frequently, should be established for each of the units that make up a task force.
Such lists would be a great aid to both the procurement
officer and the budget officer.

INITIATING OPERATIONS

A guidebook prepared by the Animal Health Division
(1971) of the United States Department of Agriculture
covers task force operation in comprehensive fashion
that even includes the qualifications for supervisors,
their tasks, and the maintenance of vehicles. The outline of the Emergency Animal Disease Eradication Guide
(somewhat simplified) is as follows:

1. Historical background of eradication programs
2. Administrative procedures (personnel, services, and
   budget)
3. Eradication procedures
   a. Investigation of cases, diagnoses, notifica-
      tions

     b. Quarantine of premises, appraisal, depopula-
         tion, disposal, cleaning, disinfection, and
         testing of clean premise
     c. Organization of task force
     d. Guidelines for infected premises, stockyards,
         packing plants, zoos, wildlife areas, and
         tracing animals
     e. Personal responsibilities and forms
4. Epidemiology, investigation, and surveillance procedures
5. Legal basis for operation
6. Information policy, responsibilities, and authority
7. Cooperating agencies

    Whether the action of the task force is to find
and eliminate diseased animals, find and protect susceptible animals, or destroy vectors of disease, the
first step is to inform the public what action will be
taken, when and where it will occur (Fig. 13.1). The
task force communication unit needs to identify the
various groups that will be affected by the program and
prepare the necessary messages. Some messages will go
to the news media, but direct contact with owners and
managers of animals and property must also be made to
tell them what to expect in terms of examination, vaccination, or even quarantine. If language or dialect
is a problem, one of the members of the team should be
native to the area and have credibility with the
people. This has been essential in such linguistically
and ethnically diverse countries as Mexico and Iran.
    The director, after taking a personal role in
initiating the effort to inform the public of the creation and purpose of the task force, must establish the
boundaries of the affected region and the points where
the effort will start (Omohundro 1972). Sometimes the
work starts at the boundary of the region and proceeds
toward the center, such as ring vaccination; at other
times it starts at the center and proceeds outward,
such as tracing the movement of infected animals.
    In most situations the region and the tasks must
be subdivided for operational reasons. Field teams are
then assigned duty in rational sequence. The unique
features of every region necessitate operation flexibility. When aggregations of poultry range from backyard flocks of four birds to commercial flocks of four
million, allowance must be made for the impact of flock
size on techniques for depopulation and disposal of
birds (Wise 1979b). Subzero weather may necessitate a
change in strategy for disposal of cattle affected with
foot-and-mouth disease, as the Canadian authorities

learned in 1952 (Wells 1952). Economic problems (Bootes and Gilchrist 1979) and public relation problems (Atwell 1975) may also lead to reappraisal of field methods. While premise cleanup and disinfection procedures are generally standardized for conventional forms of husbandry, field crews should be prepared for encountering innovative forms of husbandry. For example, slatted-floor houses with liquid-manure-handling systems, which are still uncommon in many areas, would pose problems for a crew accustomed to cleaning up concrete-floored houses and lots.

Appraisal of animals for indemnification is a very specialized job that requires prior training (Aulaqi and Sundquist 1979). If the appraiser does not establish an equitable price by considering both the quality of the animal and the current market, the resistance of the livestock community will build quickly (Bell 1972). The appraiser not only has a position of trust that requires a high level of integrity but also represents the task force in a very visible role. A system should be established to identify individuals with this specialized background to facilitate their rapid recruitment in the event of an emergency.

Targets are set and projections reviewed daily. Unforeseen problems of weather, legal resistance, or the discovery of unknown populations require adjustments in targets and reassignment or enlargement of staff. A flow of information from the field, which details progress and problems so that corrections can be made quickly, is essential for an efficient and successful operation. Some directors accomplish this with a short, daily staff meeting of unit leaders; others depend largely on the flow of paper communications.

PROCEDURE FOR TERMINATION

Since a task force is an ephemeral organization that has an assigned task to complete, the organization is no longer needed when that task is done. Criteria for defining the completion of the program must be established either before or shortly after the task force is created. The criteria should be objective, and the procedures for establishing them should be reasonable. Failure to observe overt disease is seldom an adequate criterion for declaring a disease has been eradicated because latent carriers of that disease organism may still exist. For this reason, the final stage of the task force operation may be a period of surveillance, approximately one year, during which a small staff conducts some type of systematic search for evidence of disease. After active cases of exotic Newcastle disease were eliminated in California, dead birds ("normal" mortality) were collected from sentinel farms for nine months and tested for the presence of virus. Since no virus was isolated during this period, the disease was declared eradicated.

The process of task force demobilization occurs in stages. The units that handled acute disease are phased out first, and most units are scaled down in size. The headquarters unit, which transfers the records, and the surveillance unit, which evaluates the success of the total effort, remain until completion of the project. Prior to the termination, an outside individual should be asked to prepare documents of the task force for evaluation by a study group or commission such as the groups who prepared the British Command reports. With such documentation, future task forces can profit from the program's errors as well as its success.

REFERENCES

Adlam, G. H. 1979. Planning and implementation of disease control programs: Experience in New Zealand. In Veterinary Epidemiology and Economics. Int. Symp. Vet. Epidemiol. Econ. Proc. 2:558-567. Canberra: Aust. Gov. Publ. Serv.

Advisory Committee on Foreign Animal Disease to the Secretary of Agriculture. 1976. Minutes of meeting, June 2, 3. USDA, Hyattsville, Md.

Animal Health Division. 1971. Emergency animal disease eradication guide. Agric. Res. Serv., USDA, Hyattsville, Md.

Animal Plant Health Inspection Service. 1978. Eradication of exotic Newcastle disease in southern California, 1971-74. APHIS 91-34. USDA, Hyattsville, Md.

Atwell, J. 1975. Animal protein conservation work group report. U.S. Anim. Health Assoc. Proc. 79:336-341.

Aulaqi, N. A., and Sundquist, W. B. 1979. Indemnification under animal disease control programs with special emphasis on foot-and-mouth disease. In A Study of the Potential Economic Impact of Foot-and-Mouth Disease in the United States, eds. E. H. McCauley, N. A. Aulaqi, J. C. New, Jr., W. J. Sundquist, and W. M. Miller. Tech. Rep. 12. Washington, D.C.: USGPO, pp. 201-241.

Bell, D. 1972. Southern California poultry industry reactions to the Newcastle disease eradication program. Univ. Calif. Agric. Ext., June 29, Davis, Calif.

Bootes, B. W., and Gilchrist, P. T. 1979. Economics of alternative plans for Newcastle disease eradication. In Veterinary Epidemiology and Economics. Int. Symp. Vet. Epidemiol. Econ. Proc. 2:471-475. Canberra: Aust. Gov. Publ. Serv.

Callis, J. J.; Graves, J. H.; McKercher, P. D.; and Uskavitch, P. 1975. Report on worldwide foot-and-mouth disease vaccine production, Feb. Restricted doc., Plum Island Anim. Dis. Cent., Greenport, N.Y.

Davidson, R. M. 1979a. Advisory committees in disease control schemes. In Veterinary Epidemiology and Economics. Int. Symp. Vet. Epidemiol. Econ. Proc. 2:351-353. Canberra: Aust. Gov. Publ. Serv.

————. 1979b. Administration and logistics of the brucellosis eradication scheme in New Zealand. In Veterinary Epidemiology and Economics. Int. Symp. Vet. Epidemiol. Econ. Proc. 2:633-637. Canberra: Aust. Gov. Publ. Serv.

Delbecq, A. L. 1968. The world within the "span of control." *Bus. Horiz.*, Aug., pp. 47-56.

Heyel, C., ed. 1973. The Encyclopedia of Management, 2nd ed. New York: Van Nostrand Reinhold Co.

McDaniel, H. A. 1976. Laboratory support for emergency programs. *U.S. Anim. Health Assoc. Proc.* 80:319-323.

Manger, A. J. 1972. Modern concepts of management science and their relation to the health sector. Inter-regional training course in epidemiology and control of communicable diseases held in Moscow and Alexandria, WHO, Geneva.

Mulhern, F. J. 1955. State-federal emergency programs. *U.S. Livest. Sanit. Assoc. Proc.* 59:218-223.

Northumberland, Duke of. 1968. Report of the Committee of Inquiry on Foot-and-Mouth Disease, 1968, part 2, Cmnd. 4225. London: Her Majesty's Stationery Off.

Omohundro, R. E. 1972. Exotic Newcastle disease eradication. *U.S. Anim. Health Assoc. Proc.* 76:264-268.

————. 1979. Task force approach to animal disease eradication. Paper read at Conf. Concepts Tech. Control Erad. Anim. Dis., Sept. 10-14, Auburn, Ala.

Panamericano de Fiebre Aftosa Centro. 1962. Plans of

action in the event of an outbreak of foot-and-mouth disease. Rio de Janeiro, Brazil, June 15.
————. 1975. Manual de procedimientos para la prevencion y eradicacion de las enfermedades vesiculares de los animales. Rio de Janeiro.
Scott, W. G. 1967. <u>Organization Theory: A Behavioral Analysis for Management.</u> Homewood, Ill.: Richard D. Irwin, Inc.
Sharman, R. 1973. Operation of a disease control program. Animal disease eradication: Evaluating programs. Proc. NAS Workshop, Apr. 12-13, Univ. Wis. Ext., Madison, Wis.
Wells, K. F. 1952. Foot-and-mouth disease control and eradication measures in Canada. *U.S. Livest. Sanit. Assoc. Proc.* 56:166-171.
Wise, G. H. 1979a. The conception and birth of a planned, non-emergency program. Paper read at Conf. Concepts Tech. Control Erad. Anim. Dis., Sept. 10-14, Auburn, Ala.
————. 1979b. Slaughter as a technique in disease programs. Paper read at Conf. Concepts Tech. Control Erad. Anim. Dis., Sept. 10-14, Auburn, Ala.
World Health Organization. 1973. Health project management: A manual of concepts and procedures. Proj. Syst. Anal. PSA/73.1. Geneva.
Zweigart, T. F. 1973. Task force operations: Manpower. Anim. Plant Health Insp. Serv., USDA, Hyattsville, Md., Sept. 11.

15

Program Evaluation

As pointed out in the first chapter, the final step in making a decision is assuming the responsibility for it. Because of tradition that is deeply rooted in our culture, we expect our children to acquire this capacity in their personal lives as they mature. However, it is less clearly understood what degree of responsibility should be accepted by an individual who, as a member or leader of a group, participates in making a decision that changes programs or organizations. The obligation to document the process of decision making in government agencies is neglected with impunity, and some administrators have gone so far as to destroy, conceal, and even falsify records without being censured by the public. However, this tolerance is changing, and increasing demand is being made for proper accounting. It should be understood that nothing can be accomplished without mistakes, and unless the mistakes were deliberate, the decision maker should not be subject to retribution. However, the public that lives with the mistakes and bears their costs has the right to demand that the same mistake not be repeated. Without an accounting and assessment of the workings of the decision-making process, the same mistakes are likely to be repeated many times.

There is little agreement on the methods used in evaluating programs. Standardized bookkeeping methods help the record keeper stay abreast of the organization's current financial position and trace events leading to it. Equally important, other individuals can examine those records and obtain the same information. Verification of the accuracy of financial records is done by independent auditors who examine all financial documents of both private and public institutions at regular intervals.

Unfortunately, there are no standardized record keeping methods or auditing systems for the process and criteria used in making institutional decisions. Although the minutes that are taken during most official administrative meetings identify certain decisions, there are no guidelines differentiating the sorts of decisions that are significant enough to be recorded and those that should be excluded as trivial. For that reason, it is unlikely that an independent reviewer could take official minutes of the executive body of any institution and arrive at an understanding of the decision-making process that created or sustained a given program. Even more important, the reviewer would find it difficult, if not impossible, to trace the roots of an institutional crisis, although they can be uncovered occasionally by laborious examination of correspondence and in-depth interviews of participants.

This failure to document the decision-making process is the result, in part, of a conscious or unconscious desire to avoid responsibility for actions that are or may become unpopular but still obtain credit for those actions that enable the administrator to advance personally. Consequently, most individuals decide to commit as little as possible to paper. An even larger problem than the desire to escape responsibility is the lack of understanding of the decision-making process and, particularly, the methods of documentation. Many administrators really do not know how a decision was reached and what criteria were used in its making. Small details obscure the real issues, memories of long drawn-out discussions are inadequate, and the lines of responsibility are vague. Furthermore, participants often fail to recognize that either taking or failing to take action will inevitably lead to more problems that also require decisions. Because many participants resist the realization that failure to take action is also a decision, they see no need to document it.

When a federal agency failed to assist a neighboring country in controlling a disease that was rapidly advancing toward the border of the United States, a member of Congress was provoked to talk of an investigative hearing. The agency hastily called in a committee of three to examine the agency's records and help prepare a defense. Interviews with responsible individuals and examination of documents from a professional organization to which some of those individuals belonged revealed that the problem had been discussed

at length.   However,   there   were   no   documents   in   the
agency's own files to indicate that the problem had
ever been considered.   The explanation was given that
the staff had not agreed on a course of action and
therefore nothing was recorded.   Obviously, the staff
did not understand that proper documentation was important and should have included (1) a statement regarding
the nature of the problem, (2) summaries of alternative
courses of action, and (3) a record that a decision had
been postponed.   All documents should have been dated.
If Congress had investigated that particular situation,
the agency would have been without any defense, which
is the worst possible circumstance for a government
agency.

More and more institutions around the world are
going to be asked if and when they perceived a problem,
what alternative interventions were considered, and
what actions were taken.   Documentation is essential.

ANALYSIS OF PAST PROGRAMS

Any disease-eradication program is an experiment
on a grand scale that tests concepts, technical methods, and organizational structures.   The investment of
funds and personnel in such an endeavor should be considered in terms of both the program objective and the
experience gained.   The investment of experience can be
fully realized when an adequate independent accounting
is made not only of expenditures of funds but also the
effectiveness of the infrastructure and technical methods used in surmounting problems and achieving defined
goals.   It has been proposed that this accounting responsibility should be assigned to a special group that
is privy to the entire operation from beginning to end
and has no duties other than program assessment.

No matter when the evaluation team is given its
assignment, some of the records it needs will be available but others will be lacking.   Even so, the volume
of records is apt to be staggering.   How does one sift
through the mass of data and determine what is significant?   The primary purpose of assessment is not to
ascertain whether the job was or was not done, although
that information is essential, but rather to trace the
decisions that shaped the successes and failures of the
program.   These are the elements of value to planners
and executors of future programs.   This is information
that the public has purchased, sometimes at high cost,
and it should be reviewed.   In the first chapter, deci-

sion making was defined as a six-step process, each step of which should be examined and evaluated.

1. <u>Problem definition</u>. Did the staff describe the problem in an organized fashion and identify its various components? Were the program goals clearly stated and relevant to the problem?

2. <u>Information acquisition</u>. What kinds of information were gathered (disease prevalence and incidence, property inventories, public opinion, records of meetings, correspondence, telephone memos)? Was the information gathered systematically? What systems of storage and retrieval were used?

3. <u>Data analysis</u>. What methods were used to insure both complete and accurate records? Was disease surveillance based on defensible sampling methods and sound biological assays? Were verification methods used to avoid admission of fraudulent data on inventories or personnel records? Were periodic staff performance reviews conducted and documented? Were adverse public reactions to program policies and actions gathered and maintained? Did the information obtained suggest a need to reassess timetables and goals? Were new options suggested and documented in response to this need?

4. <u>Judgement</u>. Were program strategies, goals, and standards reassessed when information revealed failure to keep to the timetables; existence of inadequacies in the staff performance; occurrence of unforeseen environmental, political, or economical problems; or availability of new research findings applicable to the program? Was a set of options considered when a need for change arose? When appropriate, were the staff and affected public allowed to participate in decisions? Were decisions made within a reasonable period?

5. <u>Execution</u>. Was authority appropriately used? Was it delegated in a systematic fashion that provided uniformity in the actions taken and assured both the staff and the public of competent leadership? Was the staff adequately trained for its tasks and used efficiently? Were the communication loops required to keep administrators and staff fully informed of decisions, accomplishments, and problems utilized at all times? Were the leaders and staff prepared for the inevitable emergencies that arose? Were program goals achieved and deadlines met?

6. <u>Responsibility bearing</u>. Was an attempt made to review the execution of the program and recommend procedures based on experience gained.

EARLY ERADICATION PROGRAMS

Rinderpest Eradication in the United Kingdom, 1866

Rinderpest was introduced into northeast England in May 1865 by cattle imported from Russia and spread to London by June (Francis 1948). The successful eradication of the 1714 epidemic by Bates and his four justices had been forgotten, and the advice of John Gamgee, a foremost British veterinarian, was ignored. The authorities sought futile cures instead of using the Act of 1847 to control animal movement. In July 1865 a Cattle Plague Order was issued that enforced notification of diseased animals and founded a veterinary department. A Royal Commission was appointed in September and issued reports in October 1865, February 1866, and May 1866 covering investigations undertaken but provided no helpful recommendations. The disease had spread throughout the country and was attacking 18,000 animals a week when the Cattle Diseases Prevention Act was put into force in February 1866. The Act compelled local authorities to slaughter all affected animals and disinfect premises, which then had to remain unoccupied for 30 days. It also empowered local authorities to slaughter healthy in-contact animals when this was considered desirable. The disease was rapidly brought under control through these measures and eradicated in September 1866.

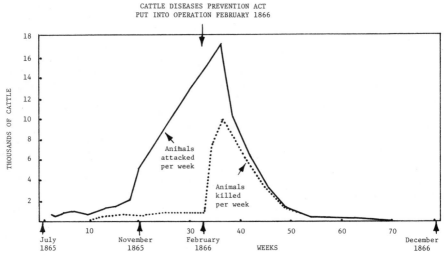

FIG. 15.1.   1865-1866 rinderpest epizootic in Great Britain: 278,943 cattle infected; 56,924 healthy contact cattle killed (Francis 1948).

In 1868 the veterinary department produced a long report with maps and tables of statistics (Fig. 15.1) that showed 278,943 cattle were attacked and an additional 56,929 healthy cattle were killed in the eradication campaign. Counties surrounding all ports were severely attacked, but Cheshire, a county with an intensive dairying industry, was the most severely affected. Over 68 percent of the cattle in Cheshire became diseased, and 86 percent of these diseased animals died. Wales and Ireland escaped the plague.

The temporary Cattle Diseases Prevention Act was replaced in 1869 by the Contagious Diseases (Animals) Act that gave wide powers to the Privy Council. Reintroduction of rinderpest in 1872 and 1877 led to almost immediate action and fewer than 350 animals were lost in the two epidemics. By 1884 an act was passed that prohibited the importation of animals from countries known to be infected with rinderpest, and the disease never reappeared in English cattle.

Pleuropneumonia Eradication in the United Kingdom, 1898

Pleuropneumonia was introduced into Great Britain about 1840 and no effort was made to control it until 1869 (Francis 1948). The disease is spread directly from animal to animal by inhalation of infective particles, its course is chronic, and recovered animals remain persistent shedders for long periods.

It is estimated that 45,000 animals were attacked prior to 1869. In 1870 when reporting was first required, 4,000 animals were listed as diseased, and this number increased to 8,000 by 1872 (Fig. 15.2).

Control began in 1873 when the slaughter of affected animals was required, and an isolation period of 28 days was imposed on a herd after the occurrence of the last case. Since these measures had only a modest effect, in 1878 more stringent measures were introduced that empowered, but did not compel, local authorities to slaughter exposed animals and also doubled the isolation period to 56 days. By 1883 the incidence had declined from about 4,000 cases a year to less than 1,000. However, by 1885 the number of cases had again doubled. In 1888, at the recommendation of a departmental committee, an order was issued enforcing the slaughter of both diseased and in-contact animals but leaving the responsibility for enforcement and compensation with local authorities. Since this did not speed eradication, the Pleuropneumonia Act was authorized in 1890. This act placed responsibility for enforcement in the hands of a central authority, the Board of Agriculture. The incidence of disease dropped

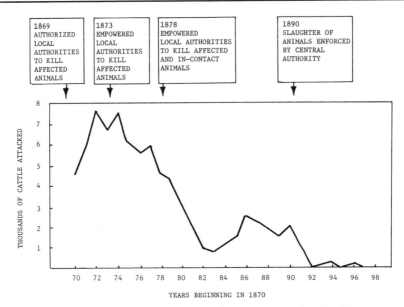

FIG. 15.2. Eradication of bovine pleuropneumonia in Great
Britain (Francis 1948).

rapidly within two years, and by 1898 pleuropneumonia
was finally eradicated from Great Britain (Fig. 15.2).

ANALYSIS OF TWENTIETH CENTURY PROGRAMS

Brucellosis Eradication in Wisconsin, 1955

　　　Brucellosis was known to be widespread in
Wisconsin dairy herds and, by the time of World War I,
had caused serious economic loss from abortions, infertility, and decreased milk production as well as debilitating disease in people (Schomisch 1967). Individual
dairy producers vaccinated calves with Strain 19 to
protect replacements to their herd and bought only
tested animals when they had to purchase animals.
Nevertheless, the disease continued to spread, particularly during World War II when demand for milk led to
rapid expansion of dairy herds (Fig. 15.3).
　　　The impetus for a statewide eradication program
was provided by Herman Bundesen, president of the
Chicago Board of Health, who announced in January 1950
that after January 1, 1955, all milk marketed in
Chicago must be from herds free of brucellosis. Loss

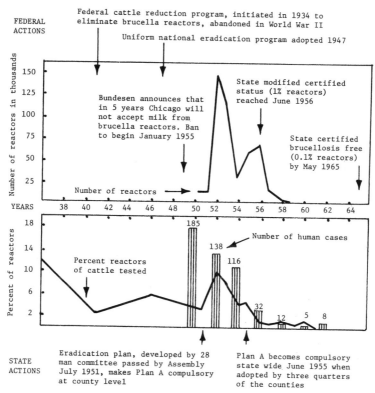

FIG. 15.3. Wisconsin brucellosis eradication program (Schomisch 1967).

of the Chicago milk shed meant severe economic consequences for Wisconsin dairy producers, and action was needed. When an eradication plan proposed by the Wisconsin Department of Agriculture was rebuffed, Director Don McDowell sought assistance from the livestock industry by appointing a 28-man committee, representative of its diverse groups, to draft an eradication program. The new program had the same control measures as the one drafted by the department, but it had social-political features that gave the dairy producers a vote on the rapidity by which the measures were implemented. For this and other reasons, the plan became politically acceptable, easily passed both houses of the legislature, and gained the governor's signature. In spite of several divisive issues, such as the proposed use of M vaccine and a proposed change in the control agency's infrastructure, the program was rapidly implemented. An important feature in the implementation was an extensive information effort, which related program objectives and methods of brucellosis eradication, that was carried out cooperatively by University Extension, the Department of Agriculture, and industry leaders. Eradication was accomplished on schedule (Fig. 15.3), and Wisconsin dairy producers have continued to supply over 90 percent of the milk to the Chicago market.

The program was not free of problems, however. A logistics problem occurred very early because not enough veterinarians were available to bleed all cattle in the state at three-month intervals. Fortunately, the milk-ring test that had been developed in Europe was tried and accepted. The use of this test identified infected herds so that only animals from the identified herds had to be bled. As eradication proceeded, nonspecific reactor herds were encountered with greater frequency. However, this difficulty also became manageable through continued research at the University of Wisconsin.

Brucellosis eradication in Wisconsin was accomplished at a cost of $46 million, which was split equally between the state and the federal governments.

Foot-and-mouth Disease Eradication in the United Kingdom, 1967

The foot-and-mouth disease epidemic in England (Northumberland 1968a, 1968b) began in October 1967 and lasted until June 4, 1968 (Fig. 15.4). Outbreaks occurred on 2,346 farms (Figs. 15.5 and 15.6) and

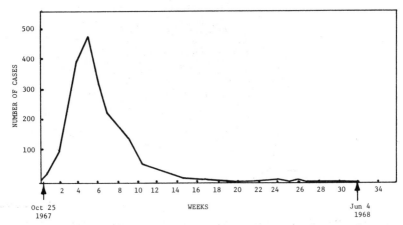

FIG. 15.4.   1967-1968 foot-and-mouth disease epidemic of type O_1 in Great Britain (Northumberland 1968a).

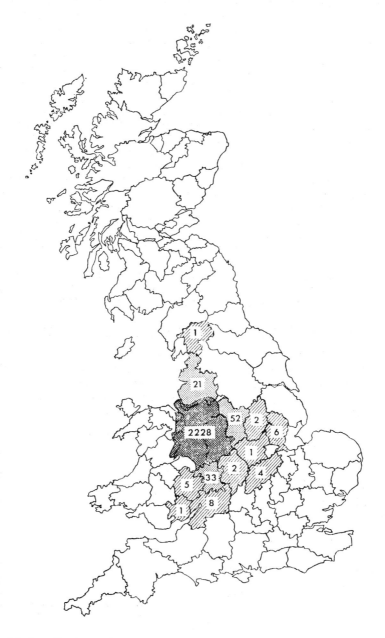

FIG. 15.5. Number of outbreaks of foot-and-mouth disease by
district during the 1967-1968 epidemic (Northumberland
1968a).

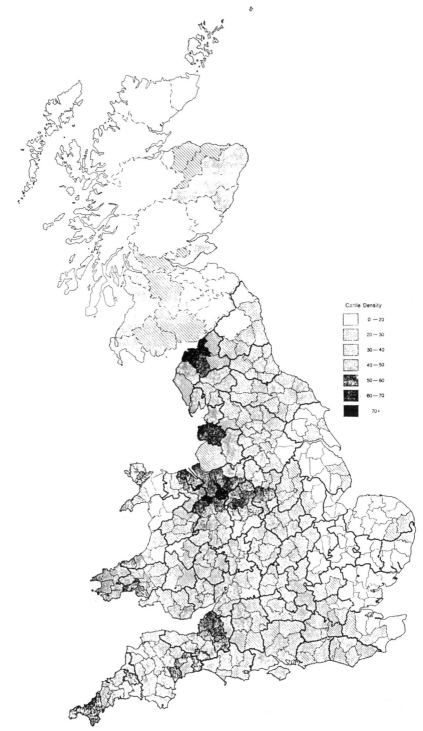

FIG. 15.6. Distribution of cattle according to density per 100 acres in 1967 (Northumberland 1968a).

resulted in the slaughter of 211,825 cattle, 113,766 pigs, 108,345 sheep, and 51 goats. The origin of the type O_1 virus, which caused the epidemic, was believed to be frozen Argentine lamb that was sold in shops in Cheshire and Shropshire, England, in September and October and initiated infection on several premises. The affected animals shed virus for varying times: cattle, five to eight days; sheep, 8 to 11 days; and swine, 7 to 13 days. The largest quantity of virus was shed from the pharynx and in the milk (10^3 to 10^5 LD_{50}), less from the vagina (10^3 LD_{50}), and still less from the rectum (10^1 to 10^2 LD_{50}). Spread was attributed to animal movement, movement of trucks and people, handling of milk (Hedger and Dawson 1970), feeding of milk to swine, and windborne aerosols (Hugh-Jones and Wright 1970)..

Direct costs of the epidemic were estimated at 35.1 million British pounds, largely borne by the Ministry of Agriculture. Compensation was estimated at 26.6 million pounds. Detection, slaughter, disposal, and disinfection amounted to 4.2 million pounds, and additional staff costs were 2.8 million pounds.

Indirect costs covered the loss of income resulting from the slaughter of animals and the disruption of services following imposition of control measures. Estimates of combined direct and indirect costs ranged from 70 million to 150 million British pounds. In addition, sporting, leisure, and other social activities were upset, particularily horse racing, fishing, hunting, car rallying, camping, canoeing, and mountaineering. Those persons who depended on these activities for their living suffered financial loss.

Newcastle Disease Eradication in California, 1971-1973

In the late 1960s, word came from the Middle East of a Newcastle disease virus that caused very high mortality in susceptible chickens and severe losses even in vaccinated flocks. Field and laboratory diagnosticians soon documented that this new form of the virus was spreading to many parts of the world, largely through traffic in caged birds. The first isolates obtained in the United States came in August 1970 from parrots that were dead on arrival at the New York International Airport. In November 1971 in Riverside California, a chicken flock adjacent to an aviary that had received imported psittacines was found to be infected. From there the disease spread into commercial and backyard poultry flocks and to a variety of associated captive birds in an eight-county area of southern California.

After consultation with federal officials, a state-federal quarantine was established on March 14, 1972, and a task force was created to carry out an eradication program. Eradication took approximately two years and cost the federal government $56 million (Fig. 15.7). The task force director was aided by a scientific advisory committee and an industry advisory committee. Technical assistance and personnel came from the U.S. Department of Agriculture; other states; the armed services; and to a limited extent, foreign governments.

The selected strategy limited the movement of in-fected birds by quarantine and eliminated the virus source by first slaughtering diseased birds and their contacts and then cleaning and disinfecting the prem-ises. In addition, a supervised vaccination program of both commercial and backyard flocks was undertaken in an effort to reduce the size of the population at risk.

The important biological problems that were encountered included: (1) differentiation of the invading exotic virus from domestic strains, (2) iden-tification of carrier flocks in which the presence of

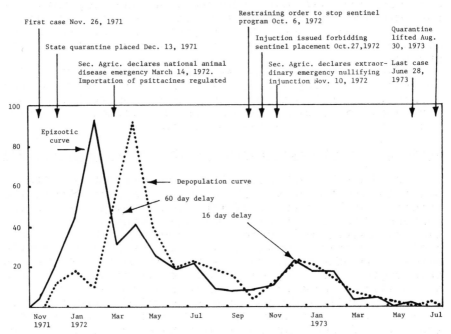

FIG. 15.7. The Newcastle disease-eradication program in California 1971-1973 (Burridge et al. 1975; Animal Plant Health Inspection Service 1978).

the disease was masked by immunity, and (3) determination of the role of migratory birds in the spread of the virus. A combination of *in vivo* and *in vitro* laboratory procedures were developed that satisfactorily established in seven to ten days whether the virus was of exotic or domestic origin. Carrier flocks were identified by use of sentinel birds or periodic sampling for virus of birds that were dying from any cause in suspect flocks. Investigation of migratory and other free-flying birds gave no evidence that they contributed to the spread of the disease.

Adverse reaction of some producers to the use of sentinel birds caused the program to be challenged in the state courts. On October 27, 1972, a restraining order was issued that was overturned on November 10, 1972 by the U.S. Secretary of Agriculture's declaration of a state of Extraordinary Emergency. The delay considerably increased the cost of the program. The demand for compensation of lost income as well as destroyed property resulted in fundamental changes in federal compensation procedures. Although the diversity and complexity of the poultry industry and its interrelations with bird fanciers, sporting groups, and bird-watchers was not understood at the beginning of the program, it was soon apparent that this knowledge was essential in establishing the epidemiology of the disease and developing an effective communication program.

The area quarantine was lifted on August 30, 1973, but the last premise in California was not removed from quarantine until September 28, 1973. Surveillance was continued for another year, and no evidence of persistence of the exotic virus was found.

National Brucellosis Program in the United States, 1978

Eradication of brucellosis in the United States began before World War II as area programs within the intensive dairy country of the north central and northeastern states. It was based upon Strain 19 vaccination of calves to reduce the population at risk, control of cattle movement, regular testing of cattle herds, and slaughter of reactor-carriers. States in this region soon adopted compulsory programs and gained a brucellosis-free status within five to ten years.

Some modifications were made in the program when it was introduced into the beef herds of the western states, and real progress was made in spite of the problems inherent in routinely testing large herds on range. Control of brucellosis in the cattle industry of the southern states proved to be far more difficult.

When it became apparent that a program of brucellosis eradication that had worked successfully in one part of the country was not working in another, the director of the federal Animal Plant Health Inspection Service appointed a commission of knowledgeable individuals (Anderson et al. 1978) and requested their evaluation of the program and recommendations. The charge to the commission asked the members to

1. Review the concept of eradication of bovine brucellosis in the United States, including the question of its ultimate feasibility. The review will include
   a. An investigation of the nature and present availability of knowledge essential to the goal of eradication.
   b. Consideration of the circumstances and realities within which the eradication concept is to be applied, such as the breeding, management, and marketing practices of the cattle industry in various parts of the country.
   c. Examination of the implications for the incidence of human brucellosis of the eradication concept and any proposed modifications of it.
2. Review the program presently authorized by the statutes as well as those projections under consideration. Consider various technical and administrative alternatives which could provide for the ultimate goal of eradication. This consideration should address the questions of cost, acceptance by all parts of industry, as well as the potential effects on incidence of human brucellosis.
3. Make an economic cost-benefit analysis of the present program with its proposed extensions, and any other alternative programs the Commission deems appropriate.

The following points have been extracted from the Commission's report.

As we followed the charge to review the concept of eradication of bovine brucellosis it became apparent, in our public hearings and in the position papers we received, that the semantic issue of the definition of eradication is a very real problem for various individuals and groups. Accordingly, we adopted a more precisely defined goal of local eradication of *Brucella abortus* from cattle, which has already been achieved in herds, states and regions of the United States, as well as in other countries, through the application of effective systems of control. This concept of local eradication is defined in the report as part of a continuum resulting from individual actions, to actions involving many groups and larger areas, until it becomes national in scope. It is our judgement that this goal is biologically feasible and that local eradication of bovine brucellosis from the United States can be achieved, in the same sense that foot-and-mouth disease has been locally eradicated in North America. It is inherent in this definition, that continuing surveillance would be necessary to assure continued freedom from the disease, and that there be an emergency plan to prevent or eliminate reintroductions.

Although it is clear that biologic knowledge essential to the goal is available, we were impressed at the extent to which important, well established facts about the disease and the program are not being distributed to those who need most to know. Furthermore, there has been a real failure to assume responsibility for adequate training and public information programs on the part of those public agencies which should have a leadership role. These deficiencies of understanding became apparent in our field trips, public hearings, the position papers we received and from data collected in a study on information and attitudes of producers conducted for us.

The major conclusions to be drawn are that the lack of understanding of brucellosis and of the elements of the program are so general as to constitute a major barrier to the achievement of the goal of local eradication.

Among other parameters of program performance monitored, one of the most significant appeared to be the outcomes of tracebacks to herds of origin of reactions in the Market Cattle Inspection, both from first point of concentration testing or from slaughter sampling. Our interpretation of the data is that program performance in some states is inadequate to achieve control leading to local eradication.

Survey of laboratory test procedures and results indicates that support, to assure quality of the laboratory procedures, backing up well trained epidemiologists and other field personnel, is inadequate. This is even more striking in relation to the large sums expended on indemnity payments, to identifying individual animals and collecting and processing blood samples in surveillance testing.

Enforcement of compliance with regulations, both at the federal and state level does not seem to have much influence on program outcomes, and does not appear to be cost effective.

The state-federal cooperative brucellosis program operates under a set of minimum standards (U.M.&R.) [Uniform Methods and Rules] for achieving and maintaining certification of herds and of areas. In addition each of the 50 states may enact legislation and regulations which impose additional standards which may be more rigorous than the minimum in the U.M.&R., and many states have done so.

The process by which the U.M.&R. are modified is a political one in which attempts are made to accommodate to the needs and desires of various geographic and industry segments. Over the years, attempts to make these accommodations have resulted in trade-offs of sound epidemiologic principles. Specially, the present U.M.&R. promotes the transfer of responsibility and accountability for acting to prevent the spread of brucellosis away from individuals engaged in the livestock and marketing industries, to the federal and state regulatory agencies. In the process, it generates a false sense of security on the part of individuals who accept animals on the basis of rules which are epidemiologically invalid. It creates rewards for systems of evasion, thus promoting the maintenance and dissemination of bovine brucellosis.

These considerations led us back to the defects we have tried to identify in the U.M.&R., and in operations under the 50 state-federal programs, in order to seek strategies which would more sharply focus efforts in achieving local eradication. We feel that some of the major defects are: a shift of responsibility and accountability from producers, handlers and the marketing sectors to the government, inadequate knowledge about the disease and the program among those who have the greatest need to know, epidemiologically unsound regulations which generate mechanisms of evasion, and a lack of high quality services to enhance the ability of individuals to develop flexible and specific programs to protect their

own herds from infection, to free them of infection and to prevent dissemination of brucellosis.

The points cited from the executive summary are
expanded in the report's text, which follow this
outline:

Findings and recommendations
Executive summary
History of the commission and charge
Definitions of eradication and control
The nature and structure of the beef cattle
industry
Structure of the dairy cattle industry
Biological factors influencing control leading to
local eradication of brucellosis
Public health factors influencing policy options
Constraints of information and the assumption of
responsibility
Political and legal constraints imposed upon the
policy options
Sociological and cultural factors influencing
policy options
Economic constraints on policy options
Benefit-cost analysis
Proposal for changes in the goals and nature of
the Uniform Methods and Rules
Research and research policy

Eight appendices provide further documentation of the
text.

SUGGESTED READINGS

Eradication Programs

Basu, R. N.; Jezek, Z.; and Ward, N. A. 1979. The
Eradication of Smallpox from India. New Dehli:
WHO South-East Asia Regional Off.
Baumhover, A. H. 1966. Eradication of the screwworm
fly. *J. Am. Med. Assoc.* 196:240-248.
Bush, G. L.; Neck, R. W.; and Kitto, G. B. 1976.
Screwworm eradication: Inadvertent selection for
non-competitive ecotypes during mass rearing.
Science 193:491-493.
Campbell, A. D. 1965. Swine fever: The eradication
programme in Great Britain, 1963-1965. *U.S.
Livest. Sanit. Assoc. Proc.* 69:390-409.

Committee on Animal Health. 1973. Animal disease
    eradication: Evaluating programs. Proc. NAS
    Workshop, Apr. 12-13, Univ. Wis. Ext., Madison,
    Wis.
Dungal, N. 1957. Eradication of hydatid disease in
    Iceland. *NZ Med. J.* 56:213-222.
du Toit, R. M. 1959. The eradication of the tsetse
    fly *Glossina pallidipes* from Zululand, Union of
    South Africa. In Advances in Veterinary Science,
    vol. 5, eds. C. A. Brandly and E. L. Jungherr.
    New York: Academic Press, pp. 227-240.
Henderson, D. A. 1976. The eradication of smallpox.
    Sci. Amer. 235(4):25-33.
Pan American Foot-and-Mouth Disease Center. 1974.
    Evaluation guide of foot-and-mouth disease control
    programs. Sci. Tech. Monogr. Ser. 2. Rio de
    Janeiro, Brazil.
Pan American Health Organization. 1966. Criteria for
    the analysis and evaluation of loan requests for
    programs for the control of foot-and-mouth dis-
    ease. Doc. 3, Aftosa, Washington, D.C., Aug. 8-9.
Richardson, R. H., ed. 1978. The Screwworm Problem:
    Evolution of Resistance to Biological Control.
    Austin, Tex.: Univ. Texas Press.
Rosenstock, I. M.; Hochbaum, G. M.; and Leventhal, H.
    1960. The impact of Asian influenza on community
    life: A study in five cities. USPHS Publ. 766.
    USDHEW, Washington, D.C.
Seddon, H. R. 1964. Eradication of sheep scab from
    New South Wales. *Aust. Vet. J.* 40:418-421.
Swann, A. I., and Sharman, R. S. 1979. History of
    disease control and eradication in Great Britain,
    North America, and Mexico. Paper read at Conf.
    Concepts Tech. Control Erad. Anim. Dis., Sept.
    10-14, Auburn, Ala.
Weisbrod, B. A.; Andreano, R. L.; Baldwin, R. E.;
    Epstein, E. H.; Kelley, A. C.; and Helmeniak, T.
    W. 1973. Disease and Economic Development: The
    Impact of Parasitic Diseases in St. Lucia.
    Madison, Wis.: Univ. Wis. Press.
World Bank. 1977. Basic issues emerging from the
    Bank's experience with animal health project
    loans. Washington, D.C.

Rinderpest

Bates, T. 1714. A brief account of the contagious
    disease which raged among the milch cows near
    London in the year 1714 and the methods that were
    taken for suppressing it. *Philos. Trans. R. Soc.
    London*.

Dorwart, R. A. 1959. Cattle disease (rinderpest?): Prevention and cure in Brandenburg, 1665-1732. *Agric. Hist.* 33:79-85.

Francis, J. 1948. The contributions that quarantine, sanitary measures, and eradication can make to preventive medicine. *Vet. Rec.* 60:361-367.

Henning, M. W. 1956. Rinderpest, cattle plague, runderpest. In Animal Diseases in South Africa, 3rd ed. South Africa: Central News Agency, Ltd., pp. 828-867.

Lane, J. 1976. Cattle plague in Conventry in the mid-eighteenth century. *Vet. Rec.* 99:218-219.

Mack, R. 1970. The great African cattle plague epidemic of the 1890's. *Trop. Anim. Health Prod.* 2:210-219.

Bovine Pleuropneumonia

Food and Agriculture Organization. 1971. Report of the fourth meeting of the FAO/OIE/OAU expert panel on contagious bovine pleuropneumonia. Paris, Mar. 15-20.

Francis, J. 1948. The contributions that quarantine, sanitary measures, and eradication can make to preventive medicine. *Vet. Rec.* 60:361-367.

Gee, R. W. 1975. The eradication of contagious bovine pleuropneumonia from Australia. *Bull. Off. Int. Episoot.* 84:477-480.

Heslop, G. G. 1973. Eradication of bovine contagious pleuropneumonia. *Aust. Vet. J.* 49:56.

Oluokun, S. B. 1976. An appraisal of the campaign against contagious bovine pleuropneumonia in Nigeria. In New Techniques in Veterinary Epidemiology and Economics. Proc. Symp., July 12-15. Reading, UK: Univ. Reading, pp. 184-191.

Brucellosis in Wisconsin

Berman, D. T. 1950. The natural course of bovine brucellosis. In Third Inter-American Congress on Brucellosis. Washington, D.C.: Pan Am. Sanit. Bur., pp. 104-114.

Schomisch, T. P. 1967. Wisconsin brucellosis campaign. M.S. thesis, Univ. Wis., Madison.

Foot-and-Mouth Disease

Argentine-United States Joint Commission on Foot-and-Mouth Disease. 1966. Studies on foot-and-mouth disease. NAS-NCR Publ. 1343. Washington, D.C.

Aulaqi, N. A. 1979. Movement of milk in the United
   States and its implications in the spread and
   control of foot-and-mouth disease. In A Study of
   the Potential Economic Impact of Foot-and-Mouth
   Disease in the United States, eds. E. H. McCauley,
   N. A. Aulaqui, J. C. New, Jr., W. B. Sundquist,
   and W. M. Miller. Tech. Rep. 10. Washington,
   D.C.: USGPO, pp. 169-184.
Casas-Olascoaga, R. 1978. Situation of the foot-and-
   mouth disease control programmes in South America.
   Brit. Vet. J. 134:16-22.
Ferguson, W. 1969. Periodicity of epidemics and cost-
   benefit of vaccination programmes. Vet. Rec. 85:
   420-421.
Hedger, R. S., and Dawson, P. S. 1970. Foot-and-mouth
   disease virus in milk: An epidemiological study.
   Vet. Rec. 87:186-188.
Hugh-Jones, M. E. 1976a. A simulation spatial model
   of the spread of foot-and-mouth disease through
   the primary movement of milk. J. Hyg. Camb. 77:
   1-9.
────────. 1976b. Epidemiological studies on the 1967-
   1968 foot-and-mouth disease epidemic: The reporting of suspected disease. J. Hyg. Camb. 77:299-
   306.
Hugh-Jones, M. E., and Tinline, R. R. 1976. Studies
   on the 1967-68 foot-and-mouth disease epidemic:
   Incubation period and herd serial interval. J.
   Hyg. Camb. 77:141-153.
Hugh-Jones, M. E., and Wright, P. B. 1970. Studies on
   the 1967-8 foot-and-mouth disease epidemic: The
   relation of weather to the spread of disease. J.
   Hyg. Camb. 68:253-271.
Hughes, H., and Jones, J. O., eds. 1969. Plague on
   the Cheshire Plain. London: Dennis Dobson.
Lowes, E. 1972. Epidemiological studies of foot-and-
   mouth disease in Great Britain. Bull. Off. Int.
   Epizoot. 77(3-4):481-486.
Nabholz, A. 1974. Lessons for the future from the
   recent outbreaks of foot-and-mouth disease in
   Europe. World Anim. Rev. 11:20-23.
Nature. 1967. Slaughter or vaccination. 216:1057-
   1059.
Northumberland, Duke of. 1968a. Report of the Commit-
   tee of Inquiry on Foot-and-Mouth Disease, 1968,
   part 1, Cmnd. 3999. London: Her Majesty's
   Stationery Off.
────────. 1968b. Report of the Committee of Inquiry on
   Foot-and-Mouth Disease, 1968, part 2, Cmnd. 4225.
   London: Her Majesty's Stationery Off.

Power, A. P., and Harris, S. A. 1973. A cost-benefit evaluation of alternative control policies for foot-and-mouth disease in Great Britain. *J. Agric. Econ.* 24:573-600.

Sellers, R. F.; Herniman, K. A. J.; and Donaldson, A. I. 1971. The effects of killing or removal of animals affected with foot-and-mouth disease on the amounts of air-borne virus present in loose-boxes. *Br. Vet. J.* 127:358-365.

Swann, A. I., and Sharman, R. S. 1979. History of disease control and eradication in Great Britain, North America, and Mexico. Paper read at Conf. Concepts Tech. Control Erad. Anim. Dis., Sept. 10-14, Auburn, Ala.

Newcastle Disease

Animal Plant Health Inspection Service. 1978. Eradication of exotic Newcastle disease in southern California, 1971-74. 91-34. USDA, Hyattsville, Md.

Bell, D. 1972. Southern California poultry industry reactions to the Newcastle disease eradication program. Univ. Calif. Agric. Ext., Davis, Calif.
————. 1973. The socio-economic impact of the VVND problem on the poultry industry of southern California. Univ. Calif. Agric. Ext., Davis, Calif.

Bickford, A. A., and Rosenwald, A. S. 1976. Peripheral avian populations and poultry disease control. *West. Poult. Dis. Conf. Proc.* 25:20-22.

Burridge, M. J., Riemann, H. P., Utterback, W. W., and Sharman, E. C. 1975. The Newcastle disease epidemic in southern California, 1971-1973: Descriptive epidemiology and effects of vaccination on the eradication program. *U.S. Anim. Health Assoc. Proc.* 79:324-333.

Chute, H. L.; Hofstad, M. S.; Ray, W. C.; Snoeyenbos, C. H.; and Tjalma, R. A. 1973. Final report of study team to review and evaluate the epidemiologic operations of the USDA Newcastle disease task force. Anim. Plant Health Insp. Serv., May 24, USDA, Hyattsville, Md.

Ferguson, A. 1972. The Newcastle problem. *Can. Poult. Rev.* 96(1):34-36.

Fraser, R. P.; Gordon, R. F.; Justice, W. M.; Kidner, G. T.; and Phillips, J. F. 1971. Fowl pest, Newcastle disease epidemic, 1970-71: Report of the review panel. Her Majesty's Stationery Off., London.

Grass, E. E. 1972. Exotic Newcastle disease in the

United States. *West. Poult. Dis. Conf. Proc.* 21:
26-30.

Hull, R. H. 1972. Exotic Newcastle disease in northern California, 1971-1972. *West. Poult. Dis.
Conf. Proc.* 21:57-59.

King, D. D. 1972. Evaluation of the NCD vaccination
program in the poultry population in southern
California during the eradication effort. *U.S.
Anim. Health Assoc. Proc.* 76:297-309.

Lancaster, J. E., and Alexander, D. J. 1975. Newcastle disease virus and spread. Monogr. 11.
Can. Dep. Agric., Ottawa.

Matulich, W. 1972. Newcastle disease eradication task
force exotic birds. *West. Poult. Dis. Conf. Proc.*
21:64-65.

Omohundro, R. E. 1972. Exotic Newcastle disease eradication. *U.S. Anim. Health Assoc. Proc.* 76:264-
268.

Pearson, G. L., and McCann, M. K. 1974. The role of
indigenous wild, semi-domestic and exotic birds in
the epizootiology of exotic Newcastle disease in
southern California. Position paper, U.S. Fish
Wildl. Serv. and Anim. Plant Health Insp. Serv.,
USDA, Hyattsville, Md.

Pierson, G. P. 1975. Problems associated with importation of exotic birds. *U.S. Anim. Health Proc.*
79:214-218.

Rivera-Cruz, E. 1976. International cooperation and
Newcastle disease surveillance. *West. Poult. Dis.
Conf. Proc.* 25:89.

Rooney, W. F., and McKeen, W. D. 1972. Extension
effort in a Newcastle quarantine area. *West.
Poult. Dis. Conf. Proc.* 21:61-63.

Sharman, E. C., and Walker, J. W. 1973. Regulatory
aspects of velogenic viscerotropic Newcastle
disease. *J. Am. Vet. Med. Assoc.* 163:1089-1093.

Swanson, M. H. 1972. The Newcastle disease eradication program and its impact on the poultry
industry of southern California. Univ. Calif.
Agric. Ext., Oct. 6, Davis, Calif.

Utterback, W. W., and Schwartz, J. H. 1973. Epizootiology of velogenic viscerotropic Newcastle disease
in southern California, 1971-1973. *J. Am. Vet.
Med. Assoc.* 163:1080-1088.

Walker, J. W. 1976. International cooperation and
Newcastle disease surveillance. *West. Poult. Dis.
Conf. Proc.* 25:30-35.

Walker, J. W.; Heron, B. R.; and Mixson, M. A. 1973.
Exotic Newcastle disease eradication program in
the United States. *Avian Dis.* 17:486-503.

Brucellosis in the United States

Anderson, R. K.; Berman, D. T.; Berry, W. T.; Hopkin,
J. A.; and Wise, R. 1978. Report National
Brucellosis Technical Commission. Anim. Plant
Health Insp. Serv., USDA, Washington, D.C.,

Berry, W. T., Jr. 1979. Lenders' guide to brucellosis. *Agric. Finance* 21(5):34.

Carpenter, T. E. 1976. The application of benefit-
cost analysis to compare alternative approaches to
the brucellosis problem in California. In New
Techniques in Veterinary Epidemiology and Economics. Proc. Int. Symp., July 12-15. Reading, UK:
Univ. Reading, pp. 122-125.

Carpenter, T. E., and Heron, B. R. 1975. Benefit-cost
study of brucellosis program: A report on the
bovine brucellosis eradication program in California. Dep. Food Agric. Health Ind. Relat.,
Sacramento, Calif., pp. 187-264.

Committee on Animal Health. 1977. Brucellosis research: An evaluation. NAS-NRC, Washington, D.C.

Hugh-Jones, M. E.; Ellis, P. R.; and Felton, M. R.
1975. An assessment of the eradication of bovine
brucellosis in England and Wales. Study 19. Dep.
Agric. and Hortic., Univ. Reading, Reading, UK.

Joint FAO/WHO expert committee on brucellosis: Fourth
report. 1964. WHO Tech. Rep. Ser. 289. Geneva.

Thomsen, A. 1957. The eradication of bovine brucel-
losis in Scandinavia. In Advances in Veterinary
Science, vol. 3, eds. C. A. Brandly and E. L.
Jungherr. New York: Academic Press, pp. 197-240.

INDEX